T0320751

Mayo Clinic
Illustrated Textbook
of Neurogastroenterology

Mayo Clinic Atlas of Regional Anesthesia and Ultrasound-Guided Nerve Blockade
Edited by James R. Hebl, MD, and Robert L. Lennon, DO

Mayo Clinic Preventive Medicine and Public Health Board Review
Edited by Prathibha Varkey, MBBS, MPH, MHPE

Mayo Clinic Infectious Diseases Board Review
Edited by Zelalem Temesgen, MD

Just Enough Physiology
By James R. Munis, MD, PhD

Mayo Clinic Cardiology: Concise Textbook, Fourth Edition
Edited by Joseph G. Murphy, MD, and Margaret A. Lloyd, MD

Mayo Clinic Electrophysiology Manual
Edited by Samuel J. Asirvatham, MD

Mayo Clinic Gastrointestinal Imaging Review, Second Edition
By C. Daniel Johnson, MD

Arrhythmias in Women: Diagnosis and Management
Edited by Yong-Mei Cha, MD, Margaret A. Lloyd, MD, and Ulrika M. Birgersdotter-Green, MD

Mayo Clinic Body MRI Case Review
By Christine U. Lee, MD, PhD, and James F. Glockner, MD, PhD

Mayo Clinic Gastroenterology and Hepatology Board Review, Fifth Edition
Edited by Stephen C. Hauser, MD

Mayo Clinic Guide to Cardiac Magnetic Resonance Imaging, Second Edition
Edited by Kiaran P. McGee, PhD, Eric E. Williamson, MD, and Matthew W. Martinez, MD

Mayo Clinic Critical Care Case Review
Edited by Rahul Kashyap, MBBS, J. Christopher Farmer, MD, and John C. O'Horo, MD

Mayo Clinic Medical Neurosciences, Sixth Edition
Edited by Eduardo E. Benarroch, MD, Jeremy K. Cutsforth-Gregory, MD, and Kelly D. Flemming, MD

Mayo Clinic Principles of Shoulder Surgery
By Joaquin Sanchez-Sotelo, MD

Mayo Clinic Essential Neurology, Second Edition
By Andrea C. Adams, MD

Mayo Clinic Antimicrobial Handbook: Quick Guide, Third Edition
Edited by John W. Wilson, MD, and Lynn L. Estes, PharmD

Mayo Clinic Critical and Neurocritical Care Board Review
Edited by Eelco F. M. Wijdicks, MD, PhD, James Y. Findlay, MB, ChB, William D. Freeman, MD, and Ayan Sen, MD

Mayo Clinic Internal Medicine Board Review, Twelfth Edition
Edited by Christopher M. Wittich, MD, PharmD, Thomas J. Beckman, MD, Sara L. Bonnes, MD, Nerissa M. Collins, MD, Nina M. Schwenk, MD, Christopher R. Stephenson, MD, and Jason H. Szostek, MD

Mayo Clinic Strategies for Reducing Burnout and Promoting Engagement
By Stephen J. Swensen, MD, and Tait D. Shanafelt, MD

Mayo Clinic General Surgery
By Jad M. Abdelsattar, MBBS, Moustafa M. El Khatib, MB, BCh, T. K. Pandian, MD, Samuel J. Allen, and David R. Farley, MD

Mayo Clinic Neurology Board Review, Second Edition
Edited by Kelly D. Flemming, MD

Mayo Clinic Illustrated Textbook of Neurogastroenterology

Michael Camilleri, MD

Consultant, Division of Gastroenterology & Hepatology
Mayo Clinic, Rochester, Minnesota
Professor of Medicine, Pharmacology, and Physiology
Mayo Clinic College of Medicine and Science

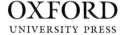

OXFORD
UNIVERSITY PRESS

Oxford University Press is a department of the University of Oxford. It furthers
the University's objective of excellence in research, scholarship, and education
by publishing worldwide. Oxford is a registered trade mark of Oxford University
Press in the UK and certain other countries.

Published in the United States of America by Oxford University Press
198 Madison Avenue, New York, NY 10016, United States of America.

© Mayo Foundation for Medical Education and Research 2021

Oxford is a registered trademark of Oxford University Press.

Library of Congress Cataloging-in-Publication Data
Names: Michael Camilleri, MD., author.
Title: Mayo Clinic illustrated textbook of neurogastroenterology / Michael Camilleri.
Other titles: Illustrated textbook of neurogastroenterology | Mayo Clinic scientific press (Series)
Description: New York, NY : Oxford University Press, [2021] |
Series: Mayo Clinic scientific press |
Includes bibliographical references and index.
Identifiers: LCCN 2021014099 (print) | LCCN 2021014100 (ebook) | ISBN 9780197512104 (hardback) |
ISBN 9780197512128 (epub) | ISBN 9780197512135 (online)
Subjects: MESH: Gastrointestinal Diseases | Gastrointestinal Motility | Gastrointestinal Tract—physiopathology |
Enteric Nervous System—physiopathology | Gastrointestinal Tract—innervation
Classification: LCC RC801 (print) | LCC RC801 (ebook) | NLM WI 195 | DDC 616.3/3—dc23
LC record available at https://lccn.loc.gov/2021014099
LC ebook record available at https://lccn.loc.gov/2021014100

Mayo Foundation does not endorse any particular products or services, and the reference to any products or services in this
book is for informational purposes only and should not be taken as an endorsement by the authors or Mayo Foundation. The
incidental appearance of brand names on any equipment or the mention of brand names in the narration in the accompanying
videos has been avoided when at all possible; any occurrences were left to preserve the educational integrity of the videos
and should not be taken as endorsement by the authors or Mayo Foundation. Care has been taken to confirm the accuracy of
the information presented and to describe generally accepted practices. However, the authors, editors, and publisher are not
responsible for errors or omissions or for any consequences from application of the information in this book and make no
warranty, express or implied, with respect to the contents of the publication. This book should not be relied on apart from the
advice of a qualified health care provider.

The authors, editors, and publisher have exerted efforts to ensure that drug selection and dosage set forth in this text are in
accordance with current recommendations and practice at the time of publication. However, in view of ongoing research,
changes in government regulations, and the constant flow of information relating to drug therapy and drug reactions, readers
are urged to check the package insert for each drug for any change in indications and dosage and for added wordings and
precautions. This is particularly important when the recommended agent is a new or infrequently employed drug.

Some drugs and medical devices presented in this publication have US Food and Drug Administration (FDA) clearance for
limited use in restricted research settings. It is the responsibility of the health care providers to ascertain the FDA status of each
drug or device planned for use in their clinical practice.

DOI: 10.1093/med/9780197512104.001.0001

9 8 7 6 5 4 3 2 1

Printed by Marquis, Canada

Foreword

Neurogastroenterology is the subdiscipline of gastroenterology that focuses on disease states characterized by neuromuscular or sensory dysfunction of the gastrointestinal tract. Patients present with a wide spectrum of symptoms from dysphagia to unexplained nausea and weight loss, abdominal distention, pain, diarrhea, and constipation. Although this area may be less recognized among gastroenterology specialties than endoscopy, inflammatory bowel disease, or hepatology, it is relevant to at least a quarter of all patients presenting for care in gastroenterology clinics. Moreover, neurogastroenterology is a multifaceted specialty with dedicated specialized techniques (motility and sensitivity studies). It also has a broad and rich interface with other specialties, such as physiology, radiology, pathology, and surgery. Thus, the scientific and pathophysiologic understanding of neurogastroenterology is built on cross-fertilization with concepts from other specialties and knowledge domains such as endocrinology, neurology, immunology, and imaging. Most of all, because the presentations and underlying mechanisms of neurogastroenterologic conditions are variable, clinical neurogastroenterologists must be creative thinkers with the ability to harness diverse disciplines to develop a highly personalized approach to each patient.

In *Mayo Clinic Illustrated Textbook of Neurogastroenterology*, Michael Camilleri, MD, covers the broad range of manifestations of disorders of gastrointestinal motility and sensation. Dr Camilleri is a true leader in this field, to which he has contributed immensely as a highly productive and innovative author of scientific publications. Because of his contributions, Dr Camilleri is a highly solicited speaker at gastroenterology meetings, where he provides an overview of emerging scientific concepts and knowledge and also always incorporates a clinical patient-oriented perspective. The same blend of high-level science and illustrated clinical case histories characterizes *Mayo Clinic Illustrated Textbook of Neurogastroenterology*. In this single-author tour-de-force, Dr Camilleri explains the physiology of motility in different regions of the gastrointestinal tract and the underlying molecular and genetic basis of the diseases and provides a state-of-the-art review of available measurement techniques. The book includes chapters on common gastrointestinal motility disorders, such as functional dyspepsia, gastroparesis, irritable bowel syndrome, constipation, and diarrhea. It also has highly specialized and well-illustrated sections on the effects of neurologic diseases on gastrointestinal motility. Indeed, in many patients with primary neurologic diseases, gastrointestinal dysmotility may be a presenting symptom. It takes a clinical research career as rich as that of Dr Camilleri's to generate a work of this scope and depth. Although the illustrations are central to the book, as they are enriched by clinical cases encountered during more than 3 decades at Mayo Clinic, important insights are also provided in the text sections.

This book will, of course, find an eager readership among clinicians and scientists with an interest in neurogastroenterology, and they will benefit from the many clinical and scientific pearls, especially in the well-documented case studies. The book is also recommended to all clinicians embarking on a career as a gastroenterologist. It will help them discover this subdiscipline that offers broad clinical diversity, stimulating supportive techniques (motility studies), and an exciting and rapidly evolving multifaceted scientific basis. This field will gain further prominence as medicine continues to evolve to individualized management based on mechanisms of chronic diseases and symptoms.

I applaud Dr Camilleri for an outstanding and impressive book, which I hope you will find an enjoyable and enriching reading and educational experience.

Jan Tack, MD, PhD
President, Rome Foundation
Head of Gastroenterology and Hepatology Division,
Leuven University Hospitals
Professor of Medicine, Leuven University
Visiting Professor, Institute of Medicine, University of
Gothenburg, Sweden

Preface

Mayo Clinic Illustrated Textbook of Neurogastro-enterology is the culmination of experiences gained in the practice of gastroenterology. Its major focuses are gastrointestinal motility disorders, the manifestations of neurologic diseases affecting the motor apparatus of the gut, and functional gastrointestinal disorders such as irritable bowel syndrome and functional dyspepsia. The book has limited text sections and is highly illustrated. The illustrations have been gathered during my 34-year clinical practice as a gastroenterologist and distinguished investigator at Mayo Clinic, during which I received research funding for more than 2 decades from the National Institutes of Health. I have been fortunate to serve in leadership roles in the field of gastroenterology and, specifically, neurogastroenterology, such as founding editor of *Clinical Gastroenterology and Hepatology*, editor of *Neurogastroenterology and Motility*, associate editor of *American Journal of Physiology (Gastroenterology and Liver)* and *Gastroenterology,* and president of the American Gastroenterological Association and the American Neurogastroenterology and Motility Society.

My career has coincided with the maturation of the field of gastrointestinal motility from studies of exotic patterns of myoelectric recordings in research laboratories to a clinical discipline with major advances in the clinical management of thousands of patients seen by gastroenterologists, primary care physicians, surgeons, or neurologists. The time span of my career has also been associated with advances in imaging, developments of ways to measure diverse motor and sensory functions from the stomach to the anorectum, introduction of genetic testing, and a plethora of novel pharmacologic and interventional therapies that have revolutionized the practice of neurogastroenterology. The book covers the spectrum of neurogastroenterologic disorders: from those that are associated with genetic and molecular disorders, through disturbances of the extrinsic neural control or the enteric neuromuscular apparatus, to dysfunction associated with disorders of the gut-brain axis.

This book has been a labor of love and reflects my desire to pass on clinical and mechanistic insights and advances in therapies that are relevant to a diverse spectrum of clinicians or clinicians in training who care for the estimated 40% of patients presenting to gastroenterologists with symptoms suggestive of disorders of stomach, intestinal, colonic, or anorectal function. The practical education offered by the extensive illustrations in every chapter is reinforced by 2 chapters that are devoted entirely to case studies of patients evaluated at Mayo Clinic. I am indebted to the patients for their consent to use their medical records in an anonymized fashion and to Mayo Clinic for the opportunity to do so for this educational endeavor.

I am indebted to my wife, Josephine, who supported me during the many days spent writing this book; to my devoted research administrative assistant, Cindy Stanislav, who helped me organize the first few drafts of the text and illustrations; and to Tracy Becker, John Hedlund, Ann Ihrke, and LeAnn Stee in Scientific Publications at Mayo Clinic for their work in editing, proofreading, and the herculean task of acquiring permissions to reproduce material from prior publications. Most of these publications originated from work performed in my laboratory by the approximately 80 research or clinical fellows and laboratory technologists with whom it has been my privilege to work.

Michael Camilleri, MD

Cover images: Left, The gut's nervous system: blue nerves are parasympathetic and brown nerves are sympathetic. Upper right, Measurement of antropyloroduodenal motility showing hypercontractility of the pylorus in a patient with gastroparesis. Lower right, Gastric volume and accommodation measured with single-photon emission computed tomography (inset, one of the 70-80 transaxial images of the stomach); an imaging algorithm reconstructs the entire stomach and estimates its volume.

Contents

Genetics and Molecular Aspects of Gastrointestinal Motility Disorders[a]

Introduction

Studying rare genetic and molecular diseases of gut motility provides an understanding of their underlying mechanisms and may provide insights on the mechanisms or management of more common illnesses. For example, constipation affects 1 in 5 people 65 years or older and 1 in 10 people younger than 65 years, and slow-transit constipation or colonic inertia is responsible for approximately 10% of referrals of patients with constipation to gastroenterologists and, among all patients with constipation, is the cause in probably 1%. Insights on the pathophysiology and mechanisms of constipation are provided by studying Hirschsprung disease (prevalence, 1:5,000 live births), mitochondrial cytopathy (1:10,000 live births), or multiple endocrine neoplasia type 2B (MEN 2B; 1:30,000 live births). These diseases are used to illustrate the congenital diseases of the enteric neuromuscular apparatus.

The Enteric Nervous System

Vast networks of ganglionated plexuses located in the wall of the gastrointestinal (GI) tract constitute the enteric nervous system (ENS), which consists of approximately the same number of neurons as are located in the spinal cord (approximately 100 million).

The most important plexuses are the myenteric (Auerbach) and submucosal (Meissner) plexuses, which include pacemakers, that is, electrically active cells, including the interstitial cells of Cajal (ICC) and fibroblast-like cells (positive for platelet-derived growth factor receptor alpha [GFRα]) that activate neuromuscular function.

There are preprogrammed functions of the ENS, and these are modulated by parasympathetic and sympathetic extrinsic nerves. In general, the parasympathetic nerves are excitatory and the sympathetic nerves inhibitory to nonsphincteric muscles in the gut; conversely, the sympathetic nerves stimulate sphincters, such as the internal anal sphincter. The basic gut motility process is the peristaltic reflex. In its simplest form, the reflex results in aboral transfer of a bolus, and it involves intrinsic primary afferent neurons (eg, calcitonin gene-related peptide neurons), an ascending excitatory nerve that stimulates contraction (eg, cholinergic and tachykininergic neurons), and a descending inhibitory nerve (eg, nitrergic, vasoactive intestinal polypeptide-ergic neurons) that mediates relaxation in the receiving segment (Figure 1.1).

The ENS originates in utero from the neural crest cells that migrate through the mesoderm into the developing alimentary canal. The processes whereby neural crest cells migrate and settle in different regions of the gut are regulated by signaling molecules. These include transcription factors, neurotrophic factors (eg, the glial-derived neurotrophic factor [GDNF] and its

[a] Portions previously published in Camilleri M. Enteric nervous system disorders: genetic and molecular insights for the neurogastroenterologist. Neurogastroenterol Motil. 2001 Aug;13(4):277-95; used with permission; and Nelson AD, Mouchli MA, Valentin N, Deyle D, Pichurin P, Acosta A, et al. Ehlers-Danlos syndrome and gastrointestinal manifestations: a 20-year experience at Mayo Clinic. Neurogastroenterol Motil. 2015 Nov;27(11):1657-66; used with permission.

Figure 1.1   Integrated Neural Control of Motility

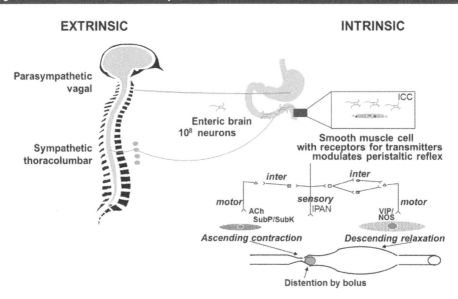

EXTRINSIC   INTRINSIC

In addition to the extrinsic and intrinsic, or enteric, neural control, mesenchymal-derived cells such as the interstitial cells of Cajal (ICCs) serve as pacemakers, transducing stimuli from the nerve to smooth muscle cells. The unit of motor function in the gut is the peristaltic reflex, consisting of an intrinsic primary afferent neuron (IPAN), interneurons and ascending excitatory neuron and descending inhibitory neurons mediating contraction and relaxation, respectively. ACh indicates acetylcholine; NOS, nitric oxide synthase; SubK, substance K; SubP, substance P; VIP, vasoactive intestinal polypeptide.

(Modified from Camilleri M. Enteric nervous system disorders: genetic and molecular insights for the neurogastroenterologist. Neurogastroenterol Motil. 2001 Aug;13(4):277-95; used with permission.)

receptor subunits), and a large group of structurally related signaling proteins, or neuregulins, that facilitate the growth, differentiation, maintenance, repair, and persistence of the migrating nerve cells in the gut. The receptors of the neuregulins are the ERBB protein tyrosine kinases, which are critical to normal cell signaling in the ENS.

Maldevelopment of the ENS may broadly result from defects in the neural crest cells themselves or from alterations in the microenvironment through which the neural crest cells migrate or settle. Such disordered development is responsible for the development of congenital neuromuscular diseases of the gut.

Ontogeny of the ENS

Migration

From 3 levels of the neural crest (vagal, rostral-truncal, and sacral levels), precursors to the ENS cells migrate and reach the developing alimentary tract. The majority of enteric neurons arise from the vagal neural crest of the developing hindbrain. When they migrate to the primordial gut, they spread in a caudal direction to settle approximately in the foregut and midgut regions that will be eventually supplied by the vagus nerve, that is, from the distal esophagus to the right side of the colon. At the same time, neurons arrive in the hindgut from the sacral level, and they colonize in a cephalocaudal manner (Figures 1.2 and 1.3).

When the migrating neural crest cells do not complete the cephalorostral migration to reach a part of the bowel, such as the end of the colon in Hirschsprung disease, the affected segment has abnormal relaxation or excessive contractility, and the colon proximal to it dilates, manifesting as megacolon. After neural crest cells reach their destination in the gut, they become neuroblasts, neuronal support cells, or glioblasts during embryonal development. Sacral neural crest cells are able to colonize, proliferate, or differentiate in the hindgut, independent of the presence of vagal-derived precursor cells. In addition to the vagal and sacral neural crest cells reaching the gut, other neural crest cells arising in the axial region of the developing nervous system enter the gut mesenchyme.

Figure 1.2   Contributions of Vagal and Sacral Neural Crests to Formation of Enteric Nervous System

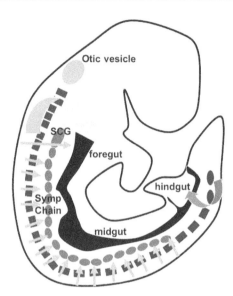

C-ret–dependent *sympathoenteric* (yellow arrow) lineage originates in vagal neural crest of the hindbrain and migrates ventrally to populate the entire gut and SCG. C-ret–independent *sympathoadrenal* (gray arrows) lineage originates in truncal crest and populates foregut and sympathetic chain. *Sacral neural crest* (orange arrow) is derived from spinal cord and colonizes mainly the hindgut. C-ret indicates the tyrosine kinase proto-oncogene; SCG, superior cervical ganglion; Symp, sympathetic.

(Modified from De Giorgio R, Camilleri M. Human enteric neuropathies: morphology and molecular pathology. Neurogastroenterol Motil. 2004 Oct;16(5):515-31; used with permission.)

Figure 1.3   Expression of Tyrosine Kinase Receptor (RET) in Progenitors of the Mammalian Enteric Nervous System (ENS) in a 9.5-Day Mouse Embryo With Specific Probe for *RET* mRNA

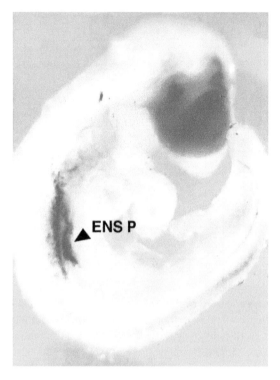

Note ENS P (RET-expressing precursors of the ENS) entering the gastrointestinal tract.

(From Pachnis V, Durbec P, Taraviras S, Grigoriou M, Natarajan D. III. Role of the RET signal transduction pathway in development of the mammalian enteric nervous system. Am J Physiol. 1998 Aug;275(2):G183-6; used with permission.)

There are other factors that control the spatial organization of the migrating and differentiating enteric nerve cell precursors, such as determination of the specific rostrocaudal sites of the cells. Two such mechanisms are 1) barriers to migration that determine whether cells migrating through the mesoderm actually enter the developing gut and 2) homeobox genes, which are highly conserved, developmental control genes necessary for correct morphogenesis in the embryonal gut.

Differentiation

After neuroblasts arrive at their final destinations in the gut, these multipotent crest cells differentiate into neurons and glial cells under influence by the microenvironment containing other cells and extracellular matrix molecules that consist of enteric growth factors and their receptors, such as GDNF-GFR-1-RET (tyrosine kinase receptor),

neurotrophin-3–tropomyosin receptor kinase, and serotonin (5-HT)-5-HT$_{2B}$ (5-hydroxytryptamine receptor 2B). When these combinations do not function correctly, genetic disorders of motility can result and may affect virtually any region because these growth-differentiation factors are present throughout the bowel (Figure 1.4).

Figure 1.4 shows examples of mutations in the tyrosine kinase receptor (RET) that are associated with specific genetic disorders. Other disorders in the combination of endothelin-3 and the endothelin B receptor, ET-3/ETB, may result in premature differentiation of enteric neurons before colonization of the GI tract has been completed. One can regard ET-3 as a brake in the differentiation process, and a different molecule, laminin-1, as an accelerator, when present in excess. Aganglionosis may result from defects in ET-3/ETB receptor in Hirschsprung disease when the defect in

Figure 1.4   Signaling Pathways Involved in Development of the Enteric Nervous System

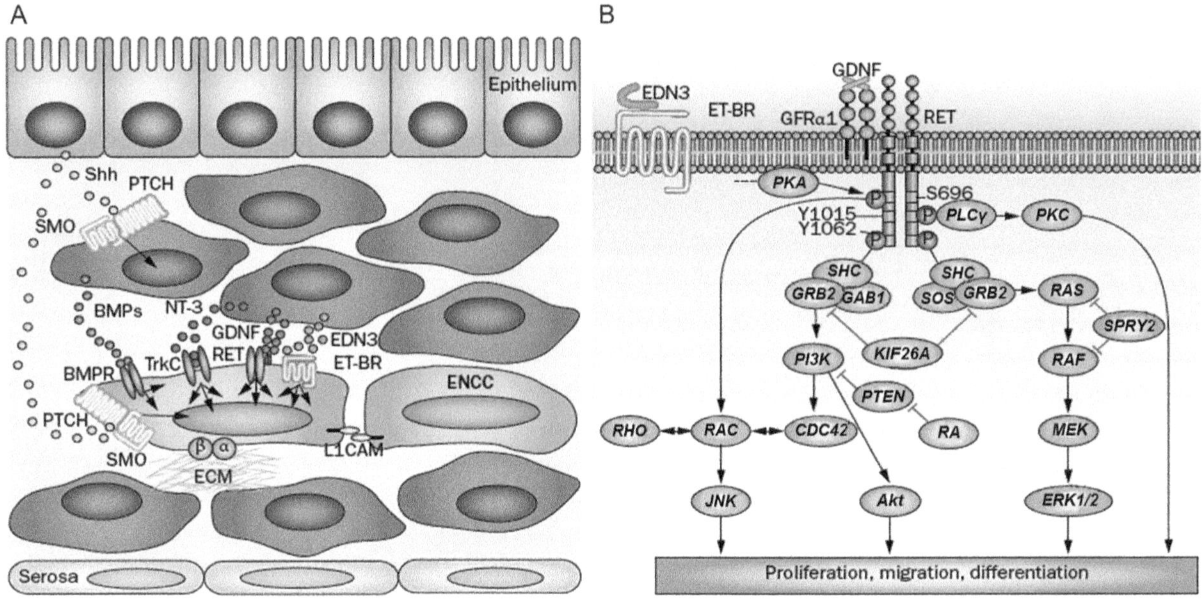

A, Pathways that influence survival, proliferation, migration, and differentiation of enteric neural crest-derived cells (ENCCs). B, Pathways activated by tyrosine kinase receptor (RET). BMPR indicates bone morphogenetic protein receptor; BMPs, bone morphogenetic protein; ECM, extracellular matrix; EDN3, endothelin 3; ET-BR, endothelin B receptor; GDNF, glial-derived neurotrophic factor; GFRα1, GDNF family receptor α-1; L1CAM, L1-cell adhesion molecule; NT-3, neurotrophin-3; PTCH, patched; Shh, sonic hedgehog; SMO, smoothened; TrkC, tropomyosin receptor kinase.

(From Obermayr F, Hotta R, Enomoto H, Young HM. Development and developmental disorders of the enteric nervous system. Nat Rev Gastroenterol Hepatol. 2013 Jan;10(1):43-57; used with permission.)

development is localized; however, a different mutation of the *ET-3* gene causes a more diffuse series of defects in Waardenburg-Shah syndrome associated with Hirschsprung disease, characterized by piebaldism, heterochromia iridis, neural deafness, pyloric stenosis, and congenital megacolon.

Another pivotal control system is provided by enteric serotonergic neurons that appear early and coexist with still-dividing neural precursors in the ganglia within the developing intestine. Serotonin (5-HT) strongly promotes development of neurons at specific times (through 5-HT$_{2B}$ receptors) and affects the development of late-arising enteric neurons.

Nuclear Transcription Factors

Several families of nuclear transcription factors are involved in neuronal differentiation in the primordial ENS and sympathetic ganglia. One example is

Phox2b, which is required for expression of RET and for switching on the genes in developing noradrenergic neurons.

Congenital Neuropathic Motility Disorders

There are 3 broad categories of congenital neuropathic motility disorders:

1. Disorders of colonization by migrating neural crest neurons, as in Hirschsprung disease, due to abnormal GDNF-RET or ET-3/ETB combinations, as described above

2. Disorders of differentiation of enteric nerves, as occurs in MEN 2B due to specific point mutations in the *RET* gene

3. Disorders of the survival or maintenance of enteric nerves, as occurs in hypoganglionosis and possibly congenital achalasia, due to dysfunctions in receptors and their ligands, such as GFRα$_2$/neurturin; GFRα$_3$/artemin; and tyrosine kinase C/neurotrophin-3, and 5HT$_{2B}$/5HT

Hirschsprung Disease

Hirschsprung disease affects 1 in 5,000 live births. It presents as intestinal obstruction in neonates and as megacolon in infants and adults (Figure 1.5). It is a result of the absence of intestinal nerve plexuses due to mutations in genes encoding GDNF-RET or ET-3/ETB (in up to 40% of patients), cRET, endothelin B system, transcription factor gene *SOX10*, and c-kit (a marker for the ICCs), among the large number of associated genetic mutations (Figure 1.6). The genetic disturbances may also result in congenital disorders in addition to the Hirschsprung disease phenotype, as occurs in Waardenburg-Shah syndrome (described above). ENS

precursors must fully colonize fetal bowel to prevent Hirschsprung disease (Figure 1.6).

Non–Hirschsprung Disease Presenting in Adolescence or Adulthood

There are several examples of chronic megacolon presenting in adulthood with proximal megacolon or hindgut dysgenesis (Figures 1.7 and 1.8) that probably arise from congenital disorders and may be associated with regional lack of innervation, as suggested by dilatation, lack of colonic haustrations, and poor colonic contractility measured intraluminally (Figure 1.9).

Chronic Megacolon in Adults: Clinical Features and Colonic Motor Disturbances

Chronic megacolon is rare in adults. It results from colonic motor dysfunction, chronic colonic dilatation, increased colonic compliance (resulting in a high

Figure 1.5   Hirschsprung Disease Presents in Neonatal Period or Infancy

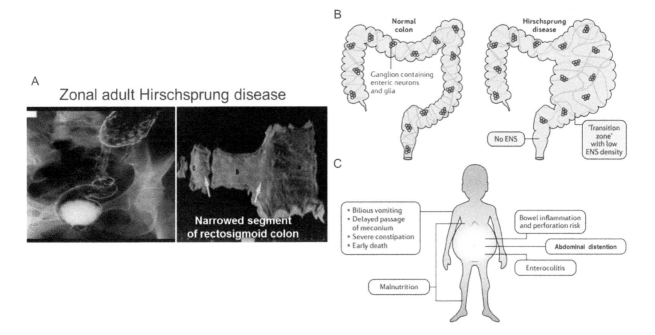

A, Radiographic images of adult Hirschsprung disease resulting in a narrowed segment of rectosigmoid colon. Resected specimen (right) includes proximal dilated part (a), stenotic part (b), and distal normal-appearing part (c) (White arrows indicated transition zones between parts.). B, Comparison of normal colon to colon with Hirschsprung disease. C, Signs and symptoms of Hirschsprung disease in an infant. ENS indicates enteric nervous system.

(Part A from Fu CG, Muto T, Masaki T, Nagawa H. Zonal adult Hirschsprung's disease. Gut. 1996 Nov;39(5):765-7; used with permission. Part C from Heuckeroth RO. Hirschsprung disease: integrating basic science and clinical medicine to improve outcomes. Nat Rev Gastroenterol Hepatol. 2018 Mar;15(3):152-167; used with permission.)

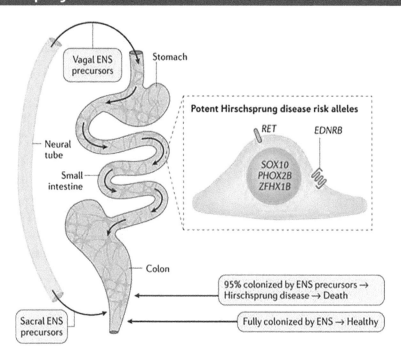

Risk alleles associated with Hirschsprung disease include *RET*, *SOX10*, *Phox2B*, and *ZFHX1B* (also denoted as *ZEB2* by the Human Genome Organisation). EDNRB indicates endothelin receptor B.

(From Heuckeroth RO. Hirschsprung disease: integrating basic science and clinical medicine to improve outcomes. Nat Rev Gastroenterol Hepatol. 2018 Mar;15(3):152-167; used with permission.)

Figure 1.7   Proximal Megacolon in an Adult

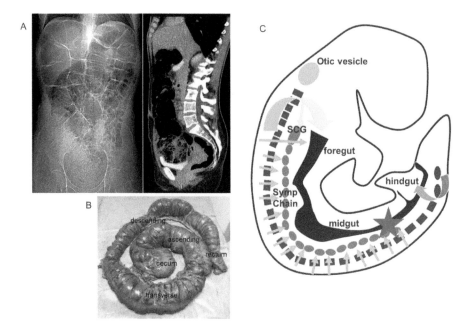

Dilatation of the proximal colon suggests failure of migration of vagal crest cells into the proximal colon, whereas sacral crest cells innervate the distal colon. A, Dilated proximal colon on abdominal radiograph (left) and normal-caliber distal colon on abdominal radiograph and sagittal computed tomographic image (right). B, Resected colon with dilated proximal region and normal-diameter distal colon. C, Failure of migration of vagal crest cells into the proximal colon. SCG indicates superior cervical ganglion; Symp, sympathetic. Red star indicates the region where neural crest cells did not colonize the developing colon. Arrows are described in the legend to Figure 1.2.

(Part B from Vijayvargiya P, Camilleri M. Proximal megacolon in an adult. Clin Gastroenterol Hepatol. 2014 Sep;12(9):e83-4; used with permission. Part C modified from De Giorgio R, Camilleri M. Human enteric neuropathies: morphology and molecular pathology. Neurogastroenterol Motil. 2004 Oct;16(5):515-31; used with permission.)

Figure 1.8   Hindgut Dysgenesis

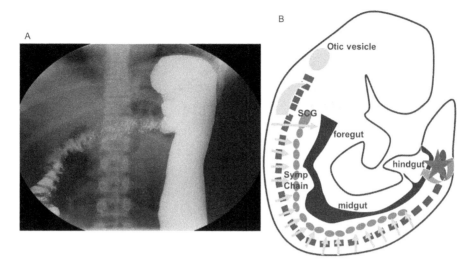

A, Ahaustral, dilated left colon, in contrast to the normal haustrations and smaller diameter of the proximal colon, which presumably are due to normal innervation by cells derived from the vagal crest. The dilated left colon is thought to be due to failure of colonization by sacral neural crest cells in the distal colon. B, SCG indicates superior cervical ganglion; Symp, sympathetic. Red star indicates the region where neural crest cells did not colonize the developing colon. Arrows are described in the legend to Figure 1.2.

Part A from Sweetser S, Camilleri M. Clinical challenges and images in GI: hindgut dysgenesis with megacolon. Gastroenterology. 2008 May;134(5):1293, 1635; used with permission. Part B modified from De Giorgio R, Camilleri M. Human enteric neuropathies: morphology and molecular pathology. Neurogastroenterol Motil. 2004 Oct;16(5):515-31; used with permission.)

Figure 1.9   Low Phasic Contractility and Tone of the Left Colon in a Patient With Hindgut Dysgenesis (shown in Figure 1.8)

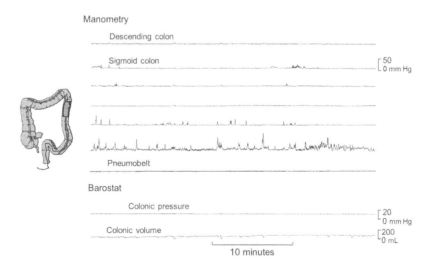

The barostatically controlled polyethylene balloon (far left) in the descending colon measures colonic tone.

(From Sweetser S, Camilleri M. Clinical challenges and images in GI: hindgut dysgenesis with megacolon. Gastroenterology. 2008 May;134(5):1293, 1635; used with permission.)

Figure 1.10   Colonic Compliance in 3 Control Groups (A-C) and in Patients With Chronic Megacolon (D)

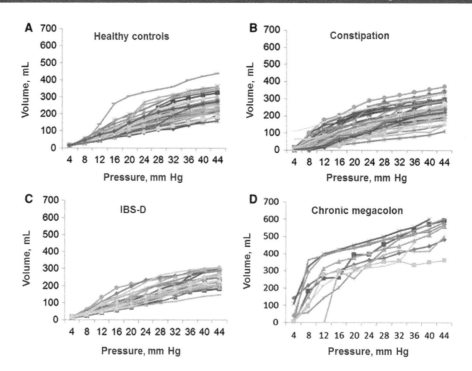

Control groups: healthy controls (A), constipation (B), and diarrhea-predominant irritable bowel syndrome (IBS-D) (C). The volume of the intracolonic balloon (10 cm long) is markedly increased in patients with megacolon compared with that in controls. Also, the volume of the intracolonic balloon is markedly increased (>300 mL) at 16 mm Hg distention in all patients with megacolon except 1 and in only 1 healthy control but none of the patients with IBS-D.

(Modified from O'Dwyer RH, Acosta A, Camilleri M, Burton D, Busciglio I, Bharucha AE. Clinical features and colonic motor disturbances in chronic megacolon in adults. Dig Dis Sci. 2015 Aug;60(8):2398-407; used with permission.)

volume in response to normal intraluminal pressures), and reduced colonic tone with retained ability to generate phasic contractions after meal ingestion (Figures 1.10 and 1.11).

For 24 patients with chronic megacolon diagnosed from 1999 to 2014 at Mayo Clinic (Table 1.1), the mean maximal colonic diameter on abdominal radiography was 12.7±0.8 cm (O'Dwyer 2015; see suggested reading). Megacolon was idiopathic in 16 patients and due to an underlying disease process in 8. Ten patients had comorbid pelvic floor dyssynergia, which was unexplained, but it did not appear related to the underlying process leading to megacolon because it was reversible with standard treatment. The colonic tonic response to feeding was generally intact, and the phasic contractile response of the colon to feeding was frequently maintained (Figure 1.12). In general, megacolon does not respond to pharmacologic treatment, and patients may require colectomy. At the time of the report of the

Mayo Clinic study in 2015, 16 patients had undergone colectomy (Table 1.2).

Multiple Endocrine Neoplasia Type 2B

MEN syndrome usually presents in families. It is suspected when there are tumors in 2 or more endocrine glands in a single patient or in close relatives. Three syndromes result from mutations of the *RET* proto-oncogene: MEN 2A, MEN 2B, and familial medullary carcinoma of the thyroid (Figure 1.13).

Among these syndromes, MEN 2B may have gastroenterologic presentations: severe constipation, diarrhea (when associated with enterocolitis), megacolon, or obstruction, often in infancy. Other characteristic manifestations are a characteristic facies, thickening of the lips from mucosal neuromas (Figure 1.14), a marfanoid habitus, and medullated

Figure 1.11   Volume in 10-cm-Long Colonic Barostat Balloon in 3 Control Groups and in Patients With Chronic Megacolon

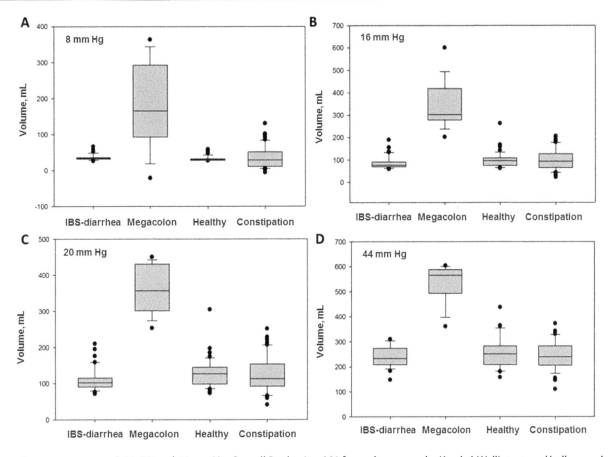

Distention pressures were 8, 16, 20, and 44 mm Hg. Overall *P* value is <.001 for each pressure by Kruskal-Wallis test, and balloon volume in megacolon is significantly higher than that in each group, *P*<.05, by Dunn test. IBS indicates irritable bowel syndrome.

(Modified from O'Dwyer RH, Acosta A, Camilleri M, Burton D, Busciglio I, Bharucha AE. Clinical features and colonic motor disturbances in chronic megacolon in adults. Dig Dis Sci. 2015 Aug;60(8):2398-407; used with permission.)

corneal nerve fibers. Medullary thyroid carcinoma develops in almost all patients, but pheochromocytomas or parathyroid tumors do not develop in all patients.

MEN 2B is an autosomal dominant disorder affecting 1 in 30,000 people, and at least 50% of patients have a de novo mutation. The precise molecular abnormality is in an intracellular tyrosine kinase domain in the *RET* proto-oncogene, which is expressed in neural crest cells that populate the enteric nervous system, adrenal medulla, parathyroid, and C cells of the thyroid. The gain of function mutations (which are constitutively active) render the patient susceptible to the endocrine tumors. A specific germline point mutation (methionine to threonine) in *RET* at codon 918 (M918T) occurs in

95% of patients; the remainder have point mutations at codon 883 (A883F) or M918V (in 50 Brazilian patients from 8 kindreds) or compound *RET* mutations with a common mutation in codon 804 in combination with a second substitution mutation in codon 781, 806, 904, or 905.

In MEN 2B, massive proliferations of neural tissues (neurons, supporting cells, and nerve fibers) appear as thickened nerve trunks among mature nerve cells (Figure 1.15), an appearance called transmural intestinal ganglioneuromatosis. Clinical and demographic features of patients with MEN 2B and megacolon evaluated at Mayo Clinic are shown in Table 1.3. In infants treated for megacolon, MEN 2B should be excluded, the most common indication being Hirschsprung

Table 1.1	Symptoms and Signs at Presentation in Patients With Chronic Megacolon[a]	
Clinical and Radiologic Features	**No. of Patients (%)[b] (N=24)**	
Bowel movement (BM)		
Average number BM/week (range)	1.5 (1-2.5)	
Straining >25% of the time	5 (21)	
Sense of incomplete evacuation	5 (21)	
Digital maneuvers to evacuate BM	1 (4)	
Abdominal pain	20 (84)	
Bloating	23 (96)	
Abdominal distention	23 (96)	
Evidence of rectal evacuation disorder		
Balloon expulsion requiring >200 g weight	8 (33)	
Abnormal resting anal sphincter pressure	12 (50)	
Treatments received before evaluation		
Fiber supplementation	3 (13)	
Osmotic laxative	12 (50)	
Prokinetic	10 (42)	
Enemas	8 (33)	
Maximal diameter of colon on radiographic examination, cm		
Mean±SEM	12.7±0.8	
Median (IQR)	12 (10.8-13)	

Abbreviations: IQR, interquartile range; SEM, standard error of the mean.

[a] Evidence of rectal evacuation disorder was based on abnormal balloon expulsion or abnormal anal manometry results.

[b] Unless otherwise indicated.

From O'Dwyer RH, Acosta A, Camilleri M, Burton D, Busciglio I, Bharucha AE. Clinical features and colonic motor disturbances in chronic megacolon in adults. Dig Dis Sci. 2015 Aug;60(8):2398-407; used with permission.

disease. Thus, an adequate full-thickness biopsy of the bowel should be performed at the time of the pull-through operation, and those with transmural intestinal ganglioneuromatosis should undergo testing by *RET* mutation analysis. If germline M918T or A883F mutations are found, patients should undergo a prophylactic thyroidectomy, periodic adrenal gland or abdominal ultrasonography, and urinary fractionated catecholamine and metanephrine tests to search for pheochromocytoma.

Mitochondrial DNA and Cytopathies

Mitochondrial disorders are characterized by mitochondrial abnormalities and manifestations in all tissues that depend on mitochondrial function: skeletal muscle, central and peripheral nervous system, gut, heart, kidney, liver, thyroid, pancreas, and bone marrow. The enzymes in the respiratory chain of mitochondria are encoded by nuclear and mitochondrial DNA. The disorders have diverse patterns of inheritance: maternal

Figure 1.12 Phasic and Tonic Contractile Activity Measured Under Constant Pressure Conditions in the Colon

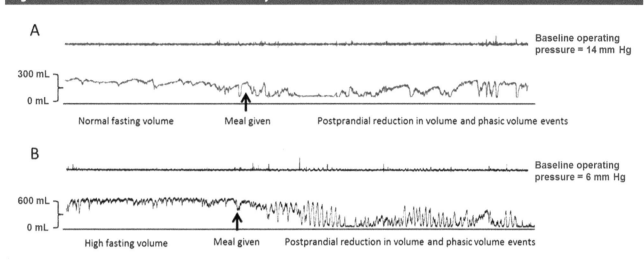

A, Patients with slow-transit constipation (operating pressure 14 mm Hg). B, Chronic megacolon (operating pressure 6 mm Hg). Note the large colonic volume (indicating low tone) during fasting and the persistence of phasic contractile activity despite the low colonic tone after ingestion of a 1,000-kcal liquid nutrient meal.

(Modified from O'Dwyer RH, Acosta A, Camilleri M, Burton D, Busciglio I, Bharucha AE. Clinical features and colonic motor disturbances in chronic megacolon in adults. Dig Dis Sci. 2015 Aug;60(8):2398-407; used with permission.)

inheritance is the more frequent, but other forms of inheritance (dominant, recessive, X-linked) and sporadic cases are documented.

Mitochondrial disorders manifest with multiple organ disturbances (Figure 1.16), typically in skeletal muscle (which shows ragged red fibers with Gomori trichrome stain) and the nervous system (leukoencephalopathy).

The mitochondrial disorders affecting the gut are mitochondrial neurogastrointestinal encephalomyopathy (MNGIE); mitochondrial myopathy with peripheral sensorimotor polyneuropathy, external ophthalmoplegia including ptosis, and pseudo-obstruction; oculogastrointestinal muscular dystrophy; or familial visceral myopathy type II. Manifestations may present

Table 1.2 Management of Megacolon After Evaluation at Mayo Clinic

Management	No. (%) (N=24)
Pyridostigmine	4 (17)
Progression to colectomy post-pyridostigmine trial (n=4)	3 (75)
Colectomy	16 (67)
With ileorectal anastomosis	15 (94)
With ileostomy	1 (6)
Outcome of colectomy (n=16)	
Alleviation of symptoms	7 (43.8)
Symptoms not alleviated	3 (18.8)
Unknown	6 (37.5)

From O'Dwyer RH, Acosta A, Camilleri M, Burton D, Busciglio I, Bharucha AE. Clinical features and colonic motor disturbances in chronic megacolon in adults. Dig Dis Sci. 2015 Aug;60(8):2398-407; used with permission.

Figure 1.13   Mutations of the *RET* Proto-oncogene Associated With MEN 2

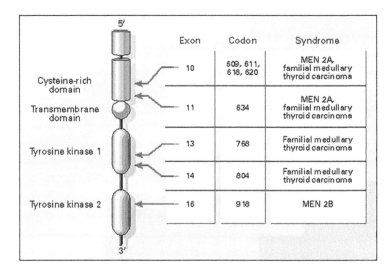

MEN 2 indicates multiple endocrine neoplasia type 2.

(From Eng C. Seminars in medicine of the Beth Israel Hospital, Boston: the RET proto-oncogene in multiple endocrine neoplasia type 2 and Hirschsprung's disease. N Engl J Med. 1996 Sep 26;335(13):943-51; used with permission.)

Figure 1.14   Clinical Manifestations of Multiple Endocrine Neoplasia Type 2B

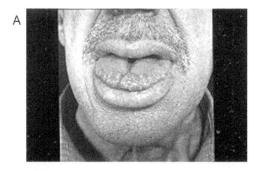

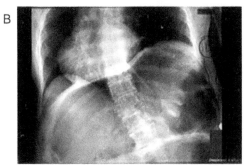
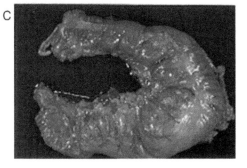

A, Thickening of the lips and tongue caused by ganglioneuromas. B, Megacolon on radiograph. C, Gross specimen of megacolon.

(From De Giorgio R, Camilleri M. Human enteric neuropathies: morphology and molecular pathology. Neurogastroenterol Motil. 2004 Oct;16(5):515-31; used with permission.)

Figure 1.15   Radiologic and Histopathologic Features of Megacolon in Multiple Endocrine Neoplasia Type 2B

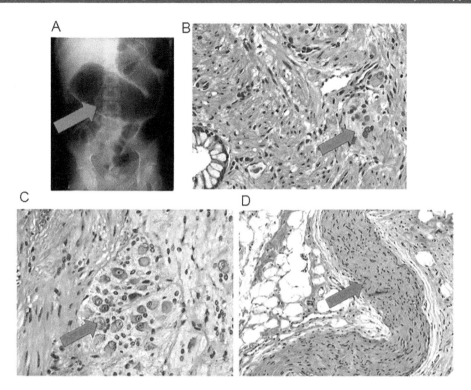

A, Megacolon (arrow) on radiograph. B, Gangliocytic nerve cell dysplasia (arrow). C, Increased number of ganglion cells (arrow). D, Subserosal nerve hypertrophy (arrow).

(From Gibbons D, Camilleri M, Nelson AD, Eckert D. Characteristics of chronic megacolon among patients diagnosed with multiple endocrine neoplasia type 2B. United European Gastroenterol J. 2016 Jun;4(3):449-54; used with permission.)

at any age: typically, hepatomegaly or hepatic failure in the neonate, seizures or diarrhea in infancy, and hepatic failure or chronic intestinal pseudo-obstruction in children or adults.

In addition to severe GI dysmotility, the small intestine is dilated or has multiple diverticula. Some patients have transfer dysphagia due to abnormal coordination and propagation of the swallow through

Table 1.3   Patient Demographics From a Mayo Clinic Series of MEN 2B and Megacolon

Characteristic	Patient A	Patient B	Patient C[a]	Patient D	Patient E[a]	Patient F[a]	Patient G[a]
Age at diagnosis of MEN 2B, y	8	20	Not known	3	31	18	51
Age at diagnosis of megacolon, y	Infancy	25	60	3	24	18	70 from autopsy
Sex	M	M	M	F	M	F	M
RET mutation	NA	M918T	M918T	M918T	NA	NA	NA
Family history of MEN	–	–	+	–	+	+	+

Abbreviations: F, female; M, male; MEN, multiple endocrine neoplasia; NA, not available; RET, rearranged during transfection proto-oncogene; –, negative; +, positive.

[a] Patients C, E, F (siblings), and G (father) are members of the same family.

From Gibbons D, Camilleri M, Nelson AD, Eckert D. Characteristics of chronic megacolon among patients diagnosed with multiple endocrine neoplasia type 2B. United European Gastroenterol J. 2016 Jun;4(3):449-54; used with permission.

Figure 1.16   Organ Involvement in Mitochondrial Cytopathy Resulting From Interaction Between Genes Encoded by Nuclear DNA and Those Encoded by Mitochondrial DNA in Oxidative Phosphorylation

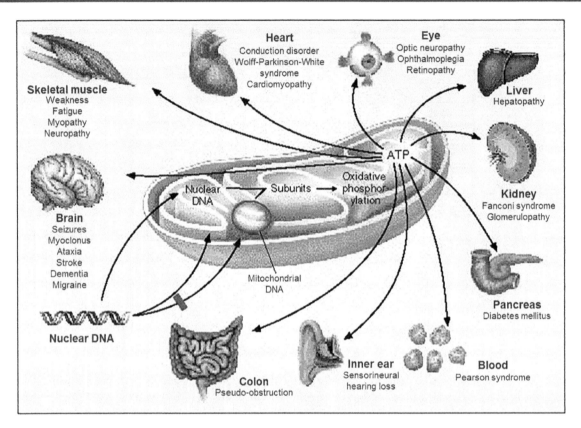

The function of the oxidative-phosphorylation complexes can be disrupted by defects in the subunits encoded by nuclear DNA and mitochondrial DNA or by defects in intergenomic communication between the 2 types of DNA. ATP indicates adenosine triphosphate.

(Modified from Johns DR. Seminars in medicine of the Beth Israel Hospital, Boston: mitochondrial DNA and disease. N Engl J Med. 1995 Sep 7;333(10):638-44; used with permission.)

the pharynx and the skeletal muscle portion of the esophagus.

As a result of skeletal muscle involvement, patients have pain and cramps in skeletal muscle, systemic (lactic) acidosis, and increased circulating muscle enzyme levels (eg, creatine phosphokinase, alanine transaminase, aldolase), and muscle biopsy shows characteristic ragged red fibers (Figure 1.17) (due to hypertrophy of mitochondria in the subsarcolemmal position) on modified Gomori stain. Paradoxically, there is a lack of mitochondria in other muscle fibers. Megamitochondria may also be identified on submucosal neurons in a rectal biopsy (Figure 1.18). On muscle biopsy, special stains for the enzymes involved in the respiratory chain within skeletal muscle can be used to identify the precise functional defect in the respiratory enzyme chain: fibers positive for 1 enzyme appear ragged blue, and an adjacent tissue section stained for another enzyme is unstained. This result indicates a deficiency in the next enzyme in the chain and signifies a specific gene defect in the complex IV respiratory chain proteins.

The intestinal abnormalities are characterized by hypertrophy of the circular muscle layer, atrophy of the longitudinal muscle, mega-mitochondria in myenteric neurons and muscle cells, and the occurrence of multiple small intestinal diverticula. Whenever a person younger than 50 years presents with multiple jejunal diverticulosis, mitochondrial cytopathy should be excluded.

Figure 1.17   Histologic and Histochemical Studies of Skeletal Muscle Biopsy From a Patient With Mitochondrial Myopathy Associated With Mitochondrial Neurogastrointestinal Encephalomyopathy

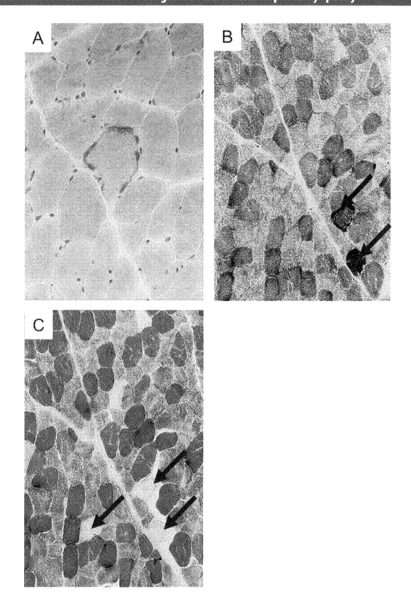

A, Modified Gomori stain (×400): ragged red fibers characterized by the subsarcolemmal location of giant mitochondria in a few fibers and paucity of mitochondria in other fibers. B, On histochemical analysis, a few fibers are succinate dehydrogenase–positive (ragged blue appearance; arrows), but the same fibers do not express cytochrome C oxidase (C, arrows), suggesting a defect in the respiratory enzyme chain that results in mitochondrial dysfunction and systemic acidosis (B and C, magnification ×180).

(Modified from Mueller LA, Camilleri M, Emslie-Smith AM. Mitochondrial neurogastrointestinal encephalomyopathy: manometric and diagnostic features. Gastroenterology. 1999 Apr;116(4):959-63; used with permission.)

Screening tests for MNGIE are measurements of serum lactic acid and muscle enzymes. The diagnosis of MNGIE in a proband is based on detection of 1 of the following: 1) biallelic pathogenic variants in thymidine phosphorylase gene, *TYMP*; 2) markedly reduced levels of TYMP enzyme activity; or 3) increased plasma concentrations of thymidine and deoxyuridine.

Figure 1.18   Submucosal Plexus Neurons Showing Megamitochondria in Rectal Biopsy From a Patient With Mitochondrial Myopathy

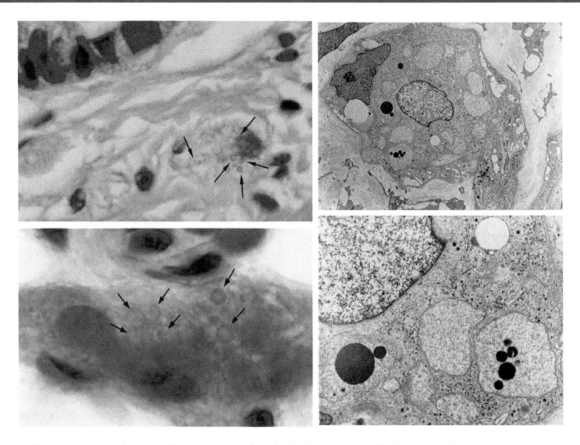

Left panels, Light microscopy. Arrows indicate megamitochondria in the cytoplasm. Right panels, Electron microscopy.

(From Perez-Atayde AR, Fox V, Teitelbaum JE, Anthony DA, Fadic R, Kalsner L, et al. Mitochondrial neurogastrointestinal encephalomyopathy: diagnosis by rectal biopsy. Am J Surg Pathol. 1998 Sep;22(9):1141-7; used with permission.)

ICCs in Maldevelopment and Acquired Diseases of the Colon

The c-kit gene encodes for a tyrosine kinase receptor that facilitates the development of the ICCs, which form close contact with smooth muscle cells through gap junctions and so permit transmission of the pacemaking activity. As in the heart, a pacemaker cell is one that has spontaneous oscillation in resting membrane potentials and is unaffected by L-type calcium channel blockers.

A relative deficiency of c-kit–positive cells has been reported in Hirschsprung disease, chronic intestinal pseudo-obstruction, and slow-transit constipation or colonic inertia. In addition, there can be delayed maturation or maldevelopment of ICCs, although this is rare. In a 1-month-old child with chronic colonic pseudo-obstruction, biopsy of the affected colon showed no peristaltic activity and no ICCs were found within the circular muscle or submuscular layer, although they were present in the myenteric plexus (Kenny 1998; see Suggested Reading). At 6 months of age, normal peristaltic activity had been restored and further full-thickness biopsy showed ICCs were fully developed in all layers of the colon. This careful case study illustrates postnatal maturation of ICCs.

Megacolon in an adult and acquired slow-transit constipation without dilatation have also been associated with abnormal morphologic and ultrastructural features of ICCs (Figure 1.19).

Figure 1.19 Histologic and Ultrastructural Studies of the Interstitial Cells of Cajal (ICCs) in Myenteric Plexus (MP) Region in an Adult With Megacolon

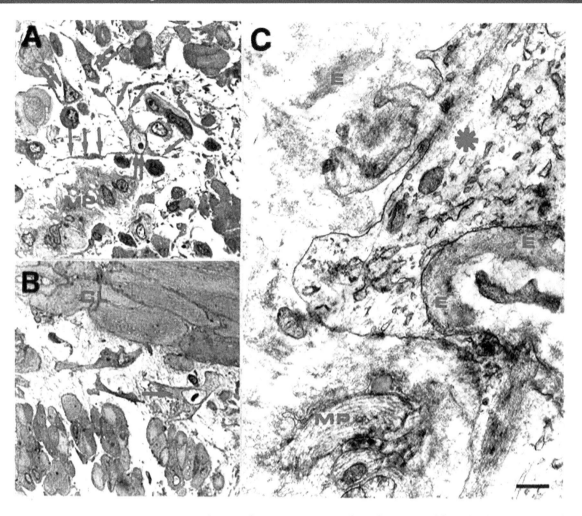

A, Three ICCs (double arrows) have multiple branches (single arrows) in the unaffected segment of dilated right transverse colon. B, ICC (arrow) between circular (CL) and longitudinal (LL) muscle layers in nondilated descending colon. (A and B: semithin section, toluidine blue, magnification ×750). C, ICC cytoplasm (asterisk) in nondilated descending colon plexus has a paucity of mitochondria, filaments, and caveolae (magnification ×25,000). E indicates elastic fibers.

(From Faussone-Pellegrini MS, Fociani P, Buffa R, Basilisco G. Loss of interstitial cells and a fibromuscular layer on the luminal side of the colonic circular muscle presenting as megacolon in an adult patient. Gut. 1999 Nov;45(5):775-9; used with permission.)

Ehlers-Danlos and Hypermobility Syndromes

Although the precise molecular or genetic defect in hypermobile Ehlers-Danlos syndrome (EDS) is not always clear, the prevalence of the association between EDS and motility or functional disorders suggests that this may, in fact, be the most important genetic or molecular disorder, although the severity of the phenotype is most often aligned with functional diseases rather than diseases associated with dilatation such as pseudo-obstruction or megacolon.

EDS results from defects in the synthesis of collagen and is a diverse group of heritable disorders of connective tissue with various degrees of skin hyperextensibility, joint hypermobility, and generalized skin fragility. The prevalence of EDS is approximately 1:5,000. Hypermobile EDS, also called joint

Box 1.1

Villefranche Diagnostic Criteria for EDS, Hypermobility Type

Inheritance

    Autosomal dominant

Major diagnostic criteria

    Skin involvement (hyperextensible or smooth and velvety)

    Generalized joint hypermobility (Beighton score ≥5/9)

Minor diagnostic criteria

    Recurring joint dislocations[a]

    Chronic joint/limb pain[a]

    Positive family history

Abbreviation: EDS, Ehlers-Danlos syndrome.

[a] Used to define musculoskeletal presentation of syndromic hypermobility.

From Beighton P, De Paepe A, Steinmann B, Tsipouras P, Wenstrup RJ. Ehlers-Danlos syndromes: revised nosology, Villefranche, 1997. Ehlers-Danlos National Foundation (USA) and Ehlers-Danlos Support Group (UK). Am J Med Genet. 1998 Apr 28;77(1):31-7; used with permission.

Table 1.4   Brighton Criteria for the Diagnosis of Joint Hypermobility Syndrome

Major criteria		
1. A Beighton score of 4 of 9 or more (either currently or historically)		
	Left	**Right**
a. Passive dorsiflexion and hyperextension of the fifth MCP joint beyond 90°	1	1
b. Passive apposition of the thumb to the flexor aspect of the forearm	1	1
c. Passive hyperextension of the elbow beyond 10°	1	1
d. Passive hyperextension of the knee beyond 10°	1	1
e. Active forward flexion of the trunk with the knees fully extended so that the palms of the hands rest flat on the floor	1	
Total	/9	
2. Arthralgia for longer than 3 months in 4 or more joints		
Minor criteria		
1. A Beighton score of 1, 2 or 3/9 (0, 1, 2, or 3 if aged >50 y)		
2. Arthralgia in 1 to 3 joints or back pain or spondylosis, spondylolysis or spondylolisthesis		
3. Dislocation in more than one joint, or in one joint on more than one occasion		
4. Three or more soft tissue lesions (eg, epicondylitis, tenosynovitis, bursitis)		
5. Marfanoid habitus (tall, slim, arm span:height >1.03; upper segment:lower segment <0.89, arachnodactyly, high arch palate)		
6. Skin striae, hyperextensibility, thin skin or abnormal scarring		
7. Eye signs: drooping eyelids or myopia or antimongoloid slant		
8. Varicose veins or hernia or uterine/rectal prolapse		

Abbreviation: MCP, metacarpophalangeal.

Modified from Grahame R, Bird HA, Child A. The revised (Brighton 1998) criteria for the diagnosis of benign joint hypermobility syndrome (BJHS). J Rheumatol. 2000 Jul;27(7):1777-9; used with permission, and Beighton P, Solomon L, Soskolne CL. Articular mobility in an African population. Ann Rheum Dis. 1973 Sep;32(5):413-8; used with permission.

hypermobility syndrome, is the most common type of EDS that is diagnosed clinically using Brighton criteria (which include Beighton scores). The precise gene involved in this type of EDS is not yet identified.

The Villefranche criteria for EDS hypermobility are listed in Box 1.1. The diagnosis requires 1 or both major criteria, and the minor criteria alone are not sufficient for diagnosis. The Brighton criteria for the diagnosis of joint hypermobility syndrome are listed in Table 1.4.

In a study of the medical records of 687 patients with EDS who were evaluated at Mayo Clinic's Medical Genetics Clinic from 1994 through 2013 (Nelson 2015; see suggested reading), 378 (55.0%) had GI manifestations (Table 1.5). The majority of patients (86.5%) were female, and the average age at diagnosis was 29.6 years. Patients also had other non-GI manifestations of EDS (Table 1.6).

GI features occurred in 58.9% (43/73) of patients with EDS classic subtype, 57.5% (271/471) of those

Table 1.5	Prevalence (Percentage) of Patients With EDS Who Had Upper and Lower GI Symptoms (N=378)						
Upper and Lower GI Symptoms	EDS Overall	EDS HM	EDS Classic	EDS Vascular	EDS Others	EDS non-HM	P Value EDS HM vs non-HM
Nausea	42.3	44.3	46.5	25.9	35.1	37.4	NS
Vomiting	23.8	24.7	30.2	14.8	16.2	21.5	NS
Globus	1.1	1.1	0.0	0.0	2.7	0.9	NS
Heartburn (reflux disease)	37.6	38.0	30.2	48.1	35.1	36.4	NS
Water brash	1.3	1.1	2.3	0.0	2.7	1.9	NS
Retrosternal chest pain	7.9	7.4	0.0	14.8	16.2	9.3	NS
Abdominal pain	56.1	56.1	51.2	81.5	43.2	56.1	NS
Dysphagia	11.4	11.1	14.0	11.1	10.8	12.1	NS
Dyspepsia	9.5	10.7	7.0	7.4	5.4	6.5	NS
Regurgitation	4.5	4.1	0.0	3.7	13.5	5.6	NS
Belching	3.2	3.3	2.3	0.0	5.4	2.8	NS
Bloating	15.1	17.0	4.7	11.1	16.2	10.3	.101
Postprandial fullness	5.8	7.0	7.0	0.0	0.0	2.8	.115
IBS-like symptoms	27.5	30.3	18.6	14.8	27.0	20.6	.057
Constipation	38.6	42.4	37.2	14.8	29.7	29.0	.015
Diarrhea	20.9	22.5	20.9	7.4	18.9	16.8	NS
Fecal urgency	1.9	1.5	0.0	7.4	2.7	2.8	NS
Fecal incontinence or perianal soiling	2.1	2.2	0.0	7.4	0.0	1.9	NS
History of rectal prolapse	2.9	3.7	2.3	0.0	0.0	1.0	NS
History of pelvic floor dysfunction	11.4	11.4	18.6	7.4	5.4	11.2	NS
History of rectocele	3.4	3.7	4.7	3.7	0.0	2.8	NS

Abbreviations: EDS, Ehlers-Danlos syndrome; GI, gastrointestinal; HM, hypermobility type; IBS, irritable bowel syndrome; NS, not significant.

From Nelson AD, Mouchli MA, Valentin N, Deyle D, Pichurin P, Acosta A, et al. Ehlers Danlos syndrome and gastrointestinal manifestations: a 20-year experience at Mayo Clinic. Neurogastroenterol Motil. 2015 Nov;27(11):1657-66; used with permission.

with EDS hypermobility subtype, and 47.3% (27/57) of patients with EDS vascular subtype. The most common GI symptoms were: abdominal pain (56.1%), nausea (42.3%), constipation (38.6%), heartburn (37.6%), and irritable bowel syndrome (27.5%). Many GI symptoms were more common in the patients with EDS hypermobility subtype than all the other subtypes combined. Among the 378 patients with GI manifestations, 143 (37.8%) underwent esophagogastroduodenoscopy: the most common findings were gastritis, hiatal hernia, and reflux esophagitis. Abnormal gastric emptying was observed in 22.3% of those who underwent that test by scintigraphy (17/76): 9 (11.8%) had delayed and 8 (10.5%) accelerated gastric emptying. Colonic transit was abnormal in 28.3% (13/46): 9 (19.6%) delayed and 4 (8.7%) accelerated (Figure 1.20). Rectal evacuation disorder was confirmed in 18 of 30 patients who underwent anorectal manometry. Angiography showed aneurysms in abdominal vessels in EDS vascular subtype (Figure 1.21).

Table 1.6   Prevalence (Percentage) of Patients With EDS Who Had Non-GI Symptoms

Non-GI Symptoms	EDS Overall	EDS HM	EDS Classic	EDS Vascular	EDS Others	EDS non-HM	P Value EDS HM vs non-HM
Skin conditions	36.0	35.4	62.8	22.2	18.9	37.4	NS
Arthralgias	74.3	83.7	65.1	33.3	45.9	50.5	<.0001
Joint dislocations	40.2	48.7	32.6	3.7	13.5	18.7	<.0001
Autonomic dysfunction[a]	36.5	43.5	20.9	3.7	27.0	18.7	<.0001
Fibromyalgia	18.3	20.7	14.0	7.4	13.5	12.1	.053
Psychopathology	37.8	37.3	41.9	29.6	43.2	39.3	NS
Chronic fatigue	30.4	35.8	18.6	11.1	18.9	16.8	.0003
Sleep disturbance	23.0	22.5	25.6	14.8	29.7	24.3	NS
Migraine headache	34.4	37.6	37.2	14.8	21.6	26.2	.034
Allergies reported	22.2	20.3	25.6	18.5	35.1	27.1	NS

Abbreviations: EDS, Ehlers-Danlos syndrome; GI, gastrointestinal; HM, hypermobility type; NS, not significant.

[a] Autonomic dysfunction: syncope, orthostatic intolerance, postural tachycardia syndrome.

From Nelson AD, Mouchli MA, Valentin N, Deyle D, Pichurin P, Acosta A, et al. Ehlers Danlos syndrome and gastrointestinal manifestations: a 20-year experience at Mayo Clinic. Neurogastroenterol Motil. 2015 Nov;27(11):1657-66; used with permission.

Figure 1.20   Gastric Emptying (A) and Colonic Transit (B) in Patients With Ehlers-Danlos Syndrome

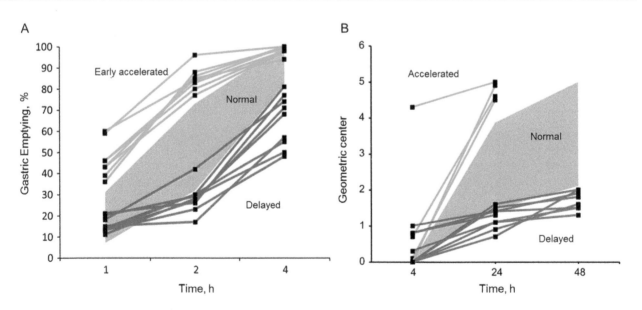

(From Nelson AD, Mouchli MA, Valentin N, Deyle D, Pichurin P, Acosta A, et al. Ehlers Danlos syndrome and gastrointestinal manifestations: a 20-year experience at Mayo Clinic. Neurogastroenterol Motil. 2015 Nov;27(11):1657-66; used with permission.)

Figure 1.21   Intra-abdominal Aneurysms in Patients With Ehlers-Danlos Syndrome Vascular Subtype

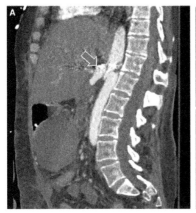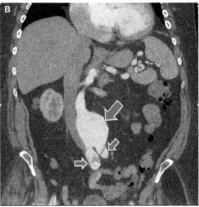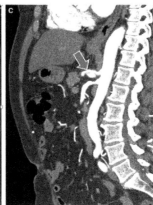

A, Computed tomogram (CT) without contrast in a 50-year-old woman. The arrow identifies coil embolization of a celiac artery aneurysm. B, CT angiogram in a 60-year-old man showing a 65-mm–diameter abdominal aortic aneurysm (large arrow) and arterial dissection with aneurysmal dilatation of both common iliac arteries measuring 27 mm on the right and 25 mm on the left (smaller arrows). C, CT angiogram in a 56-year-old woman showing celiac artery dissection with 11-mm aneurysmal dilation (arrow).

(From Nelson AD, Mouchli MA, Valentin N, Deyle D, Pichurin P, Acosta A, et al. Ehlers Danlos syndrome and gastrointestinal manifestations: a 20-year experience at Mayo Clinic. Neurogastroenterol Motil. 2015 Nov;27(11):1657-66; used with permission.)

The most commonly used medications in patients with EDS who had GI manifestations were proton pump inhibitors (38%) and drugs for constipation (23%). A minority of the patients underwent colectomy (2.9%) or small bowel surgery (4%).

Suggested Reading

Camilleri M. Enteric nervous system disorders: genetic and molecular insights for the neurogastroenterologist. Neurogastroenterol Motil. 2001 Aug;13(4):277–95. Epub 2001 Sep 29.

Gibbons D, Camilleri M, Nelson AD, Eckert D. Characteristics of chronic megacolon among patients diagnosed with multiple endocrine neoplasia type 2B. United European Gastroenterol J. 2016 Jun;4(3):449–54. Epub 2016 Jul 13.

Kenny SE, Vanderwinden JM, Rintala RJ, Connell MG, Lloyd DA, Vanderhaegen JJ, et al. Delayed maturation of the interstitial cells of Cajal: a new diagnosis for transient neonatal pseudoobstruction: report of two cases. J Pediatr Surg. 1998 Jan;33(1):94–8.

Nelson AD, Mouchli MA, Valentin N, Deyle D, Pichurin P, Acosta A, et al. Ehlers Danlos syndrome and gastrointestinal manifestations: a 20-year experience at Mayo Clinic. Neurogastroenterol Motil. 2015 Nov;27(11):1657–66. Epub 2015 Sep 18.

O'Dwyer RH, Acosta A, Camilleri M, Burton D, Busciglio I, Bharucha AE. Clinical features and colonic motor disturbances in chronic megacolon in adults. Dig Dis Sci. 2015 Aug;60(8):2398–407. Epub 2015 Apr 15.

Measurement of Gastrointestinal and Colonic Motility in Clinical Practice

Introduction

The motor functions of the gastrointestinal (GI) tract are complex, and their measurements are crucial to understanding mechanisms, achieving diagnosis, and planning treatment of diverse digestive diseases. Unlike the heart, which has a more rhythmic and patterned electrical and contractile function, the GI tract has diverse motor functions, necessitating the development, validation, and standardization of a vast repertoire of tests of GI motor functions. Measurements of motility functions have been validated and standardized and can be delivered at the point of care.

The objectives of these standardized clinical tests are to aid diagnosis of motility disorders (Figure 2.1). Motility and functional digestive disorders have relatively few symptoms, and measurements of motor functions are essential. The tests also serve to objectively document effects of treatments for motility disorders and to enhance understanding of the pathophysiologic mechanisms of these disorders or diseases.

Tests of esophageal motility are not included here. High-resolution manometry, impedance planimetry, and measurements of the diameter and distensibility of the gastroesophageal junction (usually performed during endoscopy) have become the diagnostic tools of choice and are discussed extensively in the Suggested Reading.

Gastric Capacity and Accommodation

The proximal stomach stores ingested food through accommodation of large volumes in the fundus and body, while maintaining a relatively low intragastric pressure. Although tumor infiltration (linitis plastica) may change gastric distensibility, major disturbances of gastric tone result from vagal dysfunction and effects of prior gastric surgery and are found in almost 50% of patients presenting with functional upper GI symptoms.

Barostat Balloon Measurements

In the past, the standard for measurement of tone in different gut regions was the barostat. With this device, changes in tone are reflected by the change of volume of air in an infinitely compliant polyethylene balloon maintained at a constant pressure. To ensure the volume changes reflect the tone of the viscus, the balloon has to be in apposition with the inner lining of the viscus. This is achieved by setting the intraballoon pressure at a constant low level that results in volume deflections in response to cough and a Valsalva maneuver. For example, in response to relaxation or contraction of stomach tone, the barostat maintains the constant pressure by infusion or aspiration of air from the balloon in the stomach. This method requires intubation, causes stress and discomfort (on the throat), may last 3 hours or longer (Figure 2.2), and is not used extensively in clinical practice. However, it is essential for measurements of colonic compliance and tone (discussed below).

Satiation or Nutrient Drink Test

The nutrient drink test may be an alternative, surrogate approach for estimating gastric accommodation or sensation (Figures 2.3 and 2.4). In this test, the patient ingests a liquid nutrient drink (1 kcal/mL) at a constant rate of 30 mL per minute. Satiation is measured by

Figure 2.1   Examples of the Wide Range of Tests for Motility Measurements Available for Human Studies

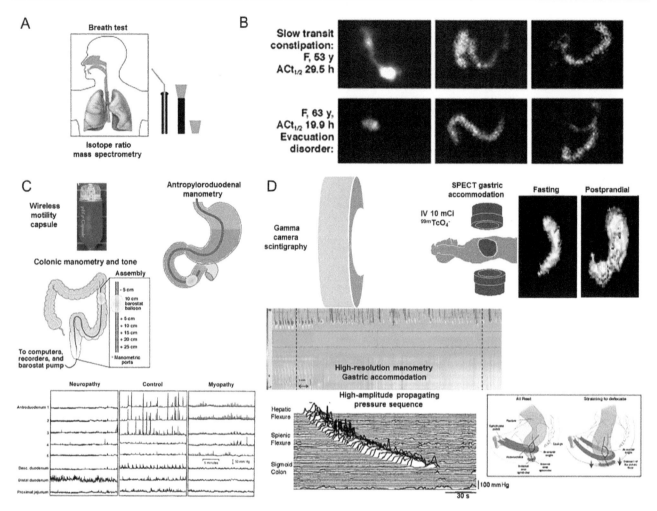

A, Stable isotope breath test. B, Scintigraphic transit. C, Intraluminal manometry with perfused manometers or strain gauges on tubes or wireless motility capsules. D, Measurement of gastric capacity and accommodation by single-photon emission computed tomography (SPECT) or high-resolution manometry. AC indicates ascending colon; Desc, descending; F, female; IV, intravenous; $t_{1/2}$, half-emptying time; $^{99m}TcO_4^-$, radiolabeled technetium.

(Modified from Camilleri M, Linden DR. Measurement of gastrointestinal and colonic motor functions in humans and animals. Cell Mol Gastroenterol Hepatol. 2016 Jul;2(4):412-28; used with permission.)

Figure 2.2   Measurement of Gastric Accommodation in Health Using Barostat Balloon

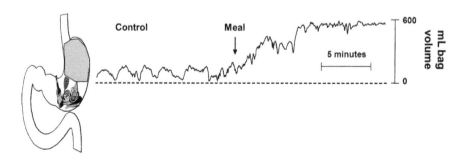

Intraballoon volume increases (under constant pressure) after the meal.

Figure 2.3   Liquid Nutrient Drink Test

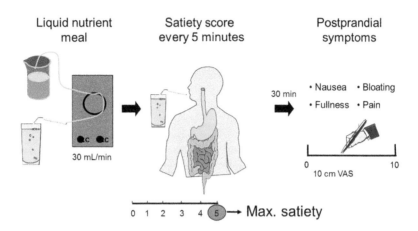

Maximum tolerable volume of liquid nutrient (1 kcal/mL) ingested at a rate of 30 mL/min, and symptoms measured 30 minutes after achieving maximum tolerable volume. Max indicates maximum; VAS, visual analog scale.

2 indices: the volume to induce a sensation of normal, comfortable fullness, and a volume that is the absolute limit before the patient feels uncomfortable or ready to vomit, called the *maximum tolerated volume*. In addition to measurement of postprandial symptoms of nausea, fullness, bloating, and pain 30 minutes after the maximum tolerated volume, this volume is a useful approximate measure of gastric accommodation. Thus, the volume of high-calorie, slowly administered liquid nutrient compares favorably with the gastric accommodation measured with a barostat balloon, especially when the maximum tolerated volume is less than 750 kcal (which is the fifth percentile for normal at Mayo Clinic) (Figure 2.4).

Single-Photon Emission Computed Tomography

Single-photon emission computed tomography (SPECT) can be performed after 10 mCi technetium Tc 99m-pertechnetate is administered intravenously and the isotope has accumulated in gastric parietal and mucin-secreting cells. Tomographic transaxial images of the stomach are acquired with the patient supine, and the images are reconstructed with a software analysis program. The calculated volume reflects the internal volume of the stomach, and total gastric volume is measured during fasting and during the first 10 minutes after 300 mL of liquid nutrient drink is ingested over up

to 5 minutes. SPECT measurements of gastric volumes during fasting and postprandially have been extensively validated in vitro and in vivo in humans, including comparison with the results obtained with the intragastric barostat balloon test (Figure 2.5).

Validation studies for gastric accommodation volumes have shown excellent performance characteristics: intraindividual and interindividual coefficients of variance from 16% to 22%, reproducibility of gastric volume with the same caloric liquid meal measured

Figure 2.4   Nutrient Drink Test as a Surrogate for Gastric Accommodation

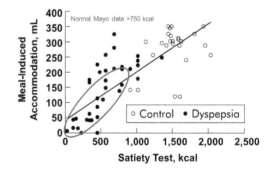

Note that in the normal range (red oval) for nutrient drink intake, there is a linear relationship between nutrient kcal ingested (satiety test) and gastric accommodation by barostat.

(Modified from Tack J, Caenepeel P, Piessevaux H, Cuomo R, Janssens J. Assessment of meal induced gastric accommodation by a satiety drinking test in health and in severe functional dyspepsia. Gut. 2003 Sep;52(9):1271-7; used with permission.)

Figure 2.5   SPECT Method to Measure Gastric Volumes

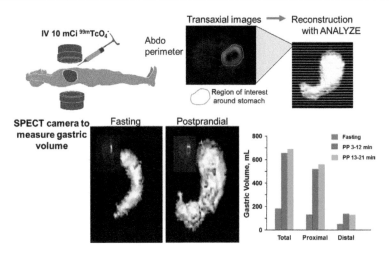

After intravenous (IV) administration of radiolabeled technetium ($^{99m}TcO_4^-$), transaxial images are obtained with SPECT, and individual slices of radiolabeled mucosa are reconstructed with a computer program (ANALYZE, Mayo Clinic) to render stomach images and estimate volumes during fasting and postprandially (PP). Abdo indicates abdominal; SPECT, single-photon emission computed tomography.

an average of 9 months apart (coefficient of variation of 10%), and similar accommodation volumes when the same person receives equicaloric liquid nutrient or solid (egg) meals.

SPECT shows effects of disease (eg, functional dyspepsia) on gastric accommodation and effects of medications such as nitrates, erythromycin, glucagon-like peptide-1 agonists and analogs, central neuromodulators, ghrelin agonist, and octreotide in health and diseases.

SPECT can also simultaneously measure gastric emptying and gastric accommodation. Advantages of SPECT measurement include its noninvasive nature, thorough validation, and extensive use in clinical practice in several thousands of patients to date. However, the test involves radiation and requires specialized equipment and analysis programs for the 3-dimensional reconstruction. The resolution of SPECT does not equal that of computed tomography or magnetic resonance imaging (MRI).

Two-Dimensional Scintigraphy

A recently introduced method assesses the area of the proximal stomach on 2-dimensional scintigraphy (during gastric emptying measurement, called *immediate meal distribution at time zero*) as an indirect method to measure gastric accommodation (Figure 2.6). However, in patients with diabetes who underwent both 2-dimensional scintigraphy and SPECT measurement of gastric accommodation, there was poor correlation between immediate meal distribution at time zero (measured as counts in or in the area of the proximal stomach, or estimated volume based on area) and SPECT measurements of gastric volume.

Three-Dimensional Ultrasonography

Gastric volume can be measured with 3-dimensional reconstruction of images acquired after ingestion of a liquid meal (that serves as a contrast medium). This method involves the use of ordinary B-mode ultrasonography assisted by magnetic scan-head tracking. This has been compared with simultaneously measured gastric volumes with SPECT. This elegant method has not been used outside research settings, in part because of the necessity for specialized equipment, challenges presented by body habitus, variation in position of the stomach relative to the rib cage, and the special training of the operators for acquiring and analyzing the data.

Figure 2.6   Intragastric Meal Distribution During Gastric-Emptying (GE) Scintigraphy for Assessment of Fundic Accommodation in the Presence of Normal GE

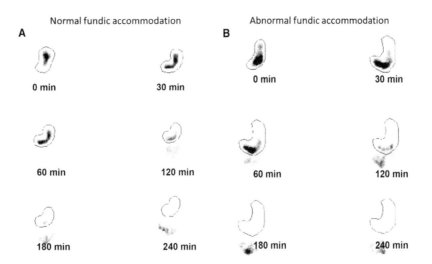

Examples of normal gastric accommodation (GA) and abnormal GA assessed by GE scintigraphy. In normal GA and normal GE (A), most radiolabeled solids appeared in proximal stomach immediately after meal ingestion (time, 0 min). Over time, solids progressed into distal stomach and GE was normal. In abnormal GA with normal GE (B), most radiolabeled solids appeared in distal stomach at 0 minute.

(From Orthey P, Yu D, Van Natta ML, Ramsey FV, Diaz JR, Bennett PA, et al; NIH Gastroparesis Consortium. Intragastric meal distribution during gastric emptying scintigraphy for assessment of fundic accommodation: correlation with symptoms of gastroparesis. J Nucl Med. 2018 Apr;59(4):691-7; used with permission.)

Magnetic Resonance Imaging

MRI records entire stomach volume, and results are notably correlated with results of SPECT. MRI demonstrates volume increases by glucagon and decreases by erythromycin and an average increase in postprandial gastric volume over ingested meal volume by 106±12 mL; under the same experimental conditions, postprandial volumes with SPECT increased by 158±18 mL. The difference may reflect the fact that SPECT volume includes the gastric wall labeled with technetium Tc 99m. With MRI, interindividual and intraindividual variation may reach 35%; however, intraindividual fasting and postprandial gastric volumes measured with MRI were generally reproducible.

MRI may have potential advantage over SPECT because of its ability to distinguish the volumes of air from fluid and the ability to measure intraluminal volume (without inclusion of the volume attributed to the wall of the stomach), which is the basis of SPECT. MRI avoids radiation, but it is not widely used to measure gastric accommodation in clinical practice or research.

High-Resolution Intragastric Manometry

High-resolution manometry is used most extensively for the measurement of esophageal motility. However, it can record a reduction in intraluminal pressure during liquid nutrient ingestion (Figure 2.7). It provides a less invasive alternative to the barostat and has been used to determine the pharmacologic effects of peppermint oil and liraglutide.

Gastrointestinal Transit

Scintigraphy to Measure Gastric Emptying

Scintigraphy, with imaging at 1, 2, and 4 hours after a standard meal, provides noninvasive quantification of gastric emptying. This protocol was developed at Mayo Clinic and was subsequently adopted by the American Neurogastroenterology and Motility Society and the

Figure 2.7   Intragastric Pressure During Food Intake Recorded With High-Resolution Manometry

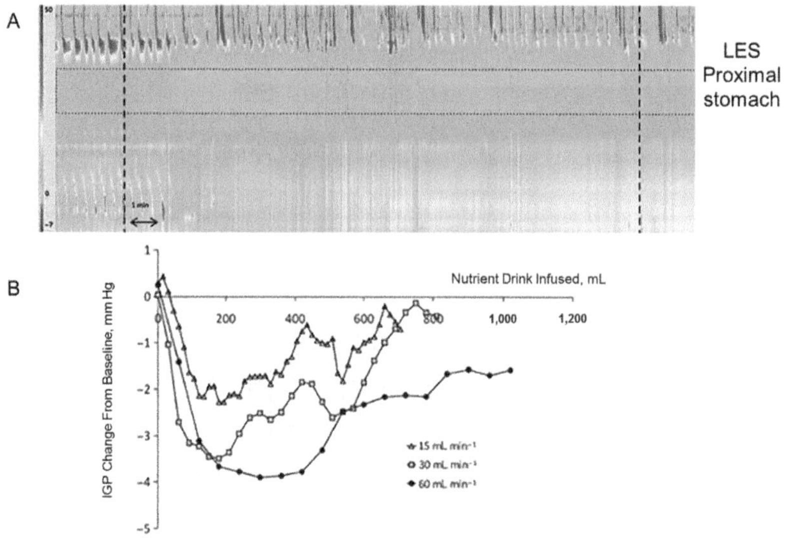

This is a physiologic and minimally invasive method to assess gastric accommodation. A, The reduced tone is reflected in the light blue coloration below the increases in pressure, yellow, from lower esophageal sphincter (LES) contraction in response to swallows, evident as yellow or red propagated contractions in the esophagus. B, Representative examples of degrees of accommodation (change in intragastric pressure [IGP] relative to baseline) in response to different rates of infusion of the same nutrient meal.

(From Janssen P, Verschueren S, Ly HG, Vos R, Van Oudenhove L, Tack J. Intragastric pressure during food intake: a physiological and minimally invasive method to assess gastric accommodation. Neurogastroenterol Motil. 2011 Apr;23(4):316-22; used with permission.)

Society of Nuclear Medicine. The meal recommended in consensus statements from these organizations is a 2% fat meal consisting of 4 ounces of egg white substitute, 2 slices of bread, strawberry jam (30 g), and 120 mL of water (total 240 kcal). However, this relatively small meal may be less sensitive for diagnosis of gastroparesis or for inducing postprandial symptoms (Figure 2.8).

The Mayo Clinic gastric emptying method uses a 320-kcal meal with 30% fat; this meal includes 2 natural scrambled eggs. It is essential to have robust normal values because the test meal determines the rate of emptying (Figure 2.9). Mayo Clinic published data from 319 healthy controls, subdivided for men and women, and these normal values can be used at other centers as long as the meal content is replicated (Camilleri 2012; see suggested reading).

The intraindividual variations in the rates of gastric emptying are considerable (12%-15%), even in healthy individuals. The following are performance characteristics of the 30% fat, 320-kcal meal: intersubject coefficients of variation for gastric emptying of half the radioactivity ($t_{1/2}$) were 24.5% overall (men, 26.0%; women, 22.5%) and 9.6% at 4 hours; intraindividual coefficients of variation for gastric emptying of $t_{1/2}$ were

23.8% overall and 12.6% at 4 hours. The normal values for gastric emptying in men and women are shown in Table 2.1.

Gastric emptying differs according to the meal substrate (Figure 2.9), that is, consistency, calorie and fat content, and proportion of solid component (homogenized or not). Emptying of a liquid nutrient meal (Figure 2.10) is similar to that of a low-fat egg-white sandwich and could be a useful alternative meal if a patient is intolerant of solids.

Measurement of gastric emptying is indicated in patients with unexplained nausea, vomiting, and upper GI or dyspeptic symptoms; for screening diabetic patients being considered for amylin- or incretin-based therapy to enhance glycemic control (eg, pramlintide and glucagon-like peptide-1 agonists or analogs); and for the assessment of patients suspected of having a generalized gut motility disorder.

In research studies, measurement of gastric emptying is useful for understanding the pathophysiologic basis of symptoms or for obtaining proof of pharmacologic efficacy with experimental agents. When the gastric emptying test is optimized (solid meal, 30% fat, 4 hours imaging), there is a significant relationship

Figure 2.8   Diabetic Gastroparesis

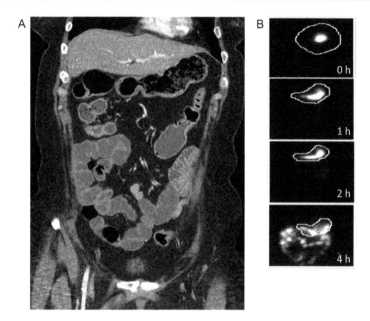

A, No outlet obstruction is seen on coronal computed tomography. B, Radioscintigraphic images show delayed emptying at 0, 1, 2, and 4 hours.

Figure 2.9   Gastric Emptying of Different Meal Substrates

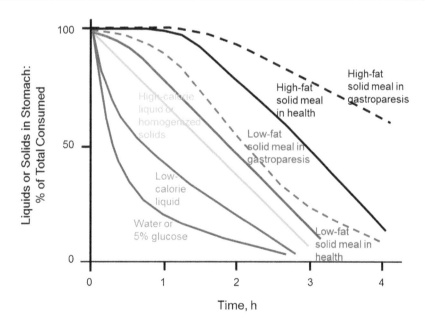

Note the phase of the meal (solid vs liquid) and calorie content determine pattern and rate of emptying. Low-calorie liquids empty exponentially. Solid emptying occurs in 2 phases: a lag phase during which food is triturated, and a postlag linear emptying phase.

(From Camilleri M, Shin A. Novel and validated approaches for gastric emptying scintigraphy in patients with suspected gastroparesis. Dig Dis Sci. 2013 Jul;58(7):1813-5; used with permission.)

Table 2.1	Results of Mayo Clinic Scintigraphic Test for Measuring Gastric Emptying			
Healthy Participants	**GE at 1 h,%**	**GE at 2 h,%**	**GE at 4 h,%**	**GE t$_{1/2}$, min**
Both sexes (N=319)				
Mean (SD)	18.1 (9.5)	51.4 (15.7)	93.2 (8.9)	121.7 (29.8)
Median (5th, 95th %)	17 (4.4, 35)	50 (25, 78.5)	96 (76.2, 100)	120 (78.4, 174)
Female (n=214)				
Mean (SD)	16.5 (8.3)	47.8 (14.3)	92.1 (9.4)	127.7 (28.7)
Median (5th, 95th %)	16 (4.3, 31.4)	47.2 (25, 71)	94.8 (76.2, 100)	125 (89, 180)
Male (n=105)				
Mean (SD)	21.3 (10.9)	58.6 (15.1)	92.1 (9.4)	109.9 (28.6)
Median (5th, 95th %)	19 (4.7, 40)	60 (28.4, 82)	98.3 (77, 100)	105 (73.2, 165)

Abbreviation: GE, gastric emptying.

Modified from Camilleri M, Iturrino J, Bharucha AE, Burton D, Shin A, Jeong ID, et al. Performance characteristics of scintigraphic measurement of gastric emptying of solids in healthy participants. Neurogastroenterol Motil. 2012 Dec;24(12):1076-e562; used with permission.

between gastric emptying and satiation and satiety (Figure 2.11) and with upper GI symptoms, particularly nausea (odds ratio [OR], 1.6; 95% CI, 1.4-1.8), vomiting (OR, 2.0; 95% CI, 1.6-2.7), abdominal pain (OR, 1.5; 95% CI, 1.0-2.2), and early satiety or fullness (OR, 1.8; 95% CI, 1.2-2.6).

Stable Isotope Breath Tests

The advantages of stable isotope breath tests to measure gastric emptying are the noninvasive approach, lack of radiation hazard, and conduct of the test and breath sample collection at the point of care. Carbon 13 (^{13}C)

Figure 2.10   Gastric Emptying of Liquid Nutrient Meal and of Solid Meal

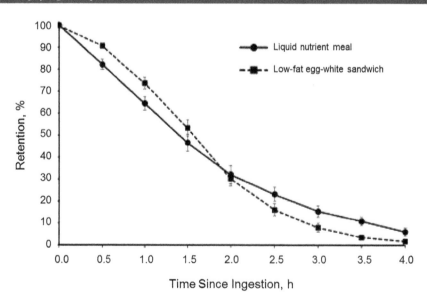

Note that the emptying rates are almost identical.

(From Sachdeva P, Kantor S, Knight LC, Maurer AH, Fisher RS, Parkman HP. Use of a high caloric liquid meal as an alternative to a solid meal for gastric emptying scintigraphy. Dig Dis Sci. 2013 Jul;58(7):2001-6; used with permission.)

Figure 2.11 Relationship of Gastric Emptying With Satiation (Liquid Nutrient Drink Test) (A) and With Satiety (Buffet Meal) (B)

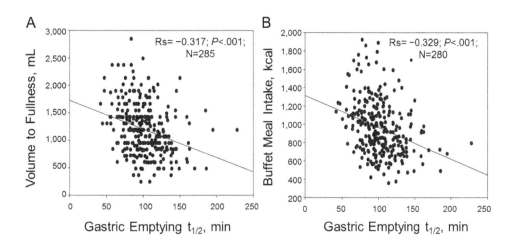

Slower gastric emptying is associated with reduced calorie intake.

(From Halawi H, Camilleri M, Acosta A, Vazquez-Roque M, Oduyebo I, Burton D, et al. Relationship of gastric emptying or accommodation with satiation, satiety, and postprandial symptoms in health. Am J Physiol Gastrointest Liver Physiol. 2017 Nov 1;313(5):G442-7.)

isotope is incorporated into a molecule that is included in a solid meal, typically, the medium-chain fatty acid octanoic acid or the blue-green algae *Spirulina platensis.* Alternatively, ^{13}C-acetate can be used to assess gastric emptying of liquids (Figure 2.12). Clearly, ^{13}C substrates cannot be used simultaneously to evaluate both solid and liquid gastric emptying. After the meal is emptied from the stomach, it is rapidly digested, absorbed, and metabolized by the liver, and the ^{13}CO$_2$ is excreted by the lungs. Because the rate-limiting step in these processes is gastric emptying, it follows that ^{13}CO$_2$ excretion reflects gastric emptying of the meal (Figure 2.12).

The gastric emptying breath test for solids is accurate compared with simultaneous scintigraphy and has similar coefficients of variation (Figure 2.13). The ^{13}C-*Spirulina platensis* test documented gastric

Figure 2.12 Principles of Gastric Emptying Breath Test

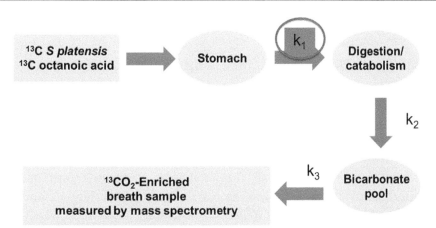

The stable isotope within a meal empties from the stomach, is absorbed in the proximal small bowel, and is metabolized, and product is excreted in breath. The rate-limiting step (red circle) for appearance of ^{13}CO$_2$ in breath is the rate of gastric emptying. S indicates *Spirulina*.

Figure 2.13   Validation of [13]C-*Spirulina platensis* Breath Test (bottom left) for Gastric Emptying by Comparing With Simultaneous Scintigraphy (top left)

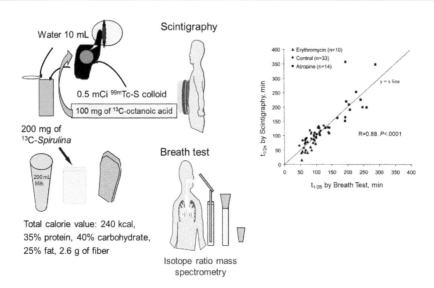

Measurements of gastric half-emptying time ($t_{1/2}$) under control conditions or pharmacologically accelerated or delayed gastric emptying fall close to the line of identity for the 2 methods (right).

(From Viramontes BE, Kim DY, Camilleri M, Lee JS, Stephens D, Burton DD, et al. Validation of a stable isotope gastric emptying test for normal, accelerated or delayed gastric emptying. Neurogastroenterol Motil. 2001 Dec;13(6):567-74; used with permission.)

emptying that was accelerated with erythromycin or delayed with atropine. The [13]C-*Spirulina platensis* test was approved by the US Food and Drug Administration in 2015; the results agreed with scintigraphy results 73% to 97% of the time when measurements were obtained at various times during the test (Figure 2.14). Accuracy could be reduced in patients with diseases affecting the absorption or digestion of the substrate or excretion in breath, that is, in diseases of intestinal mucosa, pancreas, liver, and respiratory system.

Wireless pH and Motility Capsule

Wireless motility capsules (WMC) measure pH, pressure, and temperature in the entire gut. Patients ingest the capsule with a standard meal and ingest only water over the next 6 hours. Thereafter, they can engage in normal daily activity, including ad libitum feeding. The WMC acquires data continuously for up to 5 days. The data are used to calculate regional and whole gut transit times and to measure intraluminal pressures.

There is a significant correlation between WMC and scintigraphy for measuring gastric emptying in healthy patients and in those with gastroparesis (r=0.73), and

discrimination between normal and delayed gastric emptying is highly sensitive (0.87) and specific (0.92). However, the capsule most frequently empties from the stomach (indicated by change in pH from acidic to alkaline) with the migrating motor complex (MMC) (return of fasting motility) rather than with the digestible meal.

Capsule emptying into the duodenum is usually associated with return of fasting antral phasic contractions (as part of the MMC) (Figure 2.15). In many healthy patients, estimated WMC emptying time is declared (censored) as 6 hours, which is the time of ingestion of the next meal. In only about one-third of cases has the capsule been shown to empty from the stomach with the high-amplitude antral contractions typical of the postprandial phase, before the return of the MMC.

The WMC test can be conducted anywhere, lacks radioactivity, and allows measurement of small bowel, colon, and whole-gut transit times. It also allows measurement of contractility, although the clinical application of such measurement is unclear. The WMC has documented the effects of pharmacologic agents on gastric contractility. However, although the results are correlated with those of scintigraphy, the estimated gastric emptying time with the capsule is not necessarily

Figure 2.14　Scintigraphy Compared With Gastric Emptying Breath Test (GEBT) in More Than 100 Participants

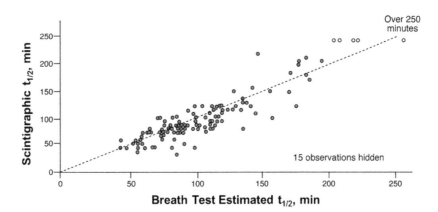

Test meal	Components	Performance characteristics*
GEBT current standardized meal	230 kcal: • 27 g egg mix • 6 saltine crackers • 6 oz water	Correlation:　r = 0.82 Sensitivity:　0.89 Specificity:　0.80

*Based on GEBT t ½ vs. scintigraphic t ½ metrics.

$t_{1/2}$ indicates half-emptying time.

(From Szarka LA, Camilleri M, Vella A, Burton D, Baxter K, Simonson J, et al. A stable isotope breath test with a standard meal for abnormal gastric emptying of solids in the clinic and in research. Clin Gastroenterol Hepatol. 2008 Jun;6(6):635-43; used with permission.)

Figure 2.15　Gastric Emptying With Wireless Motility Capsule

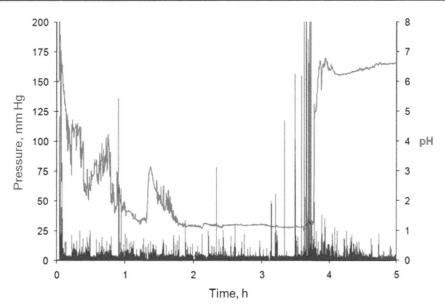

The major change in pH from acid to close to neutral approximately 3.7 hours after ingestion indicates movement of the capsule from stomach into the duodenum. The phasic pressure activity in the gastric antrum increased immediately before the major pH change.

(From Cassilly D, Kantor S, Knight LC, Maurer AH, Fisher RS, Semler J, et al. Gastric emptying of a non-digestible solid: assessment with simultaneous SmartPill pH and pressure capsule, antroduodenal manometry, gastric emptying scintigraphy. Neurogastroenterol Motil. 2008 Apr;20(4):311-9; used with permission.)

an accurate measurement of emptying of food from the stomach.

Orocecal or Small Bowel Transit

Breath Hydrogen Test

There is a basic presumption that the hydrogen excreted in the breath after ingesting a substrate (usually lactulose) results from fermentation of the unabsorbed carbohydrate by bacteria in the colon. Lactulose is the most widely used substrate for determining orocecal transit time, which is documented by a breath hydrogen increase of at least 10 parts per million above baseline. The test has a high degree of correlation with simultaneous intestinal transit of liquids measured by scintigraphy. Lactulose-breath hydrogen test documents the effects of drugs on gut motility.

The breath hydrogen test has 3 limitations. First, lactulose itself may accelerate transit because of induction of osmotic activity. Second, the test is usually performed during fasting and, therefore, may not accurately reflect postprandial small bowel transit, which is typically when patients experience symptoms. Third, the presence of small bowel bacterial overgrowth may produce a breath hydrogen signal, and this may be incorrectly diagnosed as accelerated small bowel transit time.

Stable Isotope Breath Test

The stable isotope lactose ^{13}C-ureide requires the colonic bacterial flora to free ^{13}C-ureide from binding to lactose. Subsequently, ^{13}C-ureide undergoes hydrolysis with release of $^{13}CO_2$ and excretion in breath. The lactose ^{13}C-ureide test has been validated by comparison with scintigraphy and responsiveness to pharmacologic agents. It is seldom used in clinical practice.

Small Bowel Scintigraphy

Small bowel scintigraphy is used as part of whole-gut transit tests. Small bowel transit time can be assessed by 10% or 50% of the radiolabel to arrive at the cecum, after subtracting gastric emptying of the same proportion. These measurements require multiple scans, which add inconvenience and cost. An approximate surrogate for small bowel transit time is the percentage filling of the colon at 6 hours (CF6), which measures orocecal transit and is influenced by the gastric emptying result. The diagnostic utility of this measurement is poor; in more than 200 healthy controls, the normal range was 0% to 100%; and a low value (eg, <20%) is most often due to slow right colon transit.

Wireless pH and Motility Capsule

The small bowel transit time with a WMC is defined as the interval between the increase in pH associated with gastric emptying and the time when the pH suddenly falls by more than 1 unit for at least 5 minutes as the capsule enters the cecum (Figure 2.16). Median small bowel transit times range from 4 to 6 hours in different studies. One difficulty is identifying the 1-unit pH drop, which is a signal of passage into the cecum, especially postoperatively (eg, right hemicolectomy) or in patients with an incompetent ileocecal valve, which allows bacterial colonization from the colon to the distal ileum. The use of the capsule is contraindicated with suspected mechanical obstruction, within 3 months of GI surgery, or with Crohn disease because of the risk that the nondigestible, 26×13-mm capsule may become impacted in the GI tract.

Colonic Transit

Radiopaque Markers

Several different methods with radiopaque markers can be used to evaluate total and segmental colonic transit times (Figure 2.17). Normal values are less than 5 markers retained at 5 days when patients ingest 25 markers on day 1 or measured colonic transit in hours based on the number of markers retained on the day-4 radiograph after patients ingest 24 markers on days 1 to 3. On day 4, if more than 50 markers are retained in the colon, transit time is abnormal and a second radiograph is taken on day 7 after ingestion of 24 markers on days 4

Figure 2.16   Wireless Motility Capsule (WMC) Recordings in Healthy Person (A) and Patient With Constipation (B)

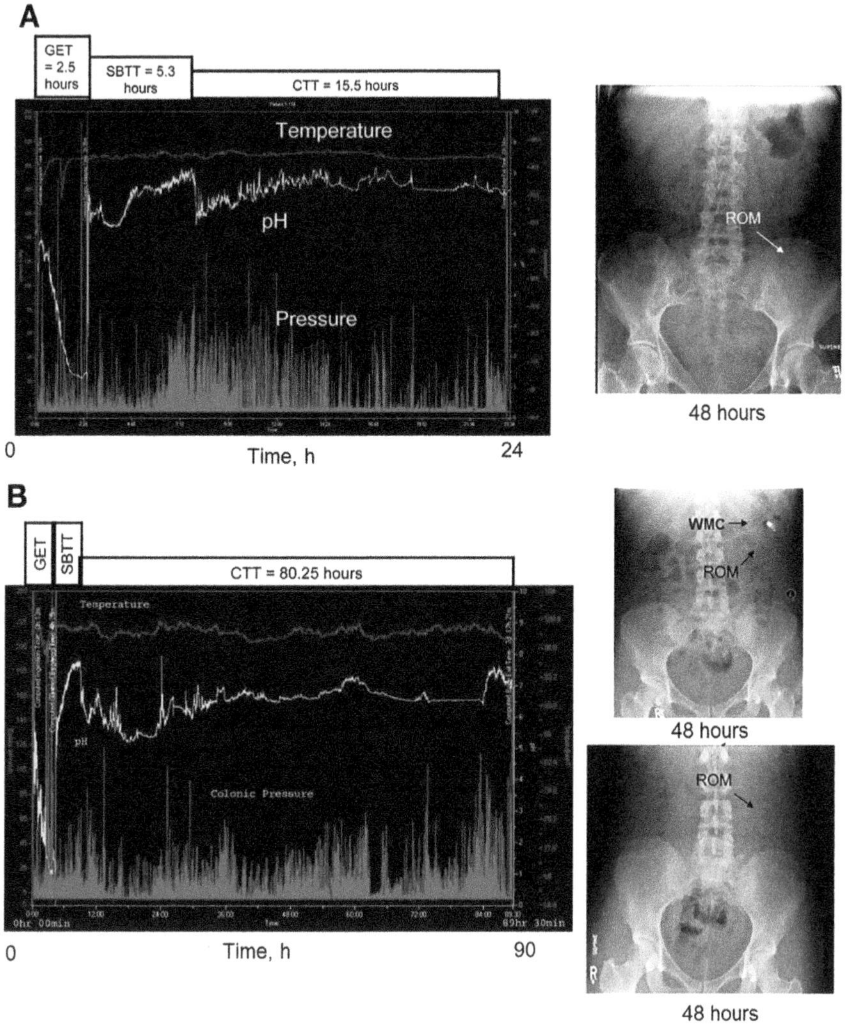

Small bowel transit time (SBTT) is the interval between a sudden increase in pH at antroduodenal transfer and a sudden drop at ileal emptying into colon. Capsule emptying times are measured in comparison with radiopaque markers (ROM) shown in the radiographs. CTT indicates colonic transit time; GET, gastric emptying time.

(From Rao SS, Kuo B, McCallum RW, Chey WD, DiBaise JK, Hasler WL, et al. Investigation of colonic and whole-gut transit with wireless motility capsule and radiopaque markers in constipation. Clin Gastroenterol Hepatol. 2009 May;7(5):537-44; used with permission.)

to 6. Again, the total number of markers retained is the value for colonic transit in hours. If total colonic transit time is more than 70 hours, transit in any segment is abnormal if it is more than 30 hours. The average and interquartile range (IQR) values estimated for 34 male volunteers were 30.7 (IQR, 13-48 h) and, for 39 females, 38.8 (IQR, 20-57 h).

Localization of retained markers may be suggestive, but not diagnostic, of the cause of constipation; predominant retention in the rectosigmoid may suggest rectal evacuation disorder, whereas distribution throughout the colon may suggest slow-transit constipation. However, a rectal evacuation disorder may inhibit colonic motility and retard proximal colonic transit, effects resulting in widespread colonic distribution of markers. Segmental transit times are measured relative to the spine and a line from the fifth lumbar vertebra to the left anterior superior iliac crest (Figure 2.17).

The radiopaque marker method has many attractive features: well-established normal values, standardization, readily available, widespread use in practice, and reasonably inexpensive.

Figure 2.17   Measurement of Colonic Transit With Radiopaque Markers (ROM) (A) or Wireless Capsule (B)

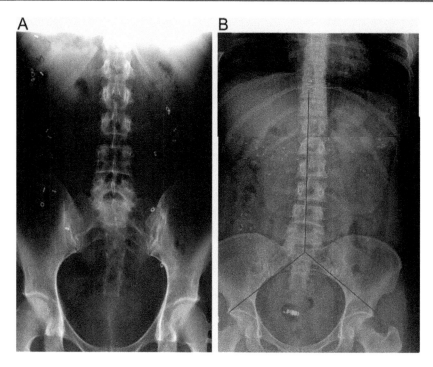

A   B

Different methods are available for measuring colonic transit using ROM, and these are best validated for documenting delayed co-lonic transit. The different methods have different normal values. When 20 markers are ingested, the presence of more than 5 markers on abdominal radiography on day 5 indicates delayed colonic transit. Alternatively, the method of Metcalf et al involves ingesting 24 markers on days 1 to 3, and the colonic transit time in hours is equal to the number of markers in the abdomen on day 4 (and day 7). ROM methods can be used to assess regional colonic transit, but they are not well validated for measuring accelerated colonic transit.

Colonic Scintigraphy

Measurement of colonic transit with scintigraphy is safe and noninvasive and correlates with radiopaque markers. Its main advantages are measurement of ascending colon emptying and overall colonic transit over 48 to 72 hours (Figure 2.18). In the most widely published method, developed and validated at Mayo Clinic, after fasting overnight, patients ingest a pH-sensitive capsule containing indium In 111-labeled activated charcoal particles and coated with a pH-sensitive polymer, methacrylate. The capsule dissolves in the neutral pH in the terminal ileum, releasing the radioisotopically labeled charcoal into the lumen. An alternative scintigraphic colonic transit test follows the transit of a radiolabeled liquid. Anterior and posterior abdominal scans of 2 minutes' duration are acquired at 4, 6, 8, 24 (Figure 2.19), and 48 hours (and 72 hours in some centers) after ingestion. Colonic transit is summarized as a geometric center (defined

as the weighted average) of radioactivity based on 5 or 7 regions.

The times of greatest interest for overall colonic transit are at 24 hours (for accelerated transit) and at 48 and 72 hours (for delayed colonic transit) (Figure 2.20). The delayed-release capsule method facilitates measurement of the time for emptying half of the radioactivity ($t_{1/2}$) from the ascending colon, which is calculated by linear interpolation of values on the ascending colon emptying curve.

Table 2.2 shows the published normal values with the delayed-release capsule method. The intraindividual coefficients of variation were 38% at 24 hours and 30% at 48 hours over a median follow-up of 2 years. This variation reflects the natural variation in colonic functions that affect stool frequency and consistency in health.

Colonic transit and ascending colon emptying determined with scintigraphy have been applied to document abnormal colonic function (which may reflect either motility or fluid secretion) in idiopathic

Figure 2.18   Gastrointestinal and Colonic Transit Test

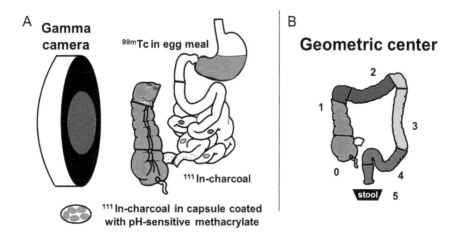

Gastric emptying and small bowel transit (A) are assessed from the transit profile of the radiolabeled technetium (^{99m}Tc) egg meal (296 kcal, 30% fat); a methacrylate-coated capsule containing indium In 111 (^{111}In)-labeled activated charcoal delivers isotope to the colon for measurement of colonic transit using the 5-region geometric center assessment (B).

constipation, functional diarrhea, carcinoid diarrhea, subtypes of irritable bowel syndrome, and bile acid diarrhea. Colonic transit has also been used to prove the efficacy of and to predict the potential clinical efficacy of diverse medications: prokinetics (eg, serotonin 4 receptor agonists, prucalopride and tegaserod), medications retarding transit (eg, serotonin 3 receptor antagonists, alosetron and ondansetron), and secretagogue medications (eg, linaclotide, plecanatide, and lubiprostone).

Figure 2.19   Colonic Transit by Scintigraphy at 24 Hours After Ingestion of Radiolabeled Charcoal

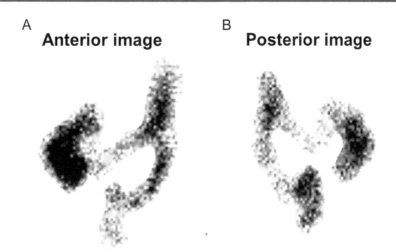

Geometric center = 3.40

Anterior (A) and posterior (B) images are used to estimate colonic geometric center. Colonic transit is weighted average of counts in the colon. In this case, the calculated colonic geometric center (0=cecum, 5=stool) is close to the mid-descending colon.

Figure 2.20   Colonic Transit Profiles at Different Intervals Showing Typical Appearances Associated With Evacuation Disorders and Slow-Transit Constipation (STC)

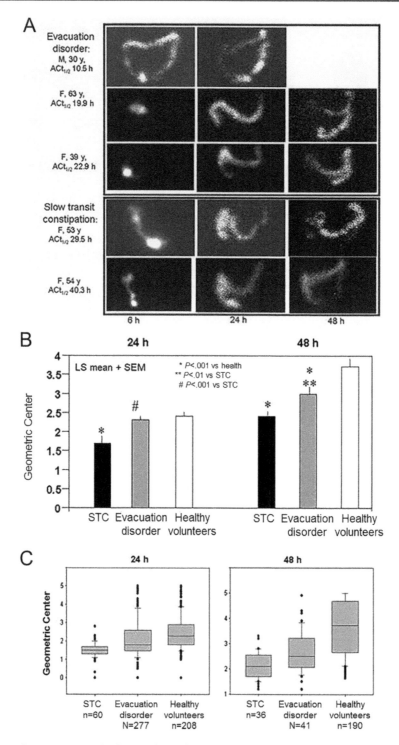

A, Images from 5 different patients at 6, 24, and 48 hours. The 48-hour images show preponderant isotope in the left colon in evacuation disorder and retention in ascending and transverse colon in STC, as indicated by longer emptying of the ascending colon (denoted by longer AC $t_{1/2}$ in hours) in STC (lower 2 rows of images) compared with patients with evacuation disorders (upper 3 rows of images), which show empty ascending colon at 24 or 48 hours. B and C, Summary data for geometric centers at 24 and 48 hours from patients with STC or evacuation disorder and from healthy volunteers summarized LS mean and SEM (B) as median, interquartile range, full range, and outliers (C). AC indicates ascending colon; F, female; LS, least square; M, male; SEM, standard error of the mean; $t_{1/2}$, half-emptying time.

(From Nullens S, Nelsen T, Camilleri M, Burton D, Eckert D, Iturrino J, et al. Regional colon transit in patients with dyssynergic defecation or slow transit in patients with constipation. Gut. 2012 Aug;61(8):1132-9; used with permission.)

Table 2.2 Normal Values With Scintigraphy Using the Delayed-Release (Methacrylate-Coated) Capsule Method			
Study Group	**GC 24[a,b]**	**GC 48[a,c]**	**AC $t_{1/2}$, h[d]**
All participants			
Mean (SD)	2.4 (0.9)	3.6 (1.1)	15.0 (7.5)
Median (5th, 95th %)	2.3 (1.3, 4.4)	3.8 (1.9, 5.0)	16.0 (4.5, 28.5)
Female			
Mean (SD)	2.3 (0.9)	3.4 (1.0)	17.8 (6.8)
Median (5th, 95th %)	2.1 (1.3, 4.4)	3.3 (1.9, 5.0)	17.8 (5.0, 28.5)
Male			
Mean (SD)	2.7 (0.9)	4.1 (1.0)	9.5 (5.7)
Median (5th, 95th %)	2.6 (1.5, 4.7)	4.5 (2.1, 5.0)	8.0 (0.5, 18.0)

Abbreviations: AC, ascending colon; GC, geometric center; $t_{1/2}$, time for emptying of half radioactivity.

[a] Definition of delayed colonic transit: GC 24 less than 1.3 in females, less than 1.5 in males; GC 48 less than 1.9 in females, less than 2.1 in males.

[b] N=220 (145 female, 75 male).

[c] N=199 (136 female, 63 male).

[d] N=36 (24 female, 12 male).

Modified from Kolar GJ, Camilleri M, Burton D, Nadeau A, Zinsmeister AR. Prevalence of colonic motor or evacuation disorders in patients presenting with chronic nausea and vomiting evaluated by a single gastroenterologist in a tertiary referral practice. Neurogastroenterol Motil. 2014 Jan;26(1):131-8; used with permission.

Wireless pH and Motility Capsule

With the WMC, colonic transit time is the time from entry into the cecum (drop in measured pH by 1 unit) to the time of capsule expulsion, evidenced by a sudden drop in the temperature and loss of pressure recordings. In one study (Rao 2009; see suggested reading), colonic transit times were 21.7 hours (median IQR, 15.5-37.3 hours; 95th percentile, 59 hours) in 87 healthy patients and 46.7 hours (median IQR, 24.0-91.9 hours) in 78 patients with constipation.

There was a significant correlation (r= −0.69) between WMC transit time and the percentage of radiopaque markers retained on day 5 in constipated patients studied simultaneously with both methods. In a separate multicenter study of 158 patients with constipation (Camilleri 2010; see suggested reading), the 2 methods agreed on the classification of slow or normal colonic transit in 87% of patients (Figure 2.21).

The WMC can measure contraction amplitude but, as a single sensor, it cannot appraise propagation of contractions in the colon. The WMC is more expensive than radiopaque markers or scintigraphy for measuring colonic or whole gut transit. However, it is convenient for patients and involves no radiation exposure.

Gastric and Small Bowel Contractility

Antroduodenal manometry is performed at few referral centers and requires transnasal or transoral placement of a catheter, typically with the aid of upper GI endoscopy. In addition, it is time consuming (6-24 hours at different centers) and requires skilled technical support. The alternative noninvasive measurement of pressure activity in the stomach and duodenum can be achieved with a WMC, which detects contractions (and their amplitudes) during passage out of the stomach and its passage through the small bowel (and colon, see below). As stated above, the capsule cannot appraise propagation or coordination of contractions.

The main indications for antroduodenal manometry are differentiation of neuropathy from myopathy

Figure 2.21   Relationship Between Colonic Transit Time (CTT) (A) and Small Bowel Transit Time (SBTT) (B) Determined With Wireless Motility Capsule (WMC) and Colonic Transit Determined With Radiopaque Markers (ROM)

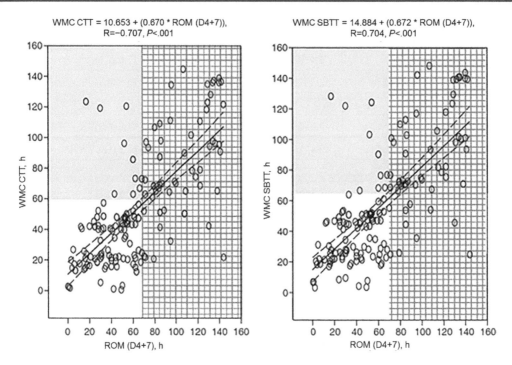

Abdominal radiographs were obtained on days 4 and 7 in patients with constipation. Correlations between WMC estimates and ROM transit time are significant. Interrupted lines are the 95% CI around the regression line. The shaded areas include the values at and above the 95th percentiles for the different methods: 67 hours for ROM transit time, 59 hours for CTT, and 65 hours for SBTT (ie, slow transit).

(Modified from Camilleri M, Thorne NK, Ringel Y, Hasler WL, Kuo B, Esfandyari T, et al. Wireless pH-motility capsule for colonic transit: prospective comparison with radiopaque markers in chronic constipation. Neurogastroenterol Motil. 2010 Aug;22(8):874-82; used with permission.)

in patients with unexplained abnormality of gastric or small bowel transit and assessment for generalized dysmotility in patients suspected to have colonic inertia who are being considered for colectomy.

The antropyloroduodenal method typically uses water-perfused manometric catheters or solid-state sensors mounted on catheters. The tube is positioned so that sensors can detect distal antral contractions; position is verified with the aid of fluoroscopy. The intragastric sensors should be 1 cm or less apart to ensure optimal measurements of distal antral contractile activity proximal to the pylorus. The pylorus is identified manometrically by the presence in the same recording of combinations of distal antral (wide and tall) peaks and duodenal (slender and small) peaks and the presence of a high-pressure zone (tone demonstrated by a tonic elevation of baseline pressure) (Figure 2.22).

A mixed meal is ingested during the test; this facilitates appraisal of the amplitude, frequency, and coordination of contractions. The physiologic responses in the postprandial period include conversion from fasting patterns (eg, MMC) to the fed pattern of irregular, but sustained, contractile responses without return of MMC for at least 2 hours after a 400-kcal or more meal. The antral component of the fed phase is characterized by consistent distal antral pressure activity (average, >40 mm Hg; average frequency of 1 contraction per minute during the first postprandial hour) and small bowel contraction amplitudes (average, >20 mm Hg).

In conditions such as scleroderma, amyloidosis, and hollow visceral myopathy (myopathic disorders), the contractions have low amplitudes, typically less than 20 mm Hg in small bowel and less than 40 mm Hg in distal antrum. In neuropathic disorders, the postprandial frequency of distal antral contractions is reduced, (typical average frequency, <1 per minute during the first hour) and fasting patterns of motility

Figure 2.22   Antropyloroduodenal Motility Tracings in the Postprandial Period With Sensors 1 cm Apart

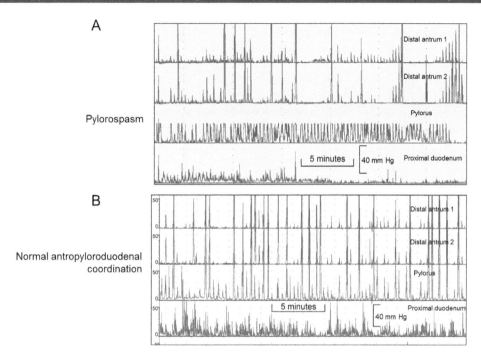

A, Consistent phasic and tonic contractions at the pylorus with intermittent loss of distal antral contractions 1 and 2 cm proximal to the pylorus. B, In contrast, consistent antropyloric coordination in the normal example.

(From Camilleri M. Novel diet, drugs, and gastric interventions for gastroparesis. Clin Gastroenterol Hepatol. 2016 Aug;14(8):1072-80; used with permission.)

return (typically a phase III MMC-like activity) within 2 hours of ingestion of a meal of more than 400 kcal (Figure 2.23).

Attempts to correlate findings on manometry with histopathologic findings are limited. In addition to the clinical indications detailed above, gastroduodenal manometry is useful for drug development programs because it can show prokinetic effects of novel medications, in addition to acceleration of gastric emptying studies, which can be conducted simultaneously.

Colonic Phasic Contractility and Tone

Colonic tone is measured exclusively with an air-filled polyethylene, infinitely compliant balloon linked to an electronic barostat, whereas phasic contractions in the colon can be measured with manometry or WMC. When colonic motility is studied in the laboratory, the tests are usually conducted over 6 hours and include measurements of colonic compliance, fasting and postprandial recordings of contractions and tone, and

responses to pharmacologic stimuli (eg, intravenous neostigmine or intraluminal bisacodyl) (Figures 2.24 and 2.25).

Ambulatory studies are usually conducted over 24 hours and involve measurement of only phasic contractions with increased numbers of solid-state sensors on a tube or a fiberoptic manometry catheter. These advanced approaches result in high-resolution measurements of antegrade and retrograde contractions. In addition, they facilitate recognition of the point of high-amplitude propagated contractions (Figure 2.26).

In clinical practice, colonic manometry (in some centers including barostat measurements of compliance and tone) is performed when severe constipation is unresponsive to medical treatment and slow colonic transit is determined (usually after exclusion of rectal evacuation disorder). This indication is often used to assess whether a patient is a candidate for colectomy, that is, to prove colonic inertia, defined as poor responses of colonic tone and phasic pressure activity to meal and pharmacologic stimulation. A second indication for intraluminal colonic

Figure 2.23   Gastroduodenal Manometry in Health

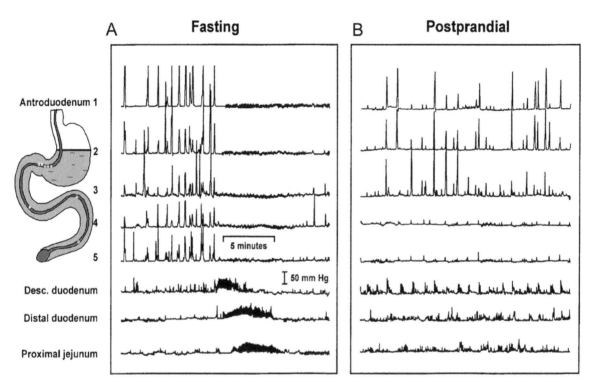

Characteristic appearances of a migrating motor complex during fasting (A) and irregular, but frequent, contractions after a meal (B). Desc. indicates descending.

(From Coulie B, Camilleri M. Intestinal pseudo-obstruction. Annu Rev Med. 1999;50:37-55; used with permission.)

motility measurement is to confirm or diagnose chronic megacolon or megarectum.

Radiologic findings may show when viscus diameters exceed 10 and 15 cm, but intraluminal measurements of colonic compliance and tone are needed for patients with borderline levels or regional differences in diameter. For these, the barostat method is currently the standard. The most useful measurements in research and clinical practice are colonic compliance, presence of high-amplitude propagated contractions, and the responses to a meal and intravenous neostigmine (see Figures 1.10 and 1.11). The performance characteristics of compliance and tone measurements have been published (Odunsi 2010; see suggested reading).

Measurements of colonic motility, tone, or compliance have documented effects of biologic agents (specifically, bile acids) and pharmacologic agents (eg, neostigmine, adrenergic agents, and the serotonin-4 receptor agonist prucalopride).

Anorectal Manometry

The evaluation of patients with constipation in gastroenterology practice requires anorectal manometry to exclude evacuation disorders. Similarly, anorectal manometry is the first-line investigation for patients with fecal incontinence. Two techniques currently dominate clinical practice and research on anorectal functions.

High-resolution anorectal manometry is performed with flexible catheters, typically with 8 to 12 longitudinal sensors spaced approximately 0.6 to 1 cm apart. The most proximal 1 or 2 sensors are located within a balloon that is attached to the uppermost part of the catheter. This balloon serves the additional purposes of rectal distention to elicit the rectoanal inhibitory reflex and sensory testing of the threshold volume for first sensation, sensation of urge to defecate, and sensation of discomfort. The most distal sensor records atmospheric pressure outside the anal canal (Figure 2.27).

Figure 2.24   Colonic Barostat and Manometric Tube in Distal Colon

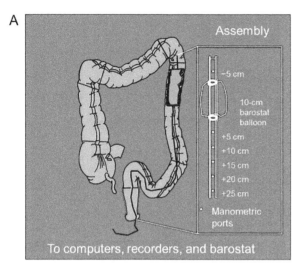

A, After flexible sigmoidoscopy without sedation, a barostat-manometry assembly is placed in the descending colon with the aid of fluoroscopy. The barostat balloon extends for 10 cm between the metal rings (upper panel). Six manometric sensors are shown at 5-cm intervals, 1 above and 5 below the barostatically controlled polyethylene balloon. B, Two radio-opaque metal markers show site of manometry sensors.

Other configurations have 12 to 36 circumferential sensors or 4 radially arranged sensors at each level, and mean pressure is recorded at each level.

Three-dimensional high-definition anorectal pressure manometry uses a rigid probe (100 mm length, 10.75 mm diameter) that includes 256 pressure sensors arranged in 16 rows spaced 4 mm apart and 16 circumferentially oriented sensors 2.1 mm apart in each row (Figure 2.28), and the area of measurement is 6.4 cm long. The test provides a detailed assessment of anal function, from which a morphologic representation of the anal sphincter forces is generated by linear interpolation of the pressures recorded. With dedicated software, this method provides 2-dimensional or 3-dimensional cylindrical topography of the anal canal (Figure 2.28).

As can be expected, normal values vary on the basis of age, sex, and body mass index. There is reasonable concordance between measurements with high-resolution anorectal manometry and 3-dimensional high-definition anorectal pressure manometry techniques.

Transanal Ultrasonography

Transanal ultrasonography is also applied in clinical practice to identify the site of anal sphincter thinning associated with weakness (documented on examination and on anorectal manometry) or tear (on anal ultrasonography) and to guide procedures such as sphincteroplasty (Figure 2.29). For example, the location of an anal sphincter tear or weakness in a female patient presenting with fecal incontinence after vaginal deliveries calls for anterior reconstruction, whereas an equivalent weakness of the anal sphincter presenting as incontinence in a homosexual man requires posterior sphincter reconstruction.

Imaging of Anorectum, Including MRI Defecography

A simple radiologic screening evaluation for rectal evacuation disorder is based on measurement of the gas and stool surface area in the rectum, defined by the lower end of the sacroiliac joints above and the upper margins of the pubis bones below. This area can be measured on

Figure 2.25   Example of Colonic Motility and Tone Measurements

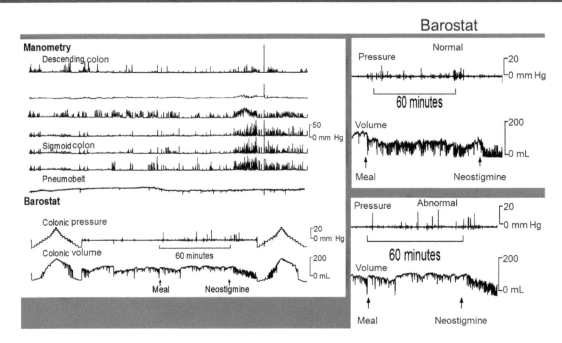

Impaired colonic response to meal and neostigmine: colonic inertia. A typical study over 6 hours includes fasting compliance, fasting colonic motility and tone measurements, and responses of all to a meal and to intravenous neostigmine, 1 mg. Colonic inertia is characterized by poor tonic and phasic response to meal ingestion and to intravenous neostigmine.

(Modified from Ravi K, Bharucha AE, Camilleri M, Rhoten D, Bakken T, Zinsmeister AR. Phenotypic variation of colonic motor functions in chronic constipation. Gastroenterology. 2010 Jan;138(1):89-97.)

Figure 2.26   Motor Patterns in a Healthy Adult Colon Recorded With High-Resolution Fiberoptic Manometry

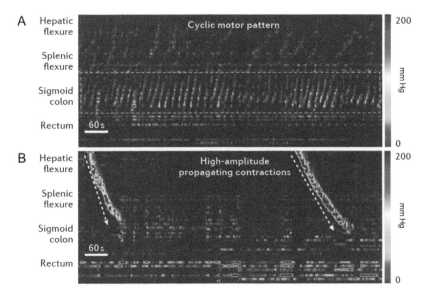

A 36-sensor catheter with an intersensor spacing of 1 cm was used. A, The cyclic motor patterns (peristalsis) prominent in the sigmoid colon are shown within the white rectangle with dashed lines. The cyclic motor pattern is prevalent after a meal and travels predominantly in a retrograde direction. B, Two high-amplitude propagating contractions originate in the proximal colon and travel to the sigmoid colon (dashed white arrows).

(From Camilleri M, Ford AC, Mawe GM, Dinning PG, Rao SS, Chey WD, et al. Chronic constipation. Nat Rev Dis Primers. 2017 Dec 14;3:17095.)

Figure 2.27   High-Resolution Anorectal Manometry (HRAM)

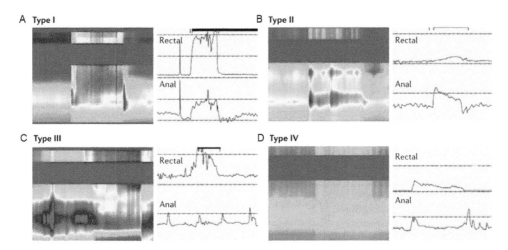

A   Type I
B   Type II
C   Type III
D   Type IV

Results of HRAM (colored panels) and conventional manometry (line graphs) in the rectum (top panels) and anus (lower panels) are shown. A normal response consists of an increase in intrarectal pressure in combination with a relaxation of the anal sphincter. Defecation patterns are abnormal. A, In dyssynergic defecation type I, intrarectal pressure increases appropriately, but the anal sphincter paradoxically contracts. B, In dyssynergic defecation type II, intrarectal pressure does not increase, and the anal sphincter paradoxically contracts. C, In dyssynergic defecation type III, intrarectal pressure increases, but the anal sphincter does not relax or inadequately relaxes. D, In dyssynergic defecation type IV, intrarectal pressure and anal sphincter relaxation are absent or inadequate.

(From Rao SS, Rattanakovit K, Patcharatrakul T. Diagnosis and management of chronic constipation in adults. Nat Rev Gastroenterol Hepatol. 2016 May;13(5):295-305; used with permission.)

Figure 2.28   Three-Dimensional Anorectal Manometry

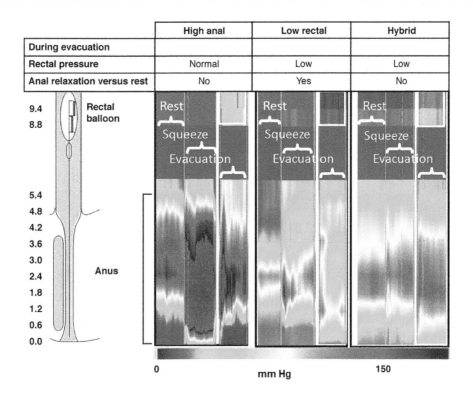

Representative examples of anorectal pressure phenotypes identified by high-resolution manometry in defecatory disorders. Pressures at rest and during squeeze and evacuation were recorded by 12 sensors (2 in the rectal balloon and 10 in the anal canal) and are depicted in color; the numbers reflect the distance in centimeters of sensors from the anal verge. High anal, low rectal, and hybrid phenotypes are defined by anal, rectal, and combined rectoanal dysfunction, respectively. During evacuation, anal relaxation was normal in the rectal phenotype but absent in the high anal and hybrid patterns. Anal resting pressure was also higher in the anal phenotype, and rectal (balloon) pressure increased, as evidenced by color change from blue to green in the rectal balloon, in the high anal phenotype only.

(From Bharucha AE, Rao SS. An update on anorectal disorders for gastroenterologists. Gastroenterology. 2014 Jan;146(1):37-45; used with permission.)

Figure 2.29   A and B, Anal Sphincter Weakness Presenting as Fecal Incontinence and Shown by Transanal Ultrasonography

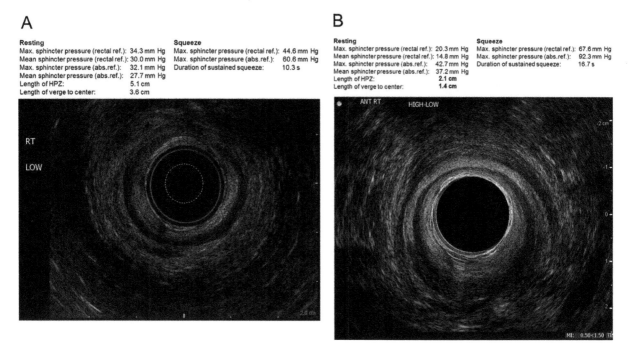

A

Resting
Max. sphincter pressure (rectal ref.): 34.3 mm Hg
Mean sphincter pressure (rectal ref.): 30.0 mm Hg
Max. sphincter pressure (abs.ref.): 32.1 mm Hg
Mean sphincter pressure (abs.ref.): 27.7 mm Hg
Length of HPZ: 5.1 cm
Length of verge to center: 3.6 cm

Squeeze
Max. sphincter pressure (rectal ref.): 44.6 mm Hg
Max. sphincter pressure (abs.ref.): 60.6 mm Hg
Duration of sustained squeeze: 10.3 s

B

Resting
Max. sphincter pressure (rectal ref.): 20.3 mm Hg
Mean sphincter pressure (rectal ref.): 14.8 mm Hg
Max. sphincter pressure (abs.ref.): 42.7 mm Hg
Mean sphincter pressure (abs.ref.): 37.2 mm Hg
Length of HPZ: 2.1 cm
Length of verge to center: 1.4 cm

Squeeze
Max. sphincter pressure (rectal ref.): 67.6 mm Hg
Max. sphincter pressure (abs.ref.): 92.3 mm Hg
Duration of sustained squeeze: 16.7 s

Weakness was confirmed by manometric sphincter pressures at rest and during squeeze and by the short high-pressure zone (HPZ) in B. Low squeeze sphincter pressure was associated with anterior anal sphincter tear in a female patient after vaginal deliveries and vaginal hysterectomy (A) and with a posterior tear in a homosexual man with incontinence (B). abs indicates absolute pressure reference; ANT, anterior; max, maximum pressure recorded; ref, reference; RT, right.

Figure 2.30   Dynamic Magnetic Resonance Imaging of Puborectalis Function During Rectal Evacuation

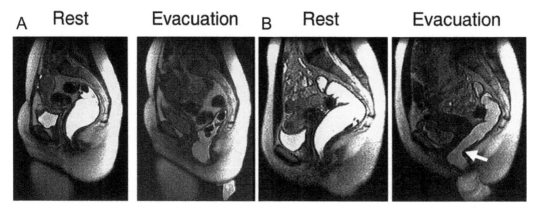

A, Normal puborectalis relaxation: perineal descent (2.6 cm) and anorectal angle increased by 36°. B, Puborectalis contraction: perineal descent 1.7 cm and anorectal angle decreased by 10°. The white arrow shows puborectalis contraction.

Figure 2.31   Dynamic Magnetic Resonance Imaging in Functional Disorders of Defecation Showing Rectal Morphologic Features at Rest (A) and During Defecation (B)

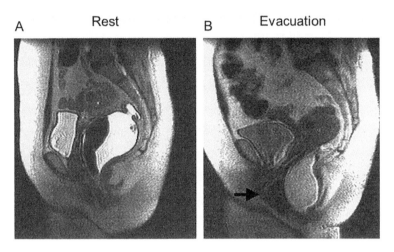

Black arrow indicates descending perineum and anterior rectocele.

(From Bharucha AE, Fletcher JG, Seide B, Riederer SJ, Zinsmeister AR. Phenotypic variation in functional disorders of defecation. Gastroenterology. 2005 May;128(5):1199-210; used with permission.)

a plain abdominopelvic radiograph or on the coronal images or scout film of a computed tomogram of the abdomen. A rectal area of more than 900 mm^2 has approximately a 75% likelihood of being associated with a rectal evacuation disorder.

Detailed imaging of the anorectum can be accomplished with contrast defecography (using barium) or functional MRI (MR defecography), and both provide information about the function (dyssynergic defecation) and anatomy (anal stenosis, enterocele, rectal intussusception, rectal prolapse and rectocele, and pelvic floor anatomy, as well as imaging other organs in the pelvis) of the anorectum (Figures 2.30 and 2.31), with the most detailed information provided by MRI. These tests have some limitations. If patients find the experience of the test embarrassing, they might not relax sufficiently to evacuate the contrast material; moreover, most MR defecography is performed in the supine position, which is not physiologic.

New MRI Applications to Measure GI Function

New approaches exploit the ability of MRI to measure volumes such as gastric volume, small bowel water content, and colonic and bowel gas volumes. A new whole gut transit method uses capsule markers filled with watery gel pellets or water doped with an MRI contrast agent. In the future, cine MRI may have potential to investigate enteric dysmotility, using motion-capture MRI, before or after an intervention such as polyethylene glycol 3350–electrolyte solution.

Suggested Reading

Camilleri M, Iturrino J, Bharucha AE, Burton D, Shin A, Jeong ID, et al. Performance characteristics of scintigraphic measurement of gastric emptying of solids in healthy participants. Neurogastroenterol Motil. 2012 Dec;24(12):1076–e562. Epub 2012 Jul 2.

Camilleri M, Linden DR. Measurement of gastrointestinal and colonic motor functions in humans and animals. Cell Mol Gastroenterol Hepatol. 2016 Jul;2(4):412–28. Epub 2016 Sep 21.

Camilleri M, Shin A. Novel and validated approaches for gastric emptying scintigraphy in patients with suspected gastroparesis. Dig Dis Sci. 2013 Jul;58(7):1813–5. Epub 2013 May 23.

Camilleri M, Thorne NK, Ringel Y, Hasler WL, Kuo B, Esfandyari T, et al. Wireless pH-motility capsule for colonic transit: prospective comparison with radiopaque markers in chronic constipation. Neurogastroenterol Motil. 2010 Aug;22(8):874–82. Epub 2010 May 11.

Fox MR, Kahrilas PJ, Roman S, Gyawali CP, Scott SM, Rao SS, et al. Clinical measurement of gastrointestinal motility and function: who, when and which test? Nat Rev Gastroenterol Hepatol. 2018 Sep;15(9):568–79. Epub 2018 Jun 07.

Metcalf AM, Phillips SF, Zinsmeister AR, MacCarty RL, Beart RW, Wolff BG. Simplified assessment of segmental colonic transit. Gastroenterology. 1987 Jan;92(1):40–7.

Odunsi ST, Camilleri M, Bharucha AE, Papathanasopoulos A, Busciglio I, Burton D, et al. Reproducibility and performance characteristics of colonic compliance, tone, and sensory tests in healthy humans. Dig Dis Sci. 2010 Mar;55(3):709–15. Epub 2009 Mar 17.

Rao SS, Kuo B, McCallum RW, Chey WD, DiBaise JK, Hasler WL, et al. Investigation of colonic and whole-gut transit with wireless motility capsule and radiopaque markers in constipation. Clin Gastroenterol Hepatol. 2009 May;7(5):537–44.

Vijayvargiya P, Jameie-Oskooei S, Camilleri M, Chedid V, Erwin PJ, Murad MH. Association between delayed gastric emptying and upper gastrointestinal symptoms: a systematic review and meta-analysis. Gut. 2019 May;68(5):804–13. Epub 2018 Jun 02.

Gastrointestinal Motility: Control Mechanisms and Pathogenesis of Disordered Function

Introduction

This chapter addresses the normal gastrointestinal (GI) motor functions and the underlying control mechanisms and how these are deranged to result in disorders of motor function. The focus of the chapter is the pathogenesis of dysmotility.

Normal GI Motility

Gastric and Small Bowel Motility

Gastric and small bowel motility are characterized by distinct repertoires of contractions during the fasting and postprandial periods. The fasting period is characterized by the interdigestive migrating motor complex (MMC), whereby this cyclical activity goes through 3 phases about once every 90 minutes: phase I, or motor quiescence; phase II, with intermittent pressure activity; and phase III, also called the activity front, during which pressure activity occurs at maximum frequencies (3 per minute in the stomach, 12 per minute in the duodenum, 8 per minute in the ileum) (see Figure 2.23). The distal small bowel has a distinct type of motility, called the giant migrating complex or power contraction. This contraction sweeps across the terminal ileum and ileocolonic junction and induces bolus transfers of residue (Figure 3.1 and see Figure 2.18).

In response to food ingestion, the vagus nerve induces a reduction in tone, which is more prominent in the proximal stomach. This reduction facilitates the accommodation of ingested food without causing an increase in intragastric pressure, which would otherwise cause postprandial symptoms (Figure 3.2).

In addition, a vagally mediated stimulation of distal antral contractions occurs at a frequency of at least 1 contraction period during the first hour after a solid-liquid meal (see Figure 2.23). This contractile response (antral fed pattern) persists for approximately 1 hour for every 200 kcal ingested.

Liquids containing low-calorie content empty from the stomach more rapidly than solids and follow an exponential trajectory; the rate of emptying of liquids varies with caloric content and viscosity of the liquid

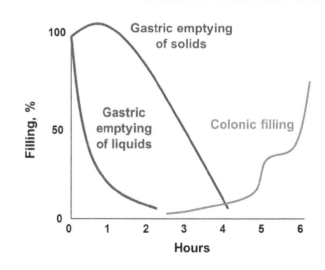

Figure 3.1   Gastric Emptying Profiles of Solids and Liquids and Intermittent Filling of Small Intestinal Content Into the Colon

phase of the meal. Nonnutrient liquids empty rapidly (exponentially) from the healthy human stomach (half-emptying time [$t_{1/2}$], <20 minutes). In contrast, solids undergo acid and peptic digestion in the stomach and shearing by forces that result from the strong antral contractions (see Figure 2.23), propelling the intragastric contents against the closed pylorus. Thus, digestible food is emptied after particle size is reduced to less than 2 mm. This time for trituration results in an initial lag period, followed by a linear post-lag emptying phase for solids (Figure 3.2).

When food substances are in the stomach and upper small bowel, several hormones are secreted that modify the motor and digestive process. For example, food in the stomach stimulates the secretion of gastrin, which, in turn, stimulates gastric acid secretion; with the entry of food into the duodenum, the duodenal mucosa releases cholecystokinin (CCK), which induces gallbladder contraction and bile and pancreatic secretion; enteric signals activate pancreatic endocrine responses (insulin, glucagon, amylin) and small bowel incretin secretion such as glucagon-like peptide (GLP)-1 for glucose regulation and glucose-stimulated insulinotropic peptide. These counter the surge in portal glycemia caused by the arrival and rapid absorption of monosaccharide in the upper small bowel. Thus, there is integrated hormonal release with the arrival of food or

chyme at different levels of the gut. These responses facilitate digestion of food and ensure glycemic control. Indeed, the CCK, incretins (GIP [glucose-stimulated insulinotropic peptide, also called gastric inhibitory polypeptide] and GLP-1), and pancreatic glucagon retard emptying of more calories from the stomach through effects mediated by vagal inhibition.

Solids and liquids are transported through the small bowel at approximately the same rate, but, because liquids are emptied more rapidly from the stomach, they typically reach the colon before the solid phase. Once solids are triturated to a particle size, less than 2 mm, they are handled like a caloric liquid and, hence, the velocity of transit through the small bowel approximates that of the liquid phase of the meal. Chyme moves from ileum to colon intermittently as bolus transfers (Figure 3.2) propelled by prolonged propagated contractions.

In the postprandial period, the stereotypical interdigestive MMC is replaced in the small bowel segments in contact with food by persistent, but irregular, contractions of variable amplitude and frequency that facilitate mixing, digestion, and absorption of food. The maximum frequency of contractions in the stomach and small bowel during the postprandial period is lower than that during phase III of the interdigestive MMC. In addition, as in the stomach, the duration of postprandial contractile activity in the small bowel is proportional to the calories consumed (about 1 hour for each 200 kcal ingested). In contrast to the minor effects of volume and carbohydrate and protein contents of the meal on gastric motility, the fat content significantly impacts the rate of gastric emptying. Nondigestible vegetable fiber does not empty with the digestible portion of the meal; it empties with phase III of the interdigestive MMC.

Integrated Response to Feeding

Ingestion of food activates gastric, pancreatic, and biliary secretions and releases GI hormones that modulate motor, secretory, and absorptive functions (Figure 3.3). The process of food ingestion results in gustatory and other visceral afferent inputs that project to different subnuclei of the nucleus of the tractus solitarus and stimulate other central circuits involving other transmitters, including neuropeptide Y and thyroid-releasing hormone, which are candidate central stimulators of the cephalic phase. The efferent path that

Figure 3.2   Gastric Accommodation in Health

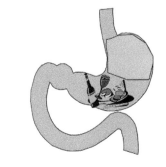

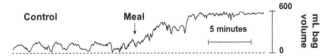

A polyethylene balloon containing air (blue area) maintained at a constant pressure (barostat) tracks the reduction in tone or accommodation after meal ingestion, as shown by the baseline volume; phasic contractions are superimposed on the tone measurements as phasic volume events.

Figure 3.3   Bowel Regulation of Gastric Emptying by Interaction of Nutrient Intake and Neurohormonal Responses

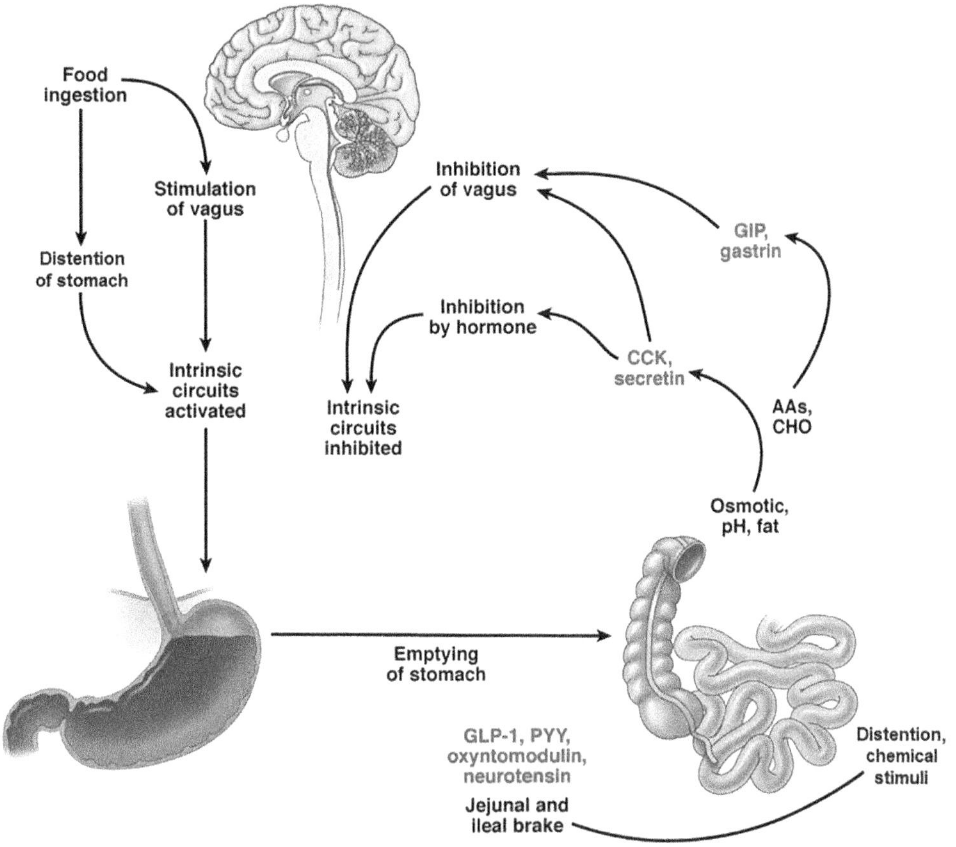

Sensing of different nutrients by enteroendocrine cells results in the release of diverse hormones and peptides. This causes gastric accommodation to the meal, stimulation of gastric contractions that lead to emptying, and, when the nutrients reach different levels of the small bowel, the release of substances that provide generally negative feedback that delays gastric emptying (eg, CCK in the duodenum, GLP-1 and PYY in the more distal small bowel and colon). AA indicates amino acid; CCK, cholecystokinin; CHO, carbohydrates; GIP, gastric inhibitory polypeptide; GLP-1, glycogen-like peptide 1; PYY, peptide tyrosine-tyrosine.

(From Camilleri M. Peripheral mechanisms in appetite regulation. Gastroenterology. 2015 May;148(6):1219-33; used with permission.)

stimulates the upper GI responses involves a vertical column of subnuclei in the dorsal motor nucleus of the vagus nerve and the efferent vagal fibers.

In addition to the reflex activation of afferents by food stimulating these vagal nuclei, there are projections from the forebrain in response to senses such as olfaction and vision in the postprandial period. Cephalically stimulated motor and secretory activities are estimated to contribute more than 50% of the overall postprandial response, a proportion indicating the overall importance of vagal innervation.

In the gastric and intestinal phases of digestion, the hormones involved include gastrin, CCK, secretin, gastric inhibitory polypeptide, ghrelin, glucagon, and pancreatic polypeptide from the upper gut and the incretins such as GLP-1 and peptide YY from the middle and distal small bowel. In general, the secretion of these diverse hormones tends to inhibit the cephalic phase, whereby stimulation of hypothalamic and brainstem nuclei, through vagal afferents activated through stretching the upper gut and chemical stimulation of sensing receptors, modulates the motor, digestive, and secretory processes. The efferent arm of these reflex responses is also mediated through vagal innervation. The dominant neurochemical transmitter in these efferent vagal functions is acetylcholine, whereas CCK and gastrin are prototypical modulators that modulate these reflexes either through effects on vagal afferents or through their paracrine or hormonal functions.

Colonic Motility

Integration of Colonic Contractility, Transit, and Fluid Balance

The normal colon contractile activity is characterized by short-duration (phasic) contractions (propagated or nonpropagated) and tone. Nonpropagated phasic contractions serve to establish segmentation of the colon, manifested by haustra. The haustra separate functional compartments in the colon and facilitate mixing, retention of residue, and formation of solid stool. There are also contractions of less than 75 mm Hg in amplitude that may propagate in an antegrade or retrograde fashion, and they also facilitate mixing. High-amplitude propagated contractions (HAPCs) are typically defined by an amplitude

more than 75 mm Hg, propagation more than at least 15 cm, and a propagation velocity of 0.15 to 2.2 cm/second. These contractions are responsible for mass movements in the colon. In healthy persons, HAPCs occur on average 6 times per day, most often postprandially and on waking in the morning (Figure 3.4).

Simultaneous contractions in the colon associated with pancolonic pressurizations have been described, and these increase significantly after a meal and are associated with a desire to evacuate gas and simultaneous anal sphincter relaxation.

Transit through the colon in healthy people is slow most of the time; residue is typically retained for approximately 24 to 30 hours in the ascending and transverse colon. Alternatively, a mass movement may deliver the contents from the proximal colon to the sigmoid colon in less than 100 seconds. Feeding stimulates colonic

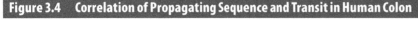

Figure 3.4   Correlation of Propagating Sequence and Transit in Human Colon

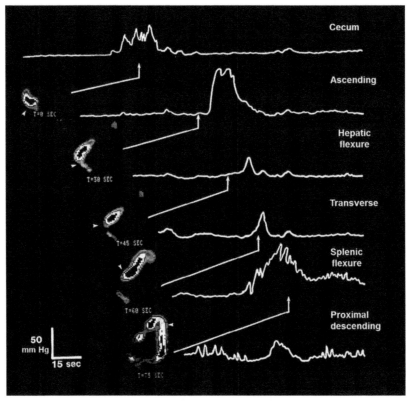

An isotope injected into the cecum traverses the entire colon in less than 2 minutes in association with a high-amplitude propagated contraction, which induces mass movements in the colon. When the pressure wave reaches the splenic flexure, the entire descending colon accommodates the isotope, with loss of lumen occlusion. Also, the propagating pressure-wave amplitudes in channels 3 and 4 are only 30 and 39 mm Hg, respectively, yet the motor pattern is clearly propulsive.

(From Cook IJ, Furukawa Y, Panagopoulos V, Collins PJ, Dent J. Relationships between spatial patterns of colonic pressure and individual movements of content. Am J Physiol Gastrointest Liver Physiol. 2000 Feb;278(2):G329-41; used with permission.)

propulsion of content through a vagally mediated reflex that involves stimulation of the colon by extrinsic pathways; thus, after food stimulates vagal afferents, an efferent reflex arm initiates from the dorsal motor nucleus of the vagus, the spinal cord and sacral nerve roots (S2-4). This is referred to as the *gastrocolonic* response. Meal calorie content affects activation of the gastrocolonic response; thus, a 500 kcal or more, fat-rich meal stimulates colonic motility and propulsion of content.

In healthy people, the average mouth-to-cecum transit time is about 6 hours, and transit times of radiopaque markers through the right colon, left colon, and combined sigmoid colon-rectum have been estimated to be about 12 hours each. Ingestion of dietary fiber accelerates colonic transit, increasing the number of daily bowel movements and softening stool form. Patients with pelvic floor dysfunction or voluntary suppression of defecation (typical of children with constipation) often have slowing of colonic transit.

Fluidity of intraluminal content affects GI transit. About 8 L of fluid enters the gut from oral intake and endogenous secretions: oral intake, gastric, pancreatic, and biliary secretions, and small bowel equilibration of osmotic gradients due to arrival of high-osmolality chyme in the small bowel and the need to equilibrate osmotic pressure across the highly permeable small bowel mucosa. However, most of that fluid load is reabsorbed in the small bowel and, therefore, only about 1.5 L of fluid is delivered to the colon, where most of the fluid is reabsorbed and a maximum of 200 mL of water is excreted in normal stool each day. In addition, the colon has significant capacitance and reserve capacity to absorb fluids; thus, at physiologic rates of delivery from the ileum to the colon, up to 3 L of fluid each day can be reabsorbed by the human colon, provided the capacitance of the proximal colon is not exceeded by large and rapid volume delivery of fluid from the small bowel. Thus, if the rate of ileocolonic flow is more rapid or if colonic motility is increased, the colon's ability to absorb fluid may be overcome, and diarrhea ensues.

Defecation and Continence

Normal defecation requires coordination of the straining effort, sometimes colorectal contractions (eg, HAPCs), and pelvic floor and anal sphincter muscles. The stimulus to initiate the process is often related to the sensation of a sufficient mass of stool filling the rectum or the induction of a mass movement by an HAPC, typically in the morning or after meal ingestion. The rectum is sufficiently sensitive to sense a volume of 10 to 20 mL, although it can accommodate 300 mL; at a volume more than 60 mL, the urge to defecate develops. Rectal distention results in relaxation of the internal anal sphincter (rectoanal inhibitory reflex); at the same time, the external anal sphincter contracts to maintain continence. The anal transition zone can differentiate and "sample" solid or liquid stool and gas, and the healthy human can then make a conscious decision whether and what to pass in the appropriate circumstances (Figure 3.5).

Continence requires sensation of intrarectal content and proper functioning of the anal sphincters; the internal sphincter has intrinsic tone (in part under adrenergic control) and is particularly relevant at night, when contraction of the external anal sphincter is suspended because of the sleep state. The voluntary contraction associated with the external anal sphincter increases pressure to prevent incontinence; however, it can be sustained for only a defined period, typically up to 20 seconds.

Mechanisms Controlling GI Motility

Extrinsic Neural Control

The gut's extrinsic innervation comprises parasympathetic vagal and sacral (S2, S3, and S4) nerves and the sympathetic outflow from the intermediolateral column between the fifth thoracic and the upper lumbar levels of the spinal cord. Sympathetic nerves synapse in the prevertebral celiac, superior mesenteric, and inferior mesenteric ganglia and course along the celiac, superior, and inferior mesenteric arteries. The neurotransmitter for the sympathetic nerve synapse in the ganglia is acetylcholine. The postganglionic sympathetic nerves are noradrenergic.

The vagus nerve innervates the GI tract from the stomach to the right colon. It is often forgotten that parasympathetic innervation of the right colon is provided by the vagal fibers coursing along ileocolonic branches of the superior mesenteric artery. The parasympathetic supply to the distal colon originates from the sacral roots S2 to S4. Sympathetic fibers to the stomach and small bowel arise from T5 to T10 levels and to the colon from T11 to L3 levels of the spinal cord.

Figure 3.5   Sagittal View of the Anorectum at Rest (A) and During Straining to Defecate (B)

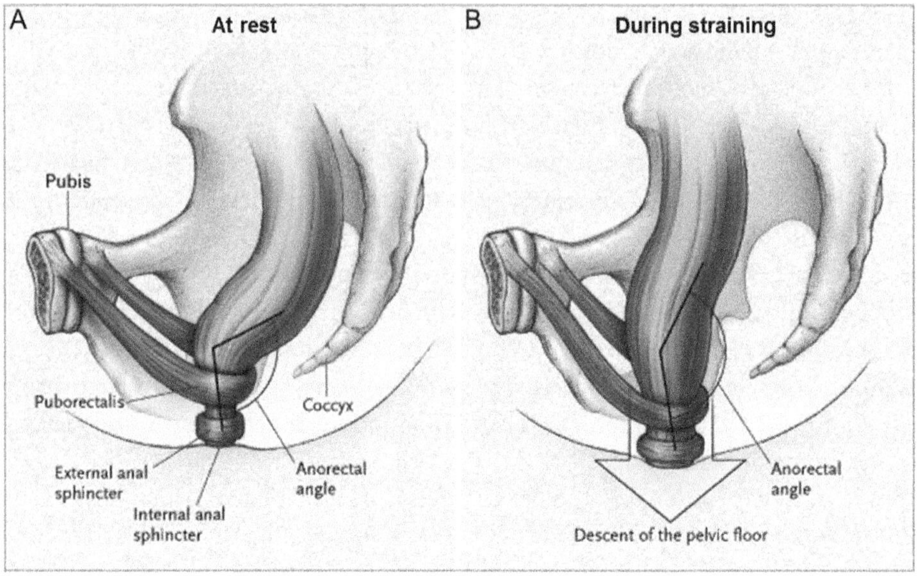

Continence is maintained by normal rectal sensation and tonic contraction of the internal anal sphincter and the puborectalis muscle, which wraps around the anorectum, maintaining an anorectal angle between 80° and 110°. During defecation, the pelvic floor muscles (including the puborectalis) relax, allowing the anorectal angle to straighten by at least 15°, and the perineum descends by 1.0 to 3.5 cm. The external anal sphincter also relaxes and reduces pressure on the anal canal.

(From Lembo A, Camilleri M. Chronic constipation. N Engl J Med. 2003 Oct 2;349(14):1360-8; used with permission.)

The prevertebral ganglia integrate afferent impulses between the gut and the spinal cord and reflexively control abdominal viscera. In general, parasympathetic preganglionic fibers (vagal and sacral) are excitatory to nonsphincteric muscle, and sympathetic fibers are inhibitory to muscle and excitatory to sphincters such as the internal anal sphincter (Figure 3.6).

There are intrinsic reflexes and synaptic pathways in the gut wall that are activated by sensory input, such as the presence of a bolus within the lumen of the gut, and that alter gut functions, independent of extrinsic control mechanisms. However, these intrinsic reflexes can be modulated by the extrinsic nervous system. Apart from these autonomous, intrinsic responses, additional reflexes are mediated at the prevertebral ganglia, spinal cord, and higher centers.

Interaction Between Extrinsic and Enteric Nerves

The efferent vagal preganglionic cholinergic fibers synapse with preprogrammed circuits in the enteric plexuses of the digestive tract. These ganglia in the enteric plexuses consist of diverse neuronal populations, including the myenteric cholinergic neurons that are excitatory to smooth muscle cells and induce contraction. Other vagal fibers act through submucous plexus neurons to alter the functions of surface enterocytes or colonocytes, affecting the absorption or secretion of fluids and electrolytes.

There is a great disparity between the limited number of extrinsic nerve fibers in the vagus (estimated 40,000 fibers, many of which are afferents) and the 100 millions of neurons in the enteric plexi. It is, therefore, believed that programmed circuits involving motor or secretory functions are under the control of command vagal preganglionic or sympathetic postganglionic fibers.

The overall effect of the sympathetic supply is to inactivate neural circuits that generate motor activity, whereas intrinsic inhibitory innervation by the enteric nerves is not affected. Thus, on simple assessment, the sympathetic nervous system is the brake of the gut. Extrinsic vagal fibers also synapse with inhibitory intramural neurons in the gut, which produce inhibitory transmitters such as nitric oxide, vasoactive intestinal peptide, and somatostatin. Loss of the sympathetic inhibitory supply (the brake) results in excessive or

Figure 3.6   The Gut's Nervous System

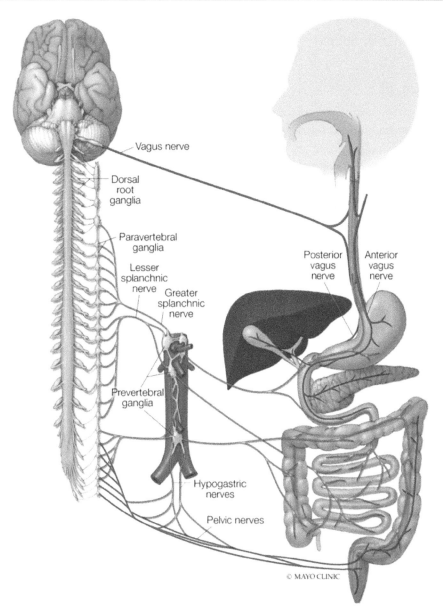

The extrinsic nervous system (parasympathetic vagal and sacral nerves and thoracolumbar sympathetic nerves) and the intrinsic or enteric nervous system are shown.

uncoordinated phasic pressure activity in the gut called *burst*, which may be propagated or nonpropagated, and may manifest gut motor overactivity, including diarrhea.

Main Functions of Extrinsic Nerves

Extrinsic nerves from the vagus control the striated muscle portion of the esophagus and the pudendal nerve (derived from S2-4 spinal roots) supply to the external anal sphincter. As stated above, parasympathetic nerve supply is excitatory to nonsphincteric muscle, whereas the thoracolumbar sympathetic supply is excitatory to sphincters and inhibitory to nonsphincteric muscle. In addition to modulating intrinsic neural circuits in the smooth muscle layer of the gut, the extrinsic nerves integrate widely separated regions of the GI tract (eg, the gastrocolonic response to food and rectocolonic inhibition). This integration is more prominent in certain regions (eg, the stomach and distal portion of the colon in response to feeding as part of the neutrally mediated gastrocolonic reflex) than in others (eg, the neural response of the small bowel to feeding).

Enteric Neural Control

The enteric nervous system (ENS) is a third component of the autonomic nervous system and functions as an independent nervous system comprising approximately 100 million neurons that are organized in ganglionated plexuses; it is also called the *little brain* to differentiate it from the *big brain,* or central nervous system. The larger myenteric or Auerbach plexus is situated between the longitudinal and circular layers of the muscularis externa. Myenteric plexus neurons control gut motility through interaction with pacemaker cells such as the interstitial cells of Cajal (ICCs) and fibroblast-like cells that express receptors for platelet-derived growth factor receptor α (PDGFRα). The submucosal, or Meissner plexus, controls transmucosal movement of fluids (absorption and secretion) and mucosal blood flow (Figure 3.7).

The ENS also functions in sensation, because the visceral afferent nerves express mechanosensitive ion channels. The ENS also interacts with both the gut endocrine and the immune systems and has roles in modifying nutrient absorption and maintaining the mucosal barrier. The vast spectrum of intrinsic neurons includes excitatory and inhibitory motor neurons, secretomotor neurons, interneurons, and intrinsic afferents that express different transmitters (Table 3.1).

The ICCs and PDGFRα fibroblast-like cells are spontaneously active pacemaker cells that coordinate muscular contraction and are mechanosensitive. They form a nonneural pacemaker system, predominantly at the interface of the circular and longitudinal muscle layers of the bowel and within the muscular layers themselves. The ICC functions are best characterized, and they serve as intermediaries between the nerves in the ENS and the muscles, which have their own intrinsic control systems. Electrical signals spread longitudinally and circumferentially through interneurons in contiguous segments of the gut. This movement occurs through neurochemical activation by transmitters that may be excitatory (eg, acetylcholine, substance P) or inhibitory (eg, nitric oxide, somatostatin) (see Figure 1.1).

Stomach and Small Bowel Pathobiology Resulting in Slow Transit

Disorders of the extrinsic nervous system and ENS and electrical syncytial elements (eg, ICCs) or smooth muscle result in GI motility disorders. These disorders

---

Figure 3.7   Organization of the Enteric Nervous System in Multiple Ganglionated Plexuses

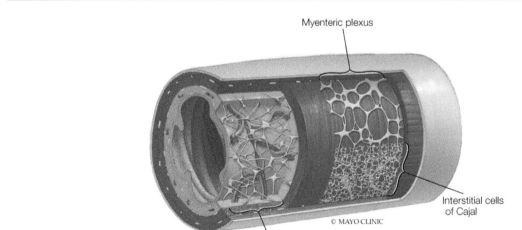

The major plexuses are the myenteric and submucosal plexuses.

Table 3.1	Intrinsic Neurons and Transmitters	
Type of Neuron	**Primary Transmitter**	**Secondary Transmitters, Modulators**
Enteric excitatory muscle motor neuron	ACh	Tachykinin, enkephalin (presynaptic inhibition)
Enteric inhibitory muscle motor neuron	Nitric oxide	VIP, ATP or ATP-like compound, CO
Ascending IN	ACh	Tachykinin, ATP
ChAT, NOS descending IN	ATP, ACh	None
ChAT, 5-HT descending IN	ACh	5-HT, ATP
ChAT, somatostatin descending IN	ACh	None
Intrinsic sensory neuron	ACh, CGRP, tachykinin	None
INs to secretomotor neurons	ACh	ATP, 5-HT
Noncholinergic secretomotor neuron	VIP	PACAP
Cholinergic secretomotor neuron	ACh	None
Motor neuron to gastrin cells	GRP, ACh	None
Motor neurons to parietal cells	ACh	Potentially VIP
Sympathetic neurons, motility inhibiting	Noradrenaline	None
Sympathetic neurons, secretion inhibiting	Noradrenaline	Somatostatin
Sympathetic neurons, vasoconstrictor	Noradrenaline, ATP	Potentially NPY
Intestinofugal neurons to sympathetic ganglia	ACh	VIP

Abbreviations: ACh, acetylcholine; ATP, adenosine trisphosphate; CGRP, calcitonin gene-related peptide; ChAT, choline acetyltransferase; CO, carbon monoxide; 5-HT, hydroxytryptamine; GRP, gastrin-releasing peptide (also called bombesin); IN, interneuron; NOS, nitric oxide synthase; NPY, neuropeptide Y; PACAP, pituitary adenylate cyclase-activating peptide; VIP, vasoactive intestinal peptide.

Modified from Furness JB. The enteric nervous system and neurogastroenterology. Nat Rev Gastroenterol Hepatol. 2012 Mar 6;9(5):286-94; used with permission.

may be genetic (including abnormalities of *RET*, the gene that encodes the tyrosine kinase receptor, and abnormalities in the endothelin B system and *KIT*, a marker of ICCs [Chapter 1, "Genetics and Molecular Aspects of Gastrointestinal Motility Disorders"]) or acquired. The most common acquired disorders are idiopathic, diabetic, and postsurgical. Neuropathic disorders are characterized by normal-amplitude, but uncoordinated, contractions, whereas myopathies are characterized by contractions of an average of less than 40 mm Hg in amplitude in the antrum and an average of less than 20 mm Hg in the small bowel (Chapter 2, "Measurement of Gastrointestinal and Colonic Motility in Clinical Practice"). Combined disorders

expressing neuropathic and myopathic features occur in systemic sclerosis, amyloidosis, and mitochondrial cytopathy, initially with neuropathic and later myopathic characteristics with disease progression. When motility disorders are suspected, an essential first step is to exclude mechanical obstruction.

Extrinsic Neuropathic Disorders

Extrinsic neuropathic processes resulting in neuropathic dysmotilities are listed in Table 3.2. The most common disorders include diabetic neuropathy, vagotomy, medication-related, Parkinson disease,

Table 3.2	Extrinsic Neuropathic Processes Resulting in Neuropathic Dysmotilities
Type	**Examples of Neuropathic Dysmotility**
Familial	Familial visceral neuropathy
Genetic	Neurofibromatosis, Hirschsprung disease (sporadic, familial)
Infiltrative neuropathy	Amyloidosis
Generalized neuropathy	Diabetes mellitus, amyloidosis, spinal cord injury, multiple sclerosis, brain stem tumor, infarct
Infectious	Chagas disease; viral (EBV, CMV, herpes zoster)
Neoplastic	Paraneoplastic
Medication-related	Narcotics, antidepressants, anticholinergics, α_2-adrenergic agonists, GLP-1 analogs or agonists
Idiopathic	Achalasia, hypertrophic pyloric stenosis, gastroparesis, pseudo-obstruction, slow-transit constipation, colonic inertia, megacolon

Abbreviations: CMV, cytomegalovirus; EBV, Epstein-Barr virus; GLP-1, glucagon-like peptide 1.

amyloidosis, and a paraneoplastic syndrome usually associated with small cell carcinoma of the lung. Medications that affect motility include α_2-adrenergic agonists, GLP-1 analogs or agonists, opiates, and anticholinergics.

Autonomic nerve involvement in disease processes such as infection, neuropathy, and neurodegeneration may lead to motor, secretory, and sensory disturbances. The most common manifestation of these extrinsic autonomic neuropathies is constipation. Spinal cord injury above the level of the sacral segments results in delayed proximal and distal colonic transit attributable to parasympathetic denervation. Fasting colonic motility, compliance, and tone are usually normal, but the response to feeding is reduced or absent because of interruption in the descending spinal fibers mediating the reflex activation of the sacral roots that supply the colon. Alternatively, spinal cord lesions involving the sacral segments or damage directly to the efferent nerves from these segments (S2-4) disrupt the neural integration of rectosigmoid expulsion and anal sphincter control. Such injuries result in loss of left colon contractility and decreased rectal tone and sensitivity, which may lead to colorectal dilatation and fecal impaction. These are higher or lower pathways that may be involved in Parkinson disease and multiple sclerosis, which are frequently associated with constipation. In addition, dopaminergic agents and anticholinergic agents used to relieve the neurologic disorders may aggravate the constipation.

Enteric and Intrinsic Neuropathic Disorders

Disorders of the ENS or the electrical syncytial elements (ICCs and PDGFRα fibroblast-like cells) are usually the result of infectious, degenerative, immune, or inflammatory processes. Virus-induced gastroparesis (eg, rotavirus, Norwalk virus, cytomegalovirus, or Epstein-Barr virus) is associated with inflammatory cell infiltration of the myenteric plexus. In idiopathic chronic intestinal pseudo-obstruction, there is usually no disturbance of the extrinsic neural control, and the main lesion is degeneration of the ICCs and inflammation with infiltration by diverse immunocytes or eosinophils. Herpes virus family infections may contribute to ENS dysfunction.

Smooth Muscle Disorders

Disturbances of smooth muscle may result in significant disorders of gastric emptying and small bowel and colonic transit. The most commonly associated conditions are systemic sclerosis, amyloidosis, metabolic muscle disorders, or metabolic disorders such as hypothyroidism and hyperparathyroidism; patients (with these conditions) more commonly present with constipation. Scleroderma may result in either localized or general dilatation, the presence of wide-mouthed diverticula, and, more commonly, delayed transit in the stomach, small bowel, and colon. The

Box 3.1

Pathophysiologic Features of Dysmotilities

Neuropathic

Acceleration or delay of transit of solids

Extrinsic vagal denervation may cause acceleration of transit of liquids

Minority have dilated bowel or air-fluid levels

Extrinsic neuropathies associated with other symptoms or signs of dysautonomia:

Orthostatic dizziness, decrease in blood pressure with posture without compensatory pulse increase

Plasma norepinephrines

Bladder and sexual dysfunction

Absence of sweating, dry mouth, mucosae

Difficulties with vision in bright lights

Myopathic

Delay of transit, usually of solids

Bacterial overgrowth common, and may cause acceleration of transit in small bowel and colon

Dilated bowel or air-fluid levels more prevalent than in neuropathies

Myopathies associated with other symptoms or signs of collagenoses:

Skin (eg, Raynaud)

Eyes (eg, uveitis)

Joints: arthralgia, arthritis

Data from Camilleri M. Diagnosis and treatment of enteric neuromuscular diseases. Clin Auton Res. 2003 Feb;13(1):10-5.

amplitude of contractions at affected levels is reduced; stasis, dilatation, and diverticula predispose to bacterial overgrowth, steatorrhea, and pneumatosis intestinalis.

Mitochondrial neurogastrointestinal encephalomyopathy, or familial visceral myopathy type II (Chapter 1, "Genetics and Molecular Aspects of Gastrointestinal Motility Disorders"), is most often inherited. It is an autosomal recessive condition, and the motility manifestation is chronic intestinal pseudo-obstruction with extensive small bowel diverticula in early adulthood. Box 3.1 summarizes the pathophysiologic features of dysmotilities, and Box 3.2 addresses the critical questions in assessment of suspected gastroduodenal dysmotility: what to look for on radiographs and on gastroduodenal manometry and selection of treatment.

Box 3.2

Critical Questions in Assessment of Suspected Gastroduodenal Dysmotility

What to Look for on Radiograph

Exclude mechanical obstruction

Evidence of bowel dilatation

Packing of valvulae conniventes (scleroderma)

Pneumatosis intestinalis

Small bowel diverticulosis

Gastric retention in scleroderma

Findings on Gastroduodenal Manometry

Amplitude in small bowel <10 mm Hg = myopathy

Antral hypomotility

Amplitude average <40 mm Hg = myopathy

Normal amplitude <1/min in 1st hour = neuropathy

Persistence of migrating motor complex activity at 15-120 min after meal = neuropathy

Simultaneous prolonged contractions = obstruction

Questions in Selecting Treatment

Are symptoms acute or chronic?

Is the disease due to a neuropathy or a myopathy?

What is the state of hydration and nutrition?

What regions of the gut are affected?

Is there severe constipation?

Stomach and Small Bowel Diseases Resulting in Rapid Transit

Dumping Syndrome and Accelerated Gastric Emptying

Dumping syndrome and accelerated gastric emptying typically result from vagal injury as a result of fundoplication for gastric esophageal reflux disease. With the widespread use of highly selective vagotomy and the advent of effective antacid secretory therapy, dumping syndrome due to surgery for peptic ulcer disease is becoming rare. Dumping syndrome may also occur in patients with vagal dysfunction from other causes, such as diabetic autonomic neuropathy. A high-calorie (usually carbohydrate) content of the liquid phase of the meal evokes a rapid insulin response with secondary hypoglycemia. Patients with vagal injury may also have gastric stasis of solids due to impaired antral contractility, which paradoxically

may result in gastroparesis (for solids) and dumping (for liquids).

Colonic Motility Disorders

Constipation

According to epidemiologic surveys, including in Olmsted County, Minnesota, constipation is reported by about 20% of the population, and 4% report needing to strain excessively to pass bowel movements. In functional constipation, colonic transit is typically normal, and there is no evidence of an evacuation disorder. Functional constipation overlaps with constipation-predominant irritable bowel syndrome when patients have pain in association with constipation that is relieved by passing a bowel movement. Although pathologic reports document diverse neurotransmitter excesses or abnormalities, the most consistent neuropathologic feature in patients

Figure 3.8   Paraneoplastic Syndrome

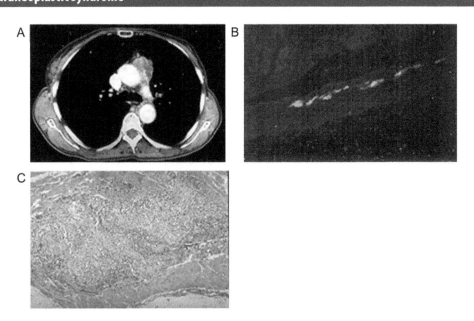

A, Computed tomographic image of paraneoplastic chronic intestinal pseudo-obstruction due to a small cell carcinoma of the lung. B, Associated circulating antineuronal nuclear or anti-Hu antibody. C, Associated inflammatory plexopathy of the myenteric plexus in the stomach (full-thickness biopsy specimen of stomach; hematoxylin-eosin, original magnification ×100).

(From Lennon VA, Sas DF, Busk MF, Scheithauer B, Malagelada JR, Camilleri M, et al. Enteric neuronal autoantibodies in pseudoobstruction with small-cell lung carcinoma. Gastroenterology. 1991 Jan;100(1):137-42; used with permission.)

Figure 3.9   Systemic Sclerosis

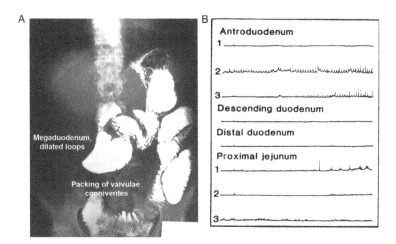

Megaduodenum (A) and low-amplitude contractions on manometry (B).

with acquired slow-transit constipation, with no colonic dilatation, is reduction in the number of ICCs in the colon compared with numbers from the colon of controls.

Megacolon and Megarectum

Idiopathic megarectum and megacolon can be either congenital or acquired and are almost invariably attributed to abnormalities in structure or function of the ENS. In megacolon, the dilated segment shows increased compliance (volume response to imposed intraluminal pressure) and normal phasic contractility but decreased colonic tone. These features are associated with abnormalities in the myenteric plexus and variable abnormalities of smooth muscle components, that is, the muscularis mucosa and the circular and longitudinal muscle layers. Congenital megacolon associated with Hirschsprung disease and acquired megacolon in adults (sporadic or associated with multiple endocrine neoplasia 2B) is discussed in Chapter 1 ("Genetics and Molecular Aspects of Gastrointestinal Motility Disorders").

Figure 3.10   Gastric Retention in Scleroderma

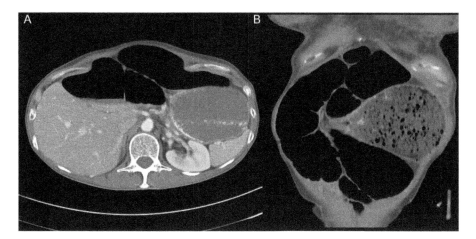

Computed tomographic images: A, transverse. B, coronal.

Box 3.3

Pathologic Features of Enteric Neuromuscular Disease

Aganglionosis

Neuronal intranuclear inclusions and apoptosis

Neural degeneration

Intestinal neuronal dysplasia

Neuronal hyperplasia and ganglioneuromas

Mitochondrial dysfunction: syndromic and nonsyndromic

Inflammatory neuropathies: cellular and humoral mechanisms

Neurotransmitter disorders

Interstitial cell abnormality

From De Giorgio R, Camilleri M. Human enteric neuropathies: morphology and molecular pathology. Neurogastroenterol Motil. 2004 Oct;16(5):515-31; used with permission.

Acquired defects in the ENS due to infection with *Trypanosoma cruzi* may result in constipation in Chagas disease, which results from the destruction of myenteric neurons. Acquired aganglionosis also has been reported with circulating antineuronal antibodies, with or without associated neoplasm (typically lung or ovarian cancers).

Examples of the pathobiologic aspects of the intrinsic and extrinsic neural control are provided in this chapter (specifically, paraneoplastic syndrome [Figure 3.8] and scleroderma [Figures 3.9 and 3.10]) and in Chapter 7 ("Neuromuscular Disorders Causing Gut Dysmotility"). Box 3.3 lists pathologic features of enteric neuromuscular disease.

Suggested Reading

Camilleri M. Integrated upper gastrointestinal response to food intake. Gastroenterology. 2006 Aug;131(2):640–58. Epub 2006 Aug 08.

Furness JB. The enteric nervous system and neurogastroenterology. Nat Rev Gastroenterol Hepatol. 2012 Mar 6;9(5):286–94. Epub 2012 Mar 07.

Gastroparesis, Chronic Intestinal Pseudo-obstruction, and Functional Dyspepsia

Introduction

Traditionally, gastroparesis is a syndrome characterized by delayed gastric emptying (GE) of solids and key upper gastrointestinal (GI) symptoms in the absence of mechanical obstruction of the stomach. However, in recent years, the spectrum has been broadened to gastroparesis and related disorders with recommendation to reconsider the syndrome a broader spectrum of gastric neuromuscular dysfunction (Pasricha 2015; see suggested reading). The principal symptoms of gastroparesis include postprandial fullness (early satiety), nausea, vomiting, bloating, belching, and upper abdominal pain. The most common causes of gastroparesis are idiopathic, diabetic (in almost one-third of cases in a tertiary referral series [Soykan 1998; see suggested reading]), and iatrogenic (medications and postsurgical). Symptoms attributable to gastroparesis are reported by 5% to 12% of patients with diabetes mellitus.

In functional dyspepsia, there is no ulcer or significant erosive disease; postprandial symptoms are chronic or recurrent, are centered in the upper abdomen, and consist of pain and discomfort such as early satiety, nausea, vomiting, or bloating. The Rome Foundation criteria III and IV classify 2 symptom complexes: postprandial distress syndrome and epigastric pain syndrome. Postprandial distress syndrome is characterized typically by postprandial fullness and early satiation, and epigastric pain syndrome is characterized by epigastric pain and burning.

Chronic intestinal pseudo-obstruction (CIPO) is often associated with gastroparesis and involves at least the small bowel and, frequently, several regions of the GI tract, including the esophagus, stomach, and colon. The prevalence and incidence of CIPO are unknown, but it is a rare disease. Approximately 100 infants are born with congenital CIPO each year in the United States. Among adults, CIPO is more prevalent in women than in men.

Gastroparesis and CIPO

Pathophysiology

This spectrum of disorders results from neuromuscular dysfunction. Vagal innervation is essential for gastric accommodation, mediated by intrinsic inhibitory mechanisms such as nitrergic neurons, and antral contractions essential for triturating solid food require innervation by the vagus and enteric excitatory nerves, particularly cholinergic nerves. Smooth muscle disorders may be infiltrative (as in scleroderma) or degenerative (as in hollow visceral myopathy, amyloidosis, and, rarely, mitochondrial cytopathy).

Screening for vagal dysfunction can be achieved by seeking the presence of sinus arrhythmia (normal) on a long-duration electrocardiogram. Myopathic disorders are invariably associated with dysmotilities affecting other regions of the gut (most often the lower two-thirds of the esophagus, lower esophageal sphincter, and small bowel), with external ophthalmoplegia or skeletal muscle involvement in mitochondrial cytopathy, and with systemic features such as CREST syndrome in scleroderma (calcinosis, Raynaud phenomenon, esophageal dysfunction, sclerodactyly, telangiectasia).

Etiopathogenesis

Box 4.1 lists the pathogenetic causes of gastroparesis and CIPO.

Acquired Diseases

The most common conditions associated with gastroparesis are idiopathic, diabetic, iatrogenic, and postviral. One of the main factors associated with delayed GE is postprandial antral hypomotility (Figure 4.1), which may result from damage or dysfunction of the vagus nerve (Figure 4.2). The dysfunction may be permanent, as after vagotomy for peptic ulceration or esophagectomy, or it may be reversible, as occurs with radiofrequency ablation of cardiac tissue in patients with atrial fibrillation (Figure 4.3) or with sclerosis of esophageal varices.

The most common medications associated with gastroparesis are μ-opioid agonists, including tramadol and tapentadol, and hypoglycemic agents such as amylin analogs (eg, pramlintide) or glucagon-like peptide-1 analogs or agonists (eg, liraglutide and exenatide), but not the dipeptidyl peptidase IV inhibitors such as vildagliptin and sitagliptin which increase glucagon-like peptide-1 and improve glycemia without delaying GE. Opioids retard GE, and chronic intake of opioids on a schedule (in contrast to opioids only as needed) has the greatest impact. In a report from Temple University (Jehangir 2017; see suggested reading), 19.3% of the 223 patients with gastroparesis on chronic scheduled opioids (median morphine equivalent dose 60 mg/day) for at least 1 month had more severe symptoms, lower employment rate, higher hospitalizations in the past year, and worse therapeutic outcomes with prokinetics or gastric electrical stimulation compared to the 70.9% not taking opioids.

Studies of the histopathologic features and expression in the intrinsic mechanisms, based on full-thickness gastric biopsies, showed reduced numbers of nitrergic neurons but no morphologic differences between diabetic and idiopathic gastroparesis (eg, nerves, glia, interstitial cells of Cajal, immune cells, and smooth muscle cells). In addition, reduction in interstitial cells of Cajal in the body of the stomach was associated with reduction in the number of CD206 (mannose receptor)-positive M2 macrophages, which normally produce heme oxygenase-1, an enzyme that enhances cell repair and reduces inflammation. Examples of these cellular abnormalities in idiopathic or diabetic gastroparesis are shown in Figures 4.4 through 4.7.

Box 4.1

Pathogenesis of Gastroparesis and Chronic Intestinal Pseudo-obstruction

Autonomic (vagal) neuropathy (eg, diabetes mellitus, orthostatic hypotension syndromes, including amyloidosis)

Intrinsic neuropathy (eg, due to acquired diseases such as diabetes mellitus, paraneoplastic process, viral infections, Chagas disease, or congenital diseases such as Hirschsprung disease, von Recklinghausen disease)

    Excitatory and inhibitory intrinsic nerves

    Interstitial cells of Cajal, oxidative stress, and altered balance of macrophages

Combined extrinsic and intrinsic neuropathy, such as diabetes mellitus, postviral (cytomegalovirus, Epstein-Barr virus, herpes family of viruses)

Myopathic (eg, scleroderma and amyloidosis)

Sequential involvement of extrinsic or enteric nervous system, followed by smooth muscle disease: scleroderma, dermatomyositis, amyloidosis, jejunal diverticulosis, radiation enteritis

Iatrogenic affecting extrinsic nerves (eg, vagotomy associated with fundoplication or esophagectomy; vagal dysfunction due to radiofrequency ablation for atrial fibrillation) or intrinsic nerves (eg, anthraquinones, dopaminergic agents, chemotherapeutic agents such as vincristine)

Inflammatory plexopathy: several rare reports document different inflammatory cells infiltrating the myenteric plexus; may be idiopathic, postinfectious, or associated with neuroblastoma

Figure 4.1   Postprandial Antroduodenal Motility in Humans

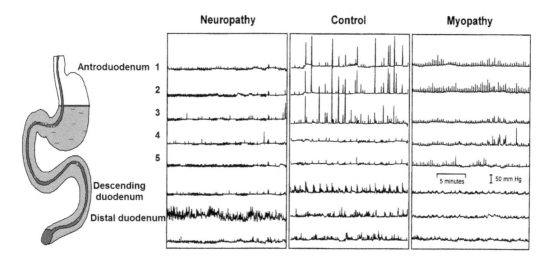

Postprandial gastric and small-bowel motility recordings in a healthy control (middle), in a patient with neuropathic chronic intestinal pseudo-obstruction (left), and in a patient with a myopathic disorder (right). The neuropathy is characterized by normal-amplitude contractions but a sustained incoordinated contractile activity in the distal duodenum and a lack of consistent antral response. In contrast, myopathic processes are associated with low-amplitude (<40 mm Hg in antrum and <10 mm Hg in the small bowel) contractions.

(Modified from Coulie B, Camilleri M. Intestinal pseudo-obstruction. Annu Rev Med. 1999;50:37-55; used with permission.)

Table 4.1 summarizes enteric or intrinsic mechanisms that may contribute to the development of gastroparesis. These include interstitial cells of Cajal, platelet-derived growth factor receptor α fibroblast-like cells, nitrergic neurons, and CD206-positive macrophages. Extrinsic neural control, particularly vagal function, may also mediate some of the anti-inflammatory effects of immune cells in the gut (Figure 4.8).

In patients followed for about 1 year, the occurrence of a prodromal viral illness before gastroparesis is generally associated with a good prognosis (relative to nonviral, idiopathic gastroparesis), unless there is virus-induced selective dysautonomia or pandysautonomia caused by Epstein-Barr virus, cytomegalovirus, and herpes virus. Postviral gastroparesis complicated by dysautonomia has a poor prognosis.

Myopathic diseases result from infiltrative disorders or muscle degeneration, as in scleroderma, hollow visceral myopathy, amyloidosis, and, rarely, mitochondrial cytopathy. GE and small bowel transit are retarded in myopathic diseases because of reduced size of bolus transfers from ileum to colon, which increase the likelihood of stasis and small bowel bacterial overgrowth. In general, the GE profile cannot differentiate neuropathic from myopathic disease, although the size of ileocolonic bolus transfers may do so (Figure 4.9). However, the assessment of size of ileocolonic transfers requires extensive detailed imaging that is not available in clinical practice.

The literature on the effects of hyperglycemia is conflicting. Epidemiologic studies show that glycemic control, assessed by patient report or by measurement of glycosylated hemoglobin, is associated with a higher prevalence of upper GI symptoms. Experimentally, acute changes in blood glucose value (typically to 180 mg/dL or 250 mg/dL) prolong GE time and inhibit antral motility (Figure 4.10).

In a study of factors contributing to hospitalization (Bharucha 2015; see suggested reading) for exacerbations of gastroparesis, 36% of patients had poor glycemic control, and, when glycemia was restored by kidney and pancreas transplants, there was significant impact on GE and associated GI symptoms. However, other studies, based on long-term glycemic control, have found that the glycosylated hemoglobin level is not a statistically significant predictor of abnormal (compared with normal) GE of solids (in a study of 129 patients) and that long-term blood glucose control had no significant effect on GE in patients with type 1 or type 2 diabetes mellitus (in a study of 30 patients) (Figure 4.11).

Figure 4.2   Vagal Innervation of Stomach

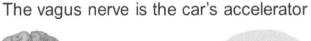

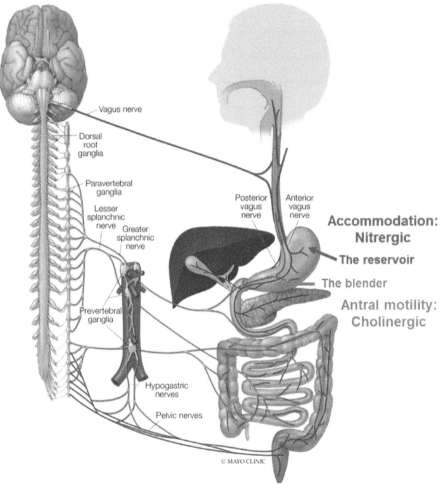

The vagus nerve supplies cholinergic intrinsic nerves that stimulate antral contractility, which sets up liquid shearing forces (the blender) that triturate solids. The vagus nerve also activates nitrergic neurons to induce gastric accommodation, providing a reservoir for food ingested. It is always important to exclude obstruction (eg, by peptic ulcer or pyloric stenosis) in patients with suspected gastroparesis.

Among the etiopathogenetic mechanisms of intrinsic neuropathies that cause gastroparesis and CIPO, immunocyte and eosinophil infiltration of the myenteric plexus is well documented (Figure 4.12) and is considered to be a significant factor in the development of neuropathic dysmotility.

Genetic Associations

Gastroparesis and CIPO are usually sporadic (Figure 4.13), but there are genetic forms (see Chapter 1, "Genetics and Molecular Aspects of Gastrointestinal Motility Disorders"), such as mitochondrial neurogastrointestinal encephalomyopathy. There are reports of homozygous CIPO (with the locus in region 8q23-q24) and 2 types of X-linked CIPO related to mutations of 2 genes mapping on chromosome Xq28: filamin A (*FLNA*) and L1 cell adhesion molecule (*L1CAM*). These present with a neuropathic disorder. Other cases of familial visceral neuropathy and myopathy also have been reported and contribute to the similarities and differences in CIPO between children and adults (Table 4.2) and to the clinical manifestations suggestive of CIPO (Box 4.2).

Figure 4.3   Vagal Dysfunction After Radiofrequency Ablation of Heart Conductivity for Atrial Fibrillation

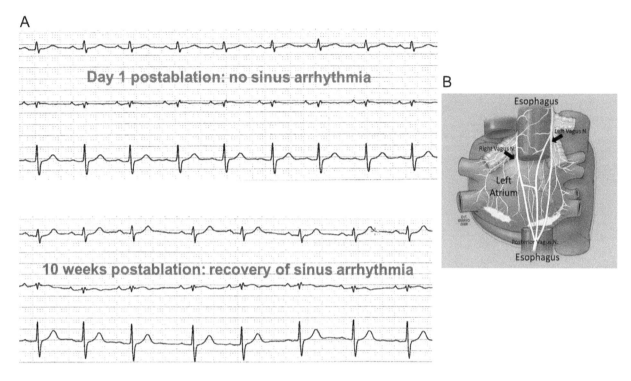

A, Day 1 postablation, there is no sinus arrhythmia, shown by the R-R interval varying by less than 120 ms (3 small squares); 10 weeks postablation, there is recovery of sinus arrhythmia, shown by the R-R interval varying by at least 120 ms. B, The vagal branches in front of the esophagus are close to the left atrium and may be temporarily or permanently damaged after radiofrequency ablation. N indicates nerve.

(Inset from Bunch TJ, Ellenbogen KA, Packer DL, Asirvatham SJ. Vagus nerve injury after posterior atrial radiofrequency ablation. Heart Rhythm. 2008 Sep;5(9):1327-30; used with permission of Mayo Foundation for Medical Education and Research.)

Figure 4.4   Cellular Changes in Idiopathic and Diabetic Gastroparesis

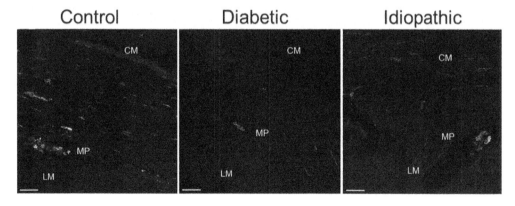

Representative images for neuronal nitric oxide synthase (nNOS). On light microscopy, there was no significant difference between diabetic and idiopathic gastroparesis, with the exception of nNOS expression, which was decreased in 40% of patients with idiopathic gastroparesis and in 20% of patients with diabetic gastroparesis, as assessed by visual grading of immunoreactivity. nNOS immunoreactivity is decreased in the circular muscle (CM), longitudinal muscle (LM), and myenteric plexus (MP). Scale bar: 100 µm.

(Modified from Grover M, Farrugia G, Lurken MS, Bernard CE, Faussone-Pellegrini MS, Smyrk TC, et al; NIDDK Gastroparesis Clinical Research Consortium. Cellular changes in diabetic and idiopathic gastroparesis. Gastroenterology. 2011 May;140(5):1575-85; used with permission.)

Figure 4.5   Smooth Muscle Cells (SMC), Interstitial Cells of Cajal (ICC), and Platelet-Derived Growth Factor Receptor α⁺ (PDGFRα⁺) Fibroblast-like Cells Are Structures of the Multicellular Electrical Syncytium

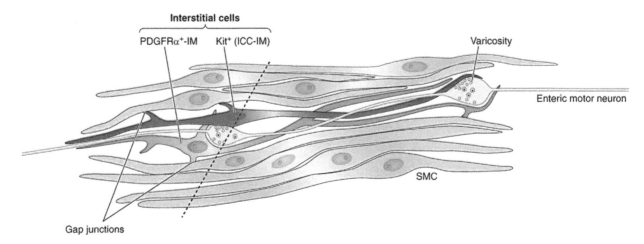

SMC, ICC, and PDGFRα⁺ cells are arranged around projections of excitatory and inhibitory enteric motor neurons. IM indicates intramuscular.

(Modified from Sanders KM, Hwang SJ, Ward SM. Neuroeffector apparatus in gastrointestinal smooth muscle organs. J Physiol. 2010 Dec 1;588[Pt 23]:4621-39; used with permission.)

Figure 4.6   Fewer Interstitial Cells of Cajal (ICCs) in the Circular Muscle Layer of Idiopathic (Id) and Diabetic (Db) Gastroparesis (Gp) Than in Controls and Diabetic Controls

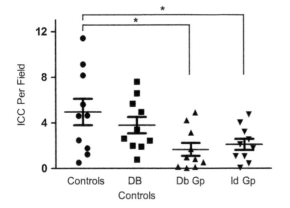

* indicates $P<.05$; DB, patients who had diabetes without gastroparesis.

(From Bernard CE, Gibbons SJ, Mann IS, Froschauer L, Parkman HP, Harbison S, et al; NIDDK Gastroparesis Clinical Research Consortium (GpCRC). Association of low numbers of CD206-positive cells with loss of ICC in the gastric body of patients with diabetic gastroparesis. Neurogastroenterol Motil. 2014 Sep;26(9):1275-84; used with permission.)

Epidemiology and Natural History of Gastroparesis

Prevalence

In view of the high prevalence and socioeconomic impact of upper GI symptoms in the United States, community studies show that the prevalence of those same symptoms is not higher in type 1 or 2 diabetes mellitus. Epidemiologic studies in Australia (Bytzer 2001; see suggested reading) documented that postprandial fullness and upper gut dysmotility symptoms of early satiety, postprandial fullness, bloating, nausea, or vomiting were more prevalent in 423 patients with diabetes mellitus than in 8,185 controls. In another Australian study, among 1,101 patients with diabetes mellitus (209 outpatients and 892 patients in the community), dyspeptic symptoms were significantly associated with the presence of neuropathy, poor glycemic control (self-reported), and female sex.

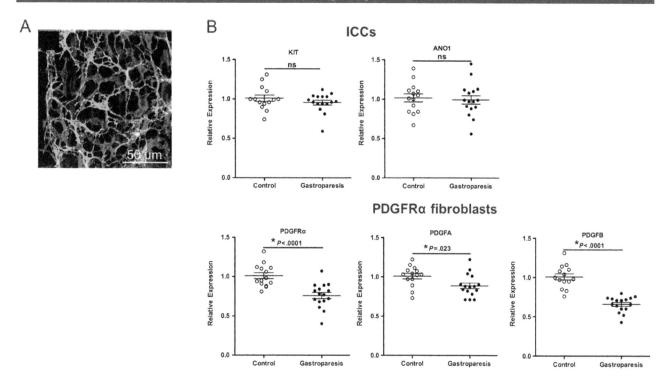

A, Intertwining of interstitial cells of Cajal (ICCs) (KIT and ANO1) and platelet-derived growth factor receptor α (PDGFRα)–positive fibroblast-like cells, which form part of the electrical syncytium of the stomach. B, Fewer PDGFRα fibroblast-like electrical cells in idiopathic gastroparesis and no differences in ICCs on basis of quantitative reverse transcriptase-polymerase chain reaction analysis of mRNA-encoding proteins characteristic of ICCs (KIT and ANO1) and PDGFRα+ fibroblasts. Levels of mRNA expression were normalized to expression of TATA binding protein (TBP) as an internal control and are shown in each plot as "relative expression." ns indicates not significant; PDGFA, platelet-derived growth factor subunit A; PDGFB, PDGF subunit B.

(A: from Sanders KM, Ward SM, Koh SD. Interstitial cells: regulators of smooth muscle function. Physiol Rev. 2014 Jul;94(3):859-907; used with permission. B: from Herring BP, Hoggatt AM, Gupta A, Griffith S, Nakeeb A, Choi JN, et al. Idiopathic gastroparesis is associated with specific transcriptional changes in the gastric muscularis externa. Neurogastroenterol Motil. 2018 Apr;30(4):e13230; used with permission.)

Table 4.1   Summary of Cellular Markers Reported in Diabetic and Idiopathic Gastroparesis and Controls

Cellular Marker	Study Group[a]			ANOVA or KW Test P Value
	DG (n=11)	IG (n=6)	Controls (n=5)	
c-kit (CM)	2.28±0.16	2.53±0.47	6.05±0.62	.004
PDGFRα staining FLC (CM)	11.03±0.96 (n=10)	11.72±0.96 (n=10)	10.75±0.87	>.05
CD45 (CM)	13.82±1.09	11.38±0.54	19.25±4.05	.07
CD45 (MP)	14.72±0.61	18.34±2.24	22.90±3.15	.09
CD206 (CM)	3.87±0.32	4.16±0.52	6.59±1.09	.04
CD206 (MP)	3.83±0.27	3.59±0.68	7.46±0.51	.004
nNOS neurons (MP)	1.85±0.12	2.00±0.34	2.07±0.30	.82
nNOS neurons (CM)	27.15±2.95	35.43±4.75	26.57±3.90	.27
Tyrosine hydroxylase (MP)	32.50±4.01	41.57±4.69	38.32±4.67	.30

Abbreviations: ANOVA, analysis of variance; c-kit, tyrosine kinase; CM, circular muscle; DG, diabetic gastroparesis; FLC, fibroblast-like cells; IG, idiopathic gastroparesis; KW, Kruskal-Wallis test; MP, myenteric plexus; nNOS, neuronal nitric oxide synthase; PDGFRα, platelet-derived growth factor receptor α.

[a] Values are mean per high-power field ± SEM; 1 hpf = 0.09 mm².

Modified from Grover M, Bernard CE, Pasricha PJ, Parkman HP, Gibbons SJ, Tonascia J, et al; NIDDK Gastroparesis Clinical Research Consortium (GpCRC). Diabetic and idiopathic gastroparesis is associated with loss of CD206-positive macrophages in the gastric antrum. Neurogastroenterol Motil. 2017 Jun;29(6):e13018; used with permission.

Figure 4.8   Vagal Function and Inflammation: Cholinergic Anti-inflammatory Effect on Immune Cells

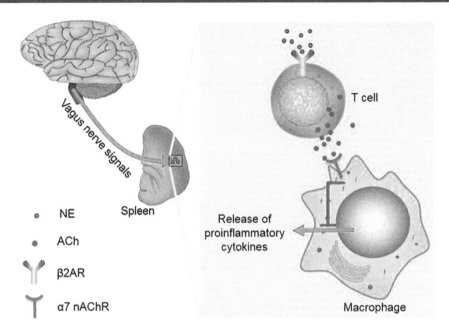

Efferent vagus nerve signals activate splenic nerves. Subsequently, norepinephrine (NE) released from splenic nerves combines with the β$_2$-adrenergic receptor (β2AR) expressed on T cells and activates acetylcholine (ACh)-synthesizing T cells. Then, T cell-derived ACh acts on the α7 nicotine acetylcholine receptor (α7 nAChR) on macrophages and other immune cells. Ultimately, the complete pathway suppresses the release of proinflammatory cytokines.

(From Han B, Li X, Hao J. The cholinergic anti-inflammatory pathway: an innovative treatment strategy for neurological diseases. Neurosci Biobehav Rev. 2017 Jun;77:358-68; used with permission.)

Incidence

In Olmsted County, Minnesota, the cumulative incidence of definite gastroparesis, determined from a combination of validated scintigraphic GE test and symptoms, was 4.8% in type 1 diabetes mellitus, 1% in type 2 diabetes mellitus, and 0.1% in controls. The crude incidence did not seem to increase from 1996 to 2000 and 2001 to 2006; diabetic gastroparesis persisted, however, despite improved glycemic control, over 12 and 25 years, and there is evidence that gastroparesis is associated with higher rates of death, emergency department visits, and hospitalizations. Diabetic gastroparesis may impair quality of life across all subscales of the 36-item Short-Form Health Survey, and this effect is independent of other factors such as age, tobacco or alcohol use, and type of diabetes mellitus.

Symptoms Associated With Gastroparesis

Clustered Symptoms, Including Nausea, Vomiting, and Postprandial Fullness

Gastroparesis typically causes a combination of symptoms. In a US national telephone interview, 483 patients with diabetes mellitus who had symptoms of gastroparesis reported clusters of symptoms, such as pain with early satiety and heartburn; heartburn with bloating, early satiety, nausea, and vomiting; and regurgitation with bloating, nausea, and vomiting. Among patients with gastroparesis, nausea, vomiting, and early satiety are more frequent with diabetic gastroparesis, and pain is more frequent with idiopathic gastroparesis.

Figure 4.9   Pathophysiology of Neuropathic and Myopathic Motility Disorders

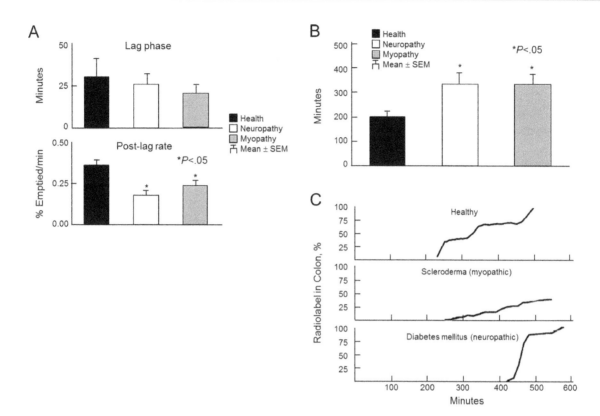

Gastric emptying profile cannot differentiate neuropathic from myopathic gastroparesis. In contrast, the size of bolus transfers from ileum to colon is greater in healthy people and people with neuropathic diseases than in those with myopathic diseases. A, Comparison of gastric emptying parameters (top, lag-phase duration; bottom, post-lag slope) in health and disease groups. Post-lag rate of emptying is reduced in both neuropathic and myopathic dysmotility groups. B, Comparison of small bowel transit time for solids (t10%). Time is delayed in both disease groups. C, Ileocolonic filling curves in health and small bowel disease. Bolus transfers and plateaus in health; onset of colonic filling is delayed in a patient with diabetes mellitus; and bolus plateau pattern of colonic filling is preserved, rate of emptying is slower, and transfers are smaller in a patient with scleroderma.

(From Greydanus MP, Camilleri M, Colemont LJ, Phillips SF, Brown ML, Thomforde GM. Ileocolonic transfer of solid chyme in small intestinal neuropathies and myopathies. Gastroenterology. 1990 Jul;99(1):158-64; used with permission.)

Pain

In a National Institutes of Health gastroparesis consortium study (Parkman 2011; see suggested reading) of 393 patients, the predominant symptoms were pain or discomfort in 21% and nausea or vomiting in 44%. Pain was rated moderate or severe in 66% of those with pain. Idiopathic gastroparesis (256 patients) was correlated with opioid and antiemetic use, depression and anxiety (with patients often receiving central neuromodulators), and poor quality of life.

A significant pain component was not associated with results of the GE test, diabetic neuropathy, or control of diabetes. An important aphorism is the following: If the patient has predominant pain, think again: it's not a motility disorder.

Early Satiety

A recent study (Parkman 2017; see suggested reading) by the National Institutes of Health gastroparesis consortium

Figure 4.10 Experimental Hyperglycemia and Effects on Gastric Functions

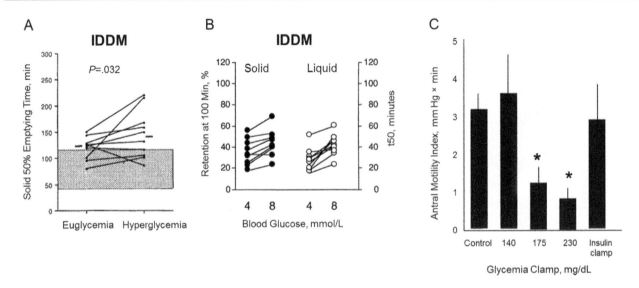

A, Individual values for solid gastric emptying expressed as 50% emptying time during euglycemia and hyperglycemia in patients with insulin-dependent diabetes mellitus (IDDM). The range for these values (mean [2SD]) obtained in 22 controls is shown in the shaded area. B, Individual values for retention at 100 minutes for solid and t50% for liquid meal components at 4 and 8 mmol/ L in patients with IDDM. C, Antral motility indices were calculated by measuring the areas under the pressure curves (that is, mm Hg × min). Hyperglycemic clamping to 140 mg/ dL did not inhibit postprandial antral motor activity. However, the threshold for motor inhibition was lower than for slow- wave disruption; decreases in antral motility index were significant at plasma glucose values of both 175 and 230 mg/ dL (denoted by * in the figure). Euglycemic, hyperinsulinemic clamping did not inhibit antral motor activity.

(Part A from Fraser RJ, Horowitz M, Maddox AF, Harding PE, Chatterton BE, Dent J. Hyperglycaemia slows gastric emptying in type 1 (insulin-dependent) diabetes mellitus. Diabetologia. 1990 Nov;33(11):675-80; used with permission. Part B from Schvarcz E, Palmer M, Aman J, Horowitz M, Stridsberg M, Berne C. Physiological hyperglycemia slows gastric emptying in normal subjects and patients with insulin-dependent diabetes mellitus. Gastroenterology. 1997 Jul;113(1):60-6; used with permission. Part C modified from Hasler WL, Soudah HC, Dulai G, Owyang C. Mediation of hyperglycemia-evoked gastric slow-wave dysrhythmias by endogenous prostaglandins. Gastroenterology. 1995 Mar;108(3):727-36; used with permission.)

Figure 4.11 Relationship Between Fasting Plasma Glucose Concentrations and Gastric Emptying (t$_{1/2}$)

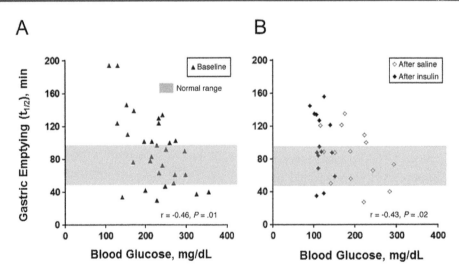

Fourteen patients had delayed (ie, t$_{1/2}$ >97 minutes) and 6 patients had rapid (ie, t$_{1/2}$ <50 minutes) gastric emptying at baseline. Gastric emptying (t$_{1/2}$) was correlated inversely with fasting plasma glucose concentrations during baseline (A, r = −0.46; P=.01) and after administration of insulin and saline (B, r = −0.43; P=.02).

(From Bharucha AE, Kudva Y, Basu A, Camilleri M, Low PA, Vella A, et al. Relationship between glycemic control and gastric emptying in poorly controlled type 2 diabetes. Clin Gastroenterol Hepatol. 2015 Mar;13(3):466-76; used with permission.)

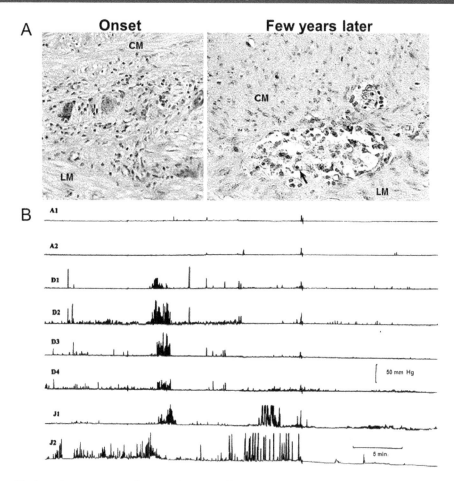

A, Photomicrographs of ileal specimens at onset of intestinal pseudo-obstruction (left) and a few years later (right). Both show inflammatory in-filtrate (hematoxylin-eosin, original magnifications ×200 in left and ×250 in right). CM indicates circular muscle; LM, longitudinal muscle; arrow, damage and loss of myenteric neurons. B, The manometric tracing is characterized by normal amplitude and propagated or nonpropagated bursts of phasic pressure activity in the small bowel. Recording ports: antrum (A1-A2), duodenum (D1-D4), proximal jejunum (J1-J2).

(From De Giorgio R, Barbara G, Stanghellini V, De Ponti F, Salvioli B, Tonini M, et al. Clinical and morphofunctional features of idiopathic myenteric ganglionitis underlying severe intestinal motor dysfunction: a study of three cases. Am J Gastroenterol. 2002 Sep;97(9):2454-9; used with permission.)

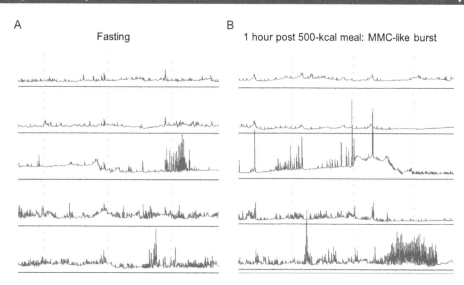

The incoordinated fasting (A) or nonpropagated postprandial phasic pressure (B) bursts are at a frequency typical of the migrating motor complex (MMC) (about 11 per minute) pressure activity.

Table 4.2   Summary of Similarities and Differences in CIPO Between Children and Adults

Factor	Children	Adults
Etiology	Mainly idiopathic	Half of cases are secondary to acquired diseases
Histopathology	Myopathies and neuropathies	Mainly neuropathies
Symptom onset	In utero, from birth or early infancy with 65%–80% of patients symptomatic by 12 mo of age	Median age at onset 17 y
Clinical features	Occlusive symptoms at birth and/or chronic symptoms without free intervals. Urologic involvement is commonly encountered ranging from 36% to 100% pediatric case series. High risk of colonic and small bowel volvulus secondary to severe gut dilatation, dysmotility, congenital bridles, or concurrent malrotation	Chronic abdominal pain and distention with superimposed acute episodes of pseudo-obstruction. Urinary bladder involvement not often reported
Natural history	Myopathic CIPO, urinary involvement, and concurrent intestinal malrotation are poor prognostic factors	The ability to restore oral feeding and the presence of symptoms <20 y of age are associated with a low mortality; systemic sclerosis and severe/diffuse esophageal and intestinal dysmotility are associated with a high mortality
Diagnostic approach	Specialized tests (eg, intestinal manometry) often difficult to perform; noninvasive, radiation-free imaging tests are warranted	Various methodologic approaches usually starting from endoscopy and radiologic tests up to more sophisticated functional exams
Nutritional therapy	To ensure normal growth, extensively hydrolyzed and elemental formulas are often empirically used to facilitate intestinal absorption	To improve nutritional status and prevent malnutrition
Pharmacologic therapy	Small number/sample size controlled trials	Small number/sample size controlled trials; few conclusions can be drawn for most drugs
Surgical therapy	Venting ostomies (although characterized by high complication rates) possibly helpful; surgery as a bridge to transplantation may be indicated in highly selected cases	Venting ostomies can be helpful; resective surgery may be indicated in accurately selected patients (with proven segmental gut dysfunction)

Abbreviation: CIPO, chronic intestinal pseudo-obstruction.

From Di Nardo G, Di Lorenzo C, Lauro A, Stanghellini V, Thapar N, Karunaratne TB, et al. Chronic intestinal pseudo-obstruction in children and adults: diagnosis and therapeutic options. Neurogastroenterol Motil. 2017 Jan;29(1): e12945; used with permission.

evaluated the symptom of early satiety in 198 patients with gastroparesis (134 idiopathic, 64 diabetic) who were receiving the following treatments: prokinetics, 35%; antiemetics, 80%; and narcotics, 35%. The study showed that, in both diabetic and idiopathic gastroparesis, early satiety and postprandial fullness are commonly severe and parallel the severity of other gastroparesis symptoms such as body weight loss, poor quality of life, delayed GE, and the volume of water that could be ingested in a water-loading test.

Functional Dyspepsia

Multiple underlying mechanisms contribute to the pathophysiology of functional dyspepsia, which manifests with diverse symptom patterns; impaired gastric accommodation to a meal, delayed GE, and hypersensitivity to gastric distention are the mechanisms classically implicated. Recent data suggest that inflammatory mechanisms in the upper small bowel also

Clinical Manifestations Suggestive of CIPO

Principal clinical and radiologic features

   Repeated, inconclusive abdominal surgery

   Recurrent episodes of abdominal pain, distention, and inability to defecate (with or without vomiting)

   Distended bowel loops and air-fluid levels in the upright position during acute episodes

   Lack of mechanical causes of gastrointestinal obstruction

Associated conditions or symptoms

   Esophageal motor disorders

   Gastroparesis

   Diarrhea/malabsorption (due to small bowel bacterial overgrowth)

   Urinary tract dysfunction (megacystis, megaureter) and related symptoms

   Underlying diseases associated with secondary CIPO

Other findings

   Family history of similar digestive disorders

   Weight loss despite dietary modifications or supplementation

   Need for parenteral nutrition

   Visible peristalsis

   Abnormal motor patterns at small bowel manometry

Abbreviation: CIPO, chronic intestinal pseudo-obstruction.

From De Giorgio R, Cogliandro RF, Barbara G, Corinaldesi R, Stanghellini V. Chronic intestinal pseudo-obstruction: clinical features, diagnosis, and therapy. Gastroenterol Clin North Am. 2011 Dec;40(4):787-807; used with permission.

redistribution to the distal stomach soon after ingestion, as well as faster GE. Hypersensitivity usually manifests as increased sensations of discomfort or fullness and bloating after a caloric meal ingestion or on distention of a balloon in the stomach. Such hypersensitivity is associated with higher intensity ratings of all epigastric symptoms, including pain, is a dominant feature in one-third of patients with dyspepsia, and is sometimes associated with evidence of increased activation on functional brain imaging studies or lack of antinociceptive responses to gastric signals. A correlate of these altered brain functions is the presence of comorbid anxiety, depression, and somatization among psychosocial disorders. Delayed GE occurs in up to one-third of patients with functional dyspepsia and is typically associated with postprandial fullness or bloating, nausea, and vomiting.

In the recent literature, impaired duodenal mucosal integrity, with low-grade mucosal inflammation characterized by eosinophils and mast cells, has been reported in functional dyspepsia (Figure 4.14), in addition to the classic mechanisms of delayed gastric emptying, impaired gastric accommodation (Figure 4.15), and hypersensitivity, in part related to cerebral dysfunction (Figures 4.16 and 4.17).

Further research is exploring how these barrier and inflammatory responses actually result in the symptoms, whether they are primary or secondary to the impaired functions (such as delayed GE), and whether there might conceivably be an association with changes in upper GI microbiota.

There is increased recognition that the symptoms of gastroparesis and functional dyspepsia may result not only from delayed GE but also from several sensory or other motor disorders of the upper gut, including impaired gastric accommodation.

In 1,287 patients presenting to Mayo Clinic (Park 2017; see suggested reading) with upper GI symptoms,

contribute to or are associated with development of symptoms of functional dyspepsia.

Up to 50% of patients with functional dyspepsia have reduced gastric accommodation to a meal, and this is associated with early satiation and weight loss. The impaired accommodation may cause meal

Figure 4.14   Pathophysiologic Mechanisms in Dyspepsia

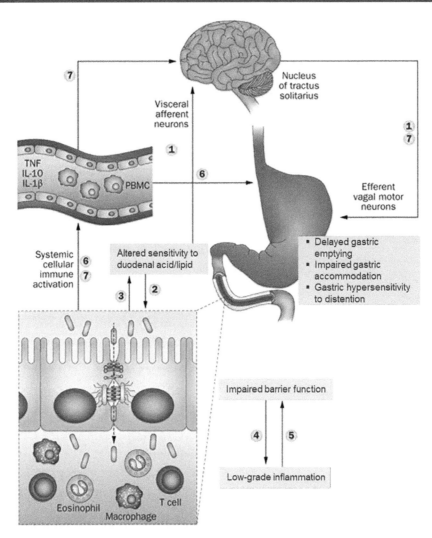

Schematic representation of the potential pathophysiologic mechanisms (numbered 1 to 7) of functional dyspepsia, including impaired gastric functions, duodenal hypersensitivity, impaired barrier function, mucosal immune responses, and inflammation. IL-10 indicates interleukin 10; IL-1β, interleukin 1β; PBMC, peripheral blood mononuclear cell; TNF, tumor necrosis factor.

(From Vanheel H, Farré R. Changes in gastrointestinal tract function and structure in functional dyspepsia. Nat Rev Gastroenterol Hepatol. 2013 Mar;10(3):142-9; used with permission.)

there were almost equal proportions with delayed GE, impaired gastric accommodation, a combination of both, or absence of both (Figure 4.18). The patients who had neither delayed GE nor impaired gastric accommodation had gastric hypersensitivity. Therefore, symptoms such as early satiety and postprandial fullness may result from impaired gastric accommodation, in addition to delayed GE. Also, among a subgroup of 108 patients with diabetes mellitus (77 [71%] type 2 and 31 [29%] type 1) in the

same cohort, nausea was the most common symptom (80.6%). There were single or combined abnormalities of gastric emptying in 56% (rapid in 37%, slow in 19%) and of gastric accommodation in 39%; gastric accommodation and emptying were normal in 28%. Of the patients with type 2 diabetes (Chedid 2019; see suggested reading), 40.3% had accelerated GE at 1 hour, which was associated with nausea or vomiting. Alternatively, fasting gastric volume was associated with bloating. These data illustrate the principle that

Figure 4.15   Gastric Accommodation in Functional Dyspepsia

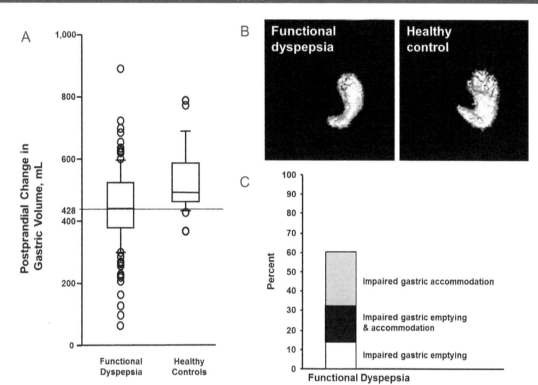

Among patients with functional dyspepsia, 40% have accommodation volumes less than 428 mL (the 5th percentile for healthy controls, panels A-C), and about 33% have impaired gastric emptying (accelerated or delayed, panel C). Some patients have both abnormal gastric emptying and gastric accommodation (panel C). Panel B shows reconstructions of stomach based on single-photon emission computed tomography after intravenous injection of technetium Tc 99m pertechnetate.

(Modified from Bredenoord AJ, Chial HJ, Camilleri M, Mullan BP, Murray JA. Gastric accommodation and emptying in evaluation of patients with upper gastrointestinal symptoms. Clin Gastroenterol Hepatol. 2003 Jul;1(4):264-72; used with permission; and B: From Camilleri M. Functional dyspepsia: mechanisms of symptom generation and appropriate management of patients. Gastroenterol Clin North Am. 2007 Sep;36(3):649-64; used with permission.)

the same upper GI symptoms may result from either accelerated or delayed GE or reduced gastric accommodation; therefore, getting the right diagnosis for the patient's symptoms based on valid physiologic or function measurements is an essential first step.

Diagnostic Tests

GE is best assessed with scintigraphy or stable isotope breath test, which are well validated and for which normal control data are available (Figure 4.19 and see Figure 2.9). GE must be assessed with optimal methods: at least 3 hours' duration, valid data analysis, use of a substrate such as fat-containing egg meal or nutrient liquid meal that can stress gastric motor function, and normal control data for comparison. With such optimal tests, the correlation between retardation of GE and symptoms is significant (Figure 4.20).

The diagnosis of impaired gastric accommodation is established with valid methods (single-photon emission computed tomography and magnetic resonance imaging), if available, or with screening tests, such as determining the size of the proximal stomach on gastric scintiscanning done immediately after radiolabeled-meal ingestion or by means of a water-loading or nutrient drink test. The nutrient drink test is reviewed in detail in Chapter 2 ("Measurement of Gastrointestinal and Colonic Motility in Clinical Practice").

The nutrient drink test could also serve as a surrogate test for gastric accommodation and sensation if the maximum tolerated volume of a nutrient drink is less than 750 mL (see Figure 2.3).

Figure 4.16   Cerebral Regions Activated During Gastric Distention

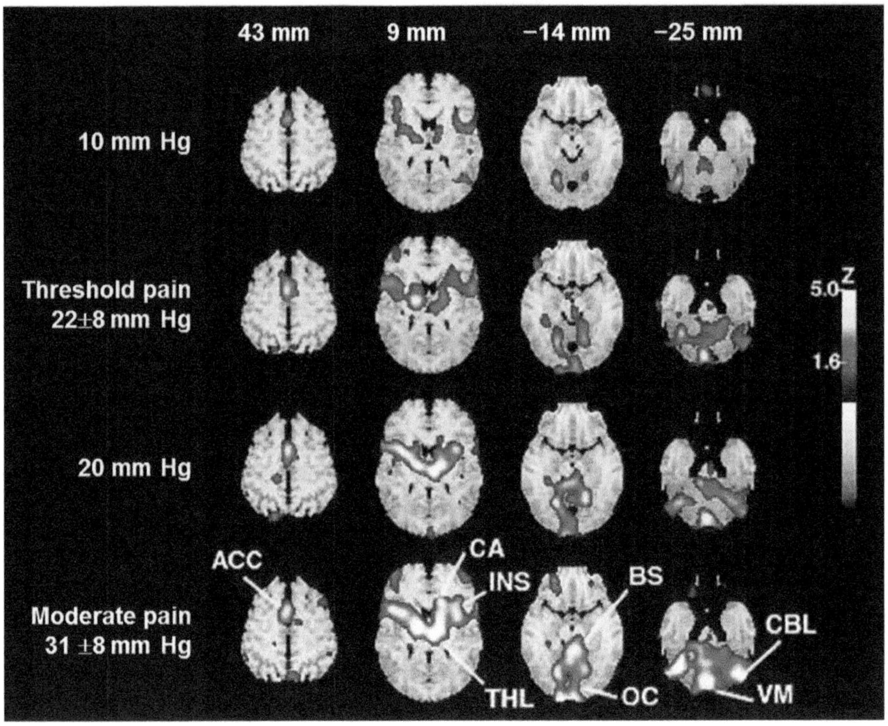

Color-coded statistical surface maps of cerebral regions activated during gastric distention under 4 pressure conditions. Maps are superimposed on a reference normal brain magnetic resonance image transformed onto the stereotactic coordinates used in this study. Z scores of 4.0 or more are considered significant. Transverse brain slices at indicated levels above (positive distances) or below (negative distances) the reference plane from the anterior to the posterior commissure. ACC indicates anterior cingulate cortex; BS, brainstem; CA, caudate nucleus; CBL, cerebellum; INS, insula; OC, occipital cortex (including fusiform and lingual gyri and cuneus); THL, thalamus; VM, cerebellar vermis.

(From Ladabaum U, Minoshima S, Hasler WL, Cross D, Chey WD, Owyang C. Gastric distention correlates with activation of multiple cortical and subcortical regions. Gastroenterology. 2001 Feb;120(2):369-76; used with permission.)

Differential Diagnosis

The main conditions that differentiate gastric neuromuscular dysfunctions are obstruction, rumination syndrome, cannabinoid hyperemesis, and cyclic vomiting syndrome. The common and uncommon causes of nausea and vomiting, the clinical features on history and examination, and pertinent blood and other investigations are discussed in detail in Chapter 2 ("Measurement of Gastrointestinal and Colonic Motility in Clinical Practice"). There is overlap between gastroparesis and functional dyspepsia with delayed GE. Indeed, symptoms with only minor delay in GE are sometimes classified as functional dyspepsia. But, in many respects, management of these conditions does not differ and, therefore, it seems more appropriate to document such symptoms as gastroparesis and declare the degree of GE delay.

Management of Gastroparesis and Pseudo-obstruction

When gastroparesis or pseudo-obstruction is suspected, it is essential to exclude mechanical obstruction, which is increasingly achieved with noninvasive imaging such as computed tomography (Figure 4.21) or enterography.

Figure 4.17   Brain Activation in Functional Dyspepsia (FD)

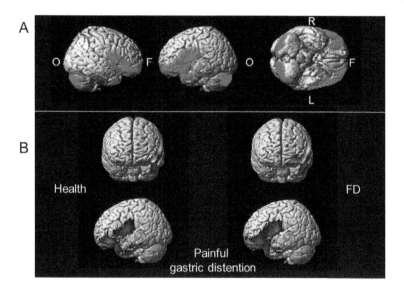

A, Proximal stomach distention in FD activates components of the lateral pain system and bilateral frontal inferior gyri, putatively involved in regulation of hunger and satiety. In hypersensitive FD, these activations occur at significantly lower distention pressures. B, Overview of cluster of gyri activated during painful gastric distention in 11 healthy volunteers (left) and 13 patients with FD (right). F indicates frontal; L, left; O, occipital; R, right.

(Part A from Vandenberghe J, Dupont P, Van Oudenhove L, Bormans G, Demyttenaere K, Fischler B, et al. Regional cerebral blood flow during gastric balloon distention in functional dyspepsia. Gastroenterology. 2007 May;132(5):1684-93; used with permission. Part B from Van Oudenhove L, Dupont P, Vandenberghe J, Geeraerts B, van Laere K, Bormans G, et al. The role of somatosensory cortical regions in the processing of painful gastric fundic distension: an update of brain imaging findings. Neurogastroenterol Motil. 2008 May;20(5):479-87; used with permission.)

Figure 4.18   Gastric Motor Dysfunction in 1,287 Patients With Functional Gastroduodenal Symptoms

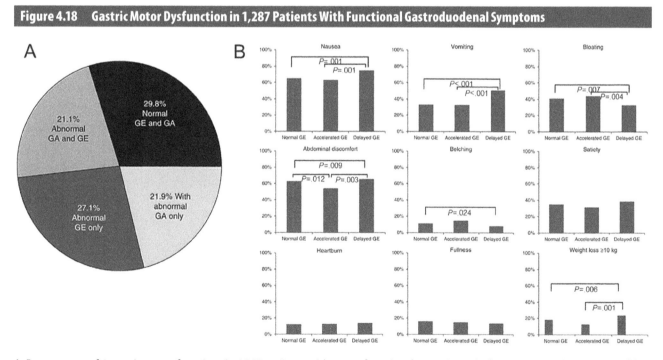

A, Percentages of 4 gastric motor functions in 1,287 patients with upper functional gastrointestinal symptoms. B, Association of dyspeptic symptoms and gastric emptying (GE). Patients with delayed GE had more frequent nausea, vomiting, and weight loss more than 10 kg than those with accelerated or normal GE (all P<.05). Patients with delayed GE had less frequent bloating than those with normal or accelerated GE (all P<.05). GA indicates gastric accommodation.

(From Park SY, Acosta A, Camilleri M, Burton D, Harmsen WS, Fox J, et al. Gastric motor dysfunction in patients with functional gastroduodenal symptoms. Am J Gastroenterol. 2017 Nov;112(11):1689-99; used with permission.)

Figure 4.19   Gastric Emptying of a Solid Meal (320 kcal, 30% Fat) Measured With Scintigraphy Over 4 Hours

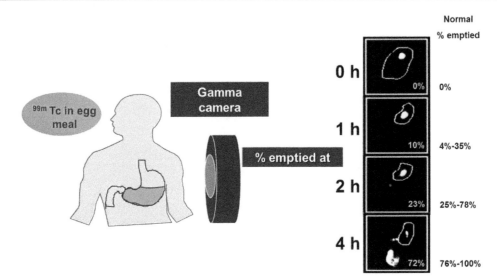

This test is cost effective for clinical practice and research, is simple and inexpensive, and can be standardized. It allows for selection of logical treatment in patients with symptoms, which are not sufficiently predictive of gastric emptying disorder. 99m Tc indicates technetium Tc 99m.

The principles of management are summarized in Box 4.3 and Figure 4.22.

Treatment is guided by the percentage of gastric retention at 4 hours and the combination of diet, nutritional support, prokinetics, antiemetics, symptom modulators, and nonpharmacologic measures. This section focuses on diet, new medical treatments relevant for gastroparesis and related disorders, off-label treatments that are used to target the underlying mechanisms, and treatments targeting the pylorus.

Diet

The 2 fundamental principles in dietary management, both based on published evidence (Homko 2015; Olausson 2014; see suggested reading), are first, a high-fat, solid meal increases overall symptoms among patients with gastroparesis and, second, a small-particle–size diet (Figure 4.23) reduces upper GI symptoms (nausea, vomiting, bloating, postprandial fullness, regurgitation, and heartburn) in patients with diabetic gastroparesis (compared with a standard meal in a controlled clinical trial).

Nutritional Support in Gastroparesis and CIPO

First-line treatment includes simpler approaches to ensure hydration and nutrition, oral nutrition, blenderized diet, or oral supplements. In patients with gastroparesis, tube feedings should be postpyloric, preferably by jejunal tube directly placed rather than by jejunal extension of a tube placed through gastrostomy. If patients cannot increase their calorie and protein intake to sustain nutritional requirements, they usually have a significant small bowel motility disorder and require parenteral nutrition or become candidates for small bowel transplant to obviate the effects of chronic intestinal dysmotility.

Standard Prokinetic Agents and Antiemetics for Gastroparesis

The algorithm for management of gastroparesis focuses on the severity of the GE delay and the degree to which nutrition is compromised. These issues are discussed in detail below. The only approved

A. Nausea

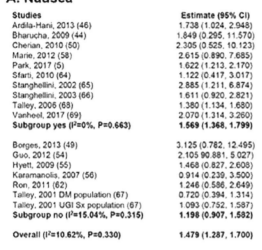
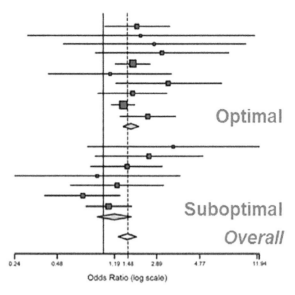

Studies	Estimate (95% CI)
Ardila-Hani, 2013 (46)	1.738 (1.024, 2.948)
Bharucha, 2009 (44)	1.849 (0.295, 11.570)
Cherian, 2010 (50)	2.305 (0.525, 10.123)
Marie, 2012 (58)	2.615 (0.890, 7.685)
Park, 2017 (5)	1.622 (1.213, 2.170)
Sfarti, 2010 (64)	1.122 (0.417, 3.017)
Stanghellini, 2002 (65)	2.885 (1.211, 6.874)
Stanghellini, 2003 (66)	1.611 (0.920, 2.821)
Talley, 2006 (68)	1.380 (1.134, 1.680)
Vanheel, 2017 (69)	2.070 (1.314, 3.260)
Subgroup yes (I²=0%, P=0.663)	**1.569 (1.368, 1.799)**
Borges, 2013 (49)	3.125 (0.782, 12.495)
Guo, 2012 (54)	2.105 90.881, 5.027)
Hyett, 2009 (55)	1.468 (0.827, 2.608)
Karamanolis, 2007 (56)	0.914 (0.239, 3.500)
Ron, 2011 (62)	1.246 (0.586, 2.649)
Talley, 2001 DM population (67)	0.720 (0.394, 1.314)
Talley, 2001 UGI Sx population (67)	1.093 (0.752, 1.587)
Subgroup no (I²=15.04%, P=0.315)	**1.198 (0.907, 1.582)**
Overall (I²=10.62%, P=0.330)	**1.479 (1.287, 1.700)**

Odds Ratio (log scale)

B. Vomiting

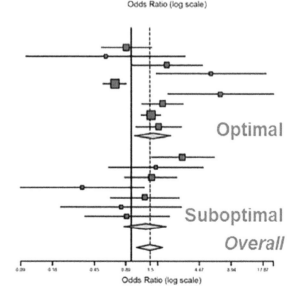

Studies	Estimate (95% CI)	Ev/Trt	Ev/Ctrl
Ardila-Hani, 2013 (46)	2.048 (1.275, 3.290)	72/127	62/159
Bharucha, 2009 (44)	1.714 (0.741, 3.964)	18/46	15/55
Marie, 2012 (58)	36.600 (2.019, 663.367)	10/27	0/30
Park, 2017 (5)	2.308 (1.773, 3.005)	186/357	213/665
Sfarti, 2010 (64)	1.773 (0.403, 7.797)	4/26	4/43
Stanghellini, 2002 (65)	0.900 (0.178, 4.548)	2/35	7/111
Stanghellini, 2003 (66)	1.341 (0.640, 2.809)	13/109	20/218
Subgroup yes (I²=14.05%, P=0.323)	**2.031 (1.555, 2.653)**	**305/727**	**321/1,281**
Boltin, 2014 (48)	1.326 (0.737, 2.383)	37/92	34/101
Guo, 2012 (54)	1.765 (0.607, 5.127)	10/44	7/49
Hyett, 2009 (55)	1.385 (0.760, 2.522)	37/94	30/94
Karamanolis, 2007 (56)	1.133 (0.317, 4.047)	5/13	16/45
Ron, 2011 (62)	2.167 (0.886, 5.299)	21/63	9/48
Talley, 2001 DM population (67)	0.570 (0.352, 0.923)	71/246	42/101
Talley, 2001 UGI Sx population (67)	1.198 (0.828, 1.735)	121/347	63/204
Subgroup no (I²=46.67%, P=0.081)	**1.173 (0.837, 1.642)**	**302/899**	**201/642**
Overall (I²=62.77%, P=0.001)	**1.479 (1.099, 1.990)**	**607/1,626**	**522/1,923**

Odds Ratio (log scale)

C. Bloating

Studies	Estimate (95% CI)
Ardila-Hani, 2013 (46)	0.906 (0.523, 1.570)
Bharucha, 2009 (44)	0.580 (0.101, 3.317)
Cuomo, 2001 (51)	2.200 (1.00, 4.840)
Marie, 2012 (58)	5.754 (1.716, 19.298)
Park, 2017 (5)	0.707 (0.539, 0.928)
Sfarti, 2010 (64)	7.087 (2.233, 22.492)
Stanghellini, 2002 (66)	1.987 (1.244, 3.174)
Talley, 2006 (68)	1.530 (1.219, 1.920)
Vanheel, 2017 (69)	1.830 (1.094, 3.060)
Subgroup yes (I²=82.01%, P=0.000)	**1.644 (1.086, 2.488)**
Boltin, 2014 (48)	3.096 (1.562, 6.137)
Guo, 2012 (54)	1.714 (0.607, 4.838)
Hyett, 2009 (55)	1.553 (0.866, 2.785)
Karamanolis, 2007 (56)	0.346 (0.089, 1.339)
Ron, 2011 (62)	1.353 (0.628, 2.913)
Talley, 2001 DM population (67)	0.806 (0.214, 3.041)
Talley, 2001 UGI Sx population (67)	0.913 (0.358, 2.327)
Subgroup no (I²=44.88%, P=0.092)	**1.357 (0.865, 2.129)**
Overall (I²=73.18%, P=0.000)	**1.504 (1.108, 2.041)**

Odds Ratio (log scale)

Relationships between gastric emptying and symptoms such as nausea, vomiting, and bloating are shown. Subgroup no indicates suboptimal method; subgroup yes, optimal method; Ctrl, control; Ev, event; Trt, treatment.

(Modified from Vijayvargiya P, Jameie-Oskooei S, Camilleri M, Chedid V, Erwin PJ, Murad MH. Association between delayed gastric emptying and upper gastrointestinal symptoms: a systematic review and meta-analysis. Gut. 2019 May;68(5):804-13; used with permission. Full reference citations for studies listed in this figure can be found in the original source.)

Figure 4.21   Staple Line Obstruction

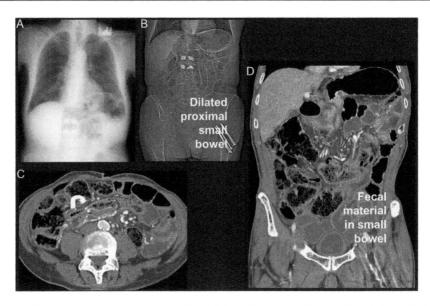

A, Chest radiograph shows dilated intestine and elevation of the left hemidiaphragm. B, Scot film of abdominal computed tomogram (CT) shows dilated small bowel loops and metal screws stabilizing a previous fracture of the neck of the left femur. C, CT transaxial image shows dilated proximal small bowel suggestive of intestinal pseudo-obstruction that is caused by staple line obstruction (white arrow) from prior surgery. D, CT coronal image confirms small bowel obstruction, which is also suggested by the presence of fecal material in the small bowel.

prokinetic for gastroparesis is metoclopramide, and the total daily dosage should not exceed 40 mg/day. Use of liquid formulation may be advantageous in

Box 4.3

Management of Gastroparesis and Psuedo-obstruction: What Treatments Work?

Restore hydration, nutrition: enteral preferable

Correct electrolyte, glycemic control

Antiemetics with caution (P450 metabolism)

Prokinetics: serotonin type 4 agonists, motilin or ghrelin agonists?

Pain relief without narcotics

Surgery and venting gastrostomy; botulinum toxin type A injections

Gastric electrical stimulation

Pyloric interventions

patients with gastroparesis to enhance pharmacokinetics. Medication is administered 15 to 30 minutes before meal ingestion and at bedtime, starting with 5-mg doses, increasing to 10-mg doses. Metoclopramide may cause involuntary movements that are totally reversible within 24 to 48 hours of cessation of medication use. Prescription databases in the United Kingdom and Sweden show that the incidence of tardive dyskinesia (irreversible involuntary movements) is probably less than 1 in 1,000. The US Food and Drug Administration's estimate of the incidence of tardive dyskinesia is 3% and is based on a neurology clinic cohort (Ganzini 1993; see suggested reading) (specializing in tremors) in the Veterans Health Administration in which the patients who were receiving metoclopramide were also receiving other medications (including central neuromodulators and analgesics) when they experienced the involuntary movements. The reports are unclear about whether the involuntary movements fulfilled criteria for irreversible tardive dyskinesia.

Motilides, such as erythromycin and azithromycin, are useful in the short term, but they are compromised

Figure 4.22　Summary of Treatment Strategy for Patients With Gastroparesis

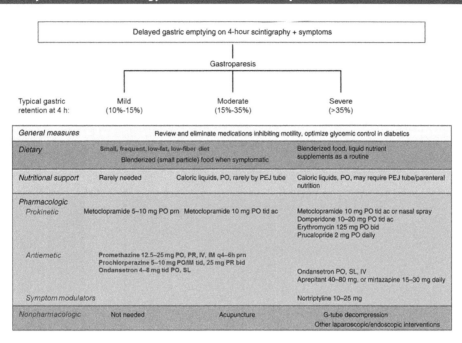

ac indicates before meals; bid, twice a day; IM, intramuscularly; IV, intravenously; PEJ, percutaneous endoscopic jejunostomy; PO, orally; PR, rectally; prn, as needed; SL, sublingually; tid, 3 times a day.

(From Lacy BE, Parkman HP, Camilleri M. Chronic nausea and vomiting: evaluation and treatment. Am J Gastroenterol. 2018 May;113(5):647-59; used with permission.)

by tachyphylaxis due to down-regulation of the motilin receptors.

New Prokinetic Drugs for Gastroparesis

Relamorelin

Relamorelin is a pentapeptide ghrelin receptor agonist that stimulates antral contractions, accelerates GE, and does not interfere with gastric accommodation. Relamorelin increased GE of solids and reduced symptoms in patients with diabetic gastroparesis, particularly nausea, fullness, bloating, and pain in mechanistic and phase 2A and 2B trials (Figures 4.24 through 4.26). Relamorelin is currently being tested in phase 3 trials, which are anticipated to clarify the optimal dose of this subcutaneous treatment.

Prucalopride

Prucalopride (1-2 mg/day), a serotonin type 4 receptor agonist, is approved for the treatment of chronic

constipation. It accelerates GE, and it was shown to also relieve symptoms in a preliminary report of 28 patients with idiopathic gastroparesis (Figure 4.27).

New Drug for Impaired Gastric Accommodation: Acotiamide

Acotiamide has fundus-relaxing and gastroprokinetic properties based on antagonism of the inhibitory muscarinic type 1 and type 2 autoreceptors on cholinergic nerve endings. It also inhibits acetylcholinesterase, enhancing gastric accommodation and emptying, and it relieves dyspeptic symptoms (Figure 4.28). It is approved in Japan for treatment of dyspepsia.

Approved Drugs for Off-Label Use

Tricyclic Antidepressants

Although nortriptyline (a tricyclic antidepressant) was not proved efficacious in a randomized

Figure 4.23   Effect of Diet in Gastroparesis

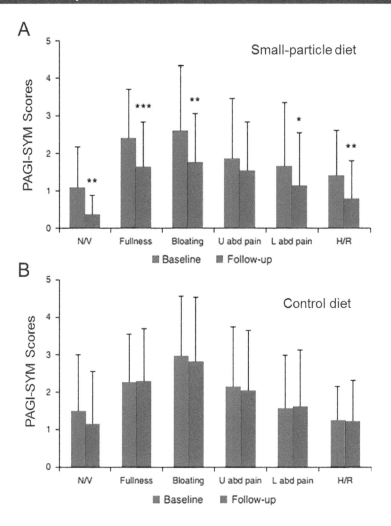

High-fat solid meals are known to increase overall symptoms in patients with gastroparesis. Additionally, a study of gastrointestinal symptom severity, as measured with the Patient Assessment of Gastrointestinal Disorders Symptom Severity Index (PAGI-SYM) at baseline and after the dietary treatment period (20 weeks) in patients who received advice to eat the intervention diet (small particle size) (A) and patients who were instructed to follow a control diet (B), found significantly greater symptom improvement in the intervention diet group than in the control group for the primary outcome variables. H/R indicates heartburn/regurgitation; L, left abdominal; N/V, nausea/vomiting; U abd, upper abdominal; * *P*<.05, ** *P*<.01, *** *P*<.001, significant differences from baseline, within-group comparisons.

(From Olausson EA, Storsrud S, Grundin H, Isaksson M, Attvall S, Simren M. A small particle size diet reduces upper gastrointestinal symptoms in patients with diabetic gastroparesis: a randomized controlled trial. Am J Gastroenterol. 2014 Mar;109(3):375-85; used with permission.)

controlled trial in patients with gastroparesis, it is sometimes used as a central neuromodulator for relief of pain. This approach appears preferable to the alternative, which is the use of opioids. It is important to recall that, at effective analgesic doses, tramadol (pure μ-opioid agonist) and tapentadol (a combined μ-opioid agonist and norepinephrine reuptake inhibitor) retard GE. In the case of tapentadol, the retardation is equivalent to that of oxycodone. In a study conducted in patients with functional dyspepsia (Talley 2015; see suggested reading), amitriptyline improved symptoms in patients who did not have delayed GE (Figure 4.29), and it modestly improved sleep quality. The typical dosages for both

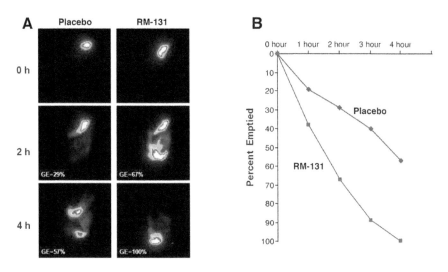

Data show median (IQR)	Placebo	RM-131	P	% Δ
Total GCSI-DD average score	0.79 (0.75, 2.08)	0.17 (0.00, 0.67)	.041	−125.0
Average score of nausea, bloating, pp fullness, upper abdominal pain	1.00 (0.50, 2.00)	0.25 (0.00, 0.50)	.041	−141.8

A, Assessment of GE of solids with scintigraphy in 1 patient. GE is delayed with placebo and normal with RM-131. B, GE is shown as the percentage emptied over time for placebo and RM-131 in the same patient. GCSI-DD indicates Gastroparesis Cardinal Symptom Index-Daily Diary; IQR, interquartile range; pp, postprandial.

(From Shin A, Camilleri M, Busciglio I, Burton D, Smith SA, Vella A, et al. The ghrelin agonist RM-131 accelerates gastric emptying of solids and reduces symptoms in patients with type 1 diabetes mellitus. Clin Gastroenterol Hepatol. 2013 Nov;11(11):1453-9; used with permission.)

Figure 4.25   Effect of Relamorelin on Antral Motility

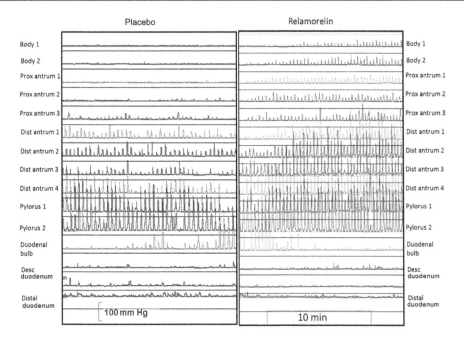

Gastroduodenal manometric tracings for healthy volunteers who were randomized to receive relamorelin or placebo; tracings are for the postprandial period from the gastric body to the duodenum. For the relamorelin group, antral contraction amplitude is normal, frequency is markedly increased, and anatomical extent where the contractions are recorded in the stomach (relative to the pylorus) is greater. Desc indicates descending; Dist, distal; prox, proximal.

(From Nelson AD, Camilleri M, Acosta A, Busciglio I, Linker Nord S, Boldingh A, et al. Effects of ghrelin receptor agonist, relamorelin, on gastric motor functions and satiation in healthy volunteers. Neurogastroenterol Motil. 2016 Nov;28(11):1705-13; used with permission.)

Figure 4.26   Effect of Relamorelin on Upper Gastrointestinal Symptoms in Patients With Diabetic Gastroparesis in a Phase 2B Placebo-Controlled Trial

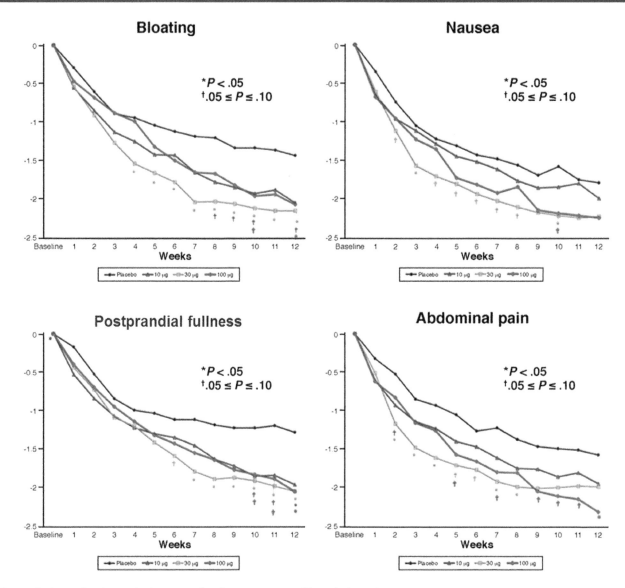

The y axis shows the change in the score of each symptom over 12 weeks in each treatment group.

(From Camilleri M, McCallum RW, Tack J, Spence SC, Gottesdiener K, Fiedorek FT. Efficacy and safety of relamorelin in diabetics with symptoms of gastroparesis: a randomized, placebo-controlled study. Gastroenterology. 2017 Nov;153(5):1240-50; used with permisison.)

amitriptyline and nortripyline are 25 mg/day. At higher dosages, the anticholinergic effects of these tricyclic agents could further inhibit GE.

Mirtazapine

Mirtazapine (15 mg/day), because of its central adrenergic and serotonergic activity, provides relief for patients with functional dyspepsia and weight loss, which may overlap with gastroparesis (Figure 4.30).

An open-label study with mirtazapine, 15 mg orally at bedtime, improved nausea, vomiting, retching, and anorexia in patients with gastroparesis.

Buspirone

Buspirone (7.5-15 mg daily or twice daily), a serotonin type 1A agonist, enhances gastric accommodation and reduces postprandial symptoms in patients with functional dyspepsia (Figure 4.31).

Figure 4.27   Effect of Prucalopride on Gastric Emptying (GE) (A) and Symptoms (B)

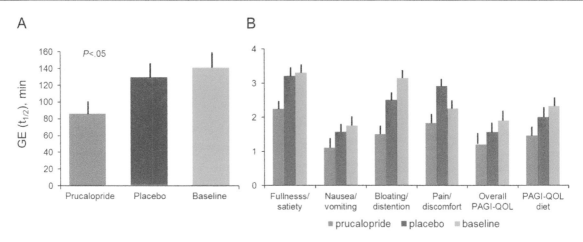

Twenty-eight patients with idiopathic gastroparesis underwent a $_{13}$C-octanoic acid solid GE breath test and symptom severity assessment with Gastroparesis Cardinal Symptom Index at run-in and at the end of 4 weeks. Prucalopride treatment significantly enhanced GE (A) and improved symptoms (based on severity grade 0-4 scale, as shown in B) and quality of life compared with placebo. PAGI-QOL indicates Patient Assessment of Upper Gastrointestinal Disorders-Quality of Life.

(Data plotted from Carbone F, Rotondo A, Andrews CN, Holvoet L, Van Oudenhove L, Vanuytsel T, et al. A controlled cross-over trial shows benefit of prucalopride for symptom control and gastric emptying enhancement in idiopathic gastroparesis. Gastroenterology. 2016;150(4):S213-4.)

Figure 4.28   Change in Postprandial Distress Syndrome Symptom Score From Baseline With Acotiamide

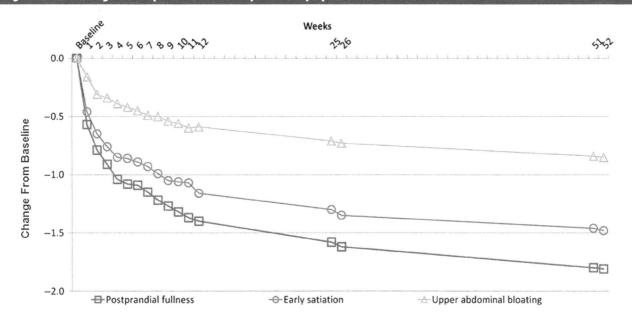

(From Tack J, Pokrotnieks J, Urbonas G, Banciu C, Yakusevich V, Bunganic I, et al. Long-term safety and efficacy of acotiamide in functional dyspepsia (postprandial distress syndrome)-results from the European phase 3 open-label safety trial. Neurogastroenterol Motil. 2018 Jun;30(6):e13284; open access article distributed under the Creative Commons Attribution Non-Commercial No Derivatives License [https://creativecommons.org/licenses/by-nc-nd/4.0/].)

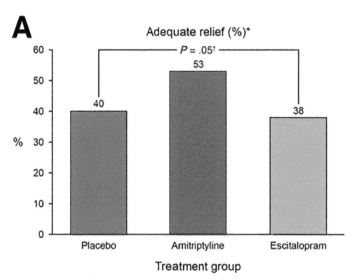

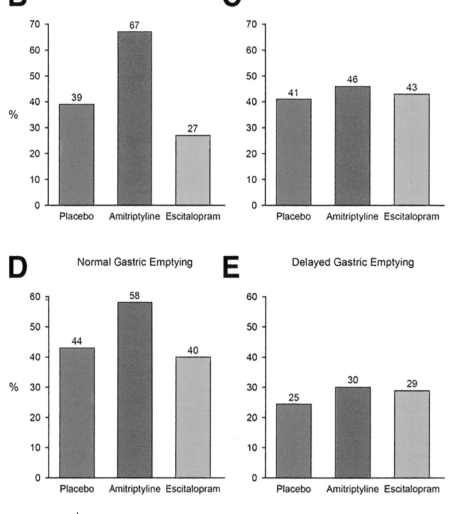

Primary end point was adequate relief. Response to amitriptyline was greatest in patients with ulcer-like FD and those with normal gastric emptying at baseline, whereas escitalopram was ineffective in all groups.

(From Talley NJ, Locke GR, Saito YA, Almazar AE, Bouras EP, Howden CW, et al. Effect of amitriptyline and escitalopram on functional dyspepsia: a multicenter, randomized controlled study. Gastroenterology. 2015 Aug;149(2):340-9; used with permission.)

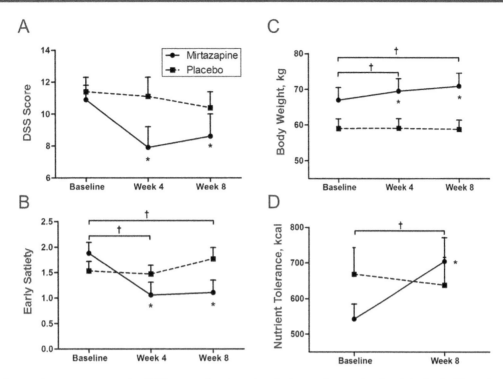

A, Change in dyspepsia symptom severity (DSS) score after 8 weeks of mirtazapine or placebo. B, Individual line plots of changes in severity ratings of early satiety. C, Change in body weight after 4 and 8 weeks of treatment with placebo or mirtazapine. D, Change in meal volume tolerance during nutrient challenge test after 8 weeks of treatment with placebo or mirtazapine. *P<.05 compared with baseline within the mirtazapine arm. †P<.05 change from baseline between treatments.

(From Tack J, Ly HG, Carbone F, Vanheel H, Vanuytsel T, Holvoet L, et al. Efficacy of mirtazapine in patients with functional dyspepsia and weight loss. Clin Gastroenterol Hepatol. 2016 Mar;14(3):385-92; used with permission.)

Figure 4.31   Effect of Buspirone in Functional Dyspepsia

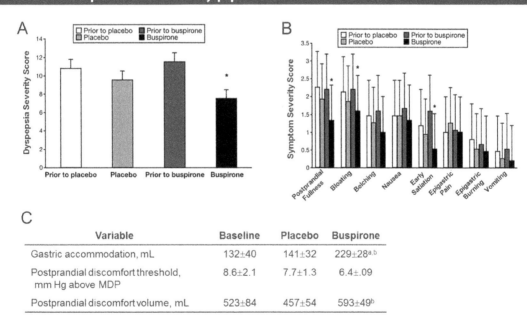

Variable	Baseline	Placebo	Buspirone
Gastric accommodation, mL	132±40	141±32	229±28[a,b]
Postprandial discomfort threshold, mm Hg above MDP	8.6±2.1	7.7±1.3	6.4±.09
Postprandial discomfort volume, mL	523±84	457±54	593±49[b]

A, Influence of buspirone and placebo on dyspepsia severity score. B, Influence of buspirone and placebo on severity scores of individual dyspeptic symptoms. * (for both A and B) P<.05 compared with baseline. C, Influence of placebo and buspirone on different parameters of gastric sensorimotor function testing. a indicates P=.05 compared with baseline; b, P<.05 compared with placebo; MDP, minimal distending pressure.

(From Tack J, Janssen P, Masaoka T, Farre R, Van Oudenhove L. Efficacy of buspirone, a fundus-relaxing drug, in patients with functional dyspepsia. Clin Gastroenterol Hepatol. 2012 Nov;10(11):1239-45; used with permission.)

Figure 4.32   Effect of Aprepitant on Symptoms in Gastroparesis

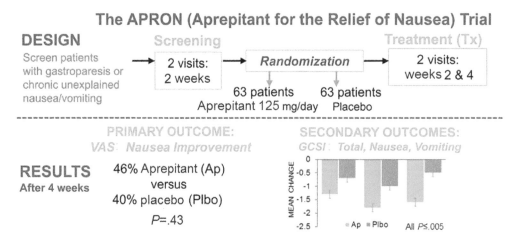

GCSI indicates Gastroparesis Cardinal Symptom Index; VAS, visual analog scale.

(From Pasricha PJ, Yates KP, Sarosiek I, McCallum RW, Abell TL, Koch KL, et al; NIDDK Gastroparesis Clinical Research Consortium (GpCRC). Aprepitant has mixed effects on nausea and reduces other symptoms in patients with gastroparesis and related disorders. Gastroenterology. 2018 Jan;154(1):65-76; used with permission.)

Figure 4.33   Effect of Aprepitant and Placebo on Fasting and Postprandial Gastric Volumes

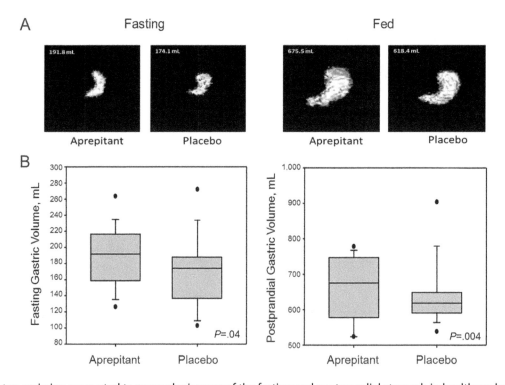

A, Single-photon emission computed tomography images of the fasting and postprandial stomach in healthy volunteers during aprepitant and placebo treatment. B, Fasting and postprandial gastric volumes for groups of healthy volunteers randomized to aprepitant and placebo treatment. Data are median, interquartile range, 5th-95th percentile range, and outliers, adjusted for body mass index and sex. Note that there is marked increase in these volumes in the aprepitant group as compared with the placebo group.

(From Jacob D, Busciglio I, Burton D, Halawi H, Oduyebo I, Rhoten D, et al. Effects of NK1 receptors on gastric motor functions and satiation in healthy humans: results from a controlled trial with the NK1 antagonist aprepitant. Am J Physiol Gastrointest Liver Physiol. 2017 Nov 1;313(5):G505-10.)

Figure 4.34   Pylorospasm Shown on Manometry in Patients With Diabetes

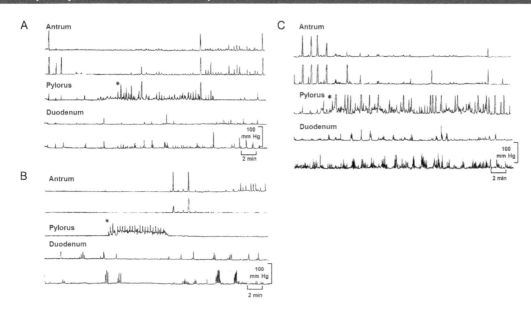

A, Phasic pattern (*) of pyloric activity (mixed antral-type and duodenal-type pressure waves) in a patient with diabetes. Example obtained during the postcibal period. B, Episode of pylorospasm (*) in a patient with diabetes during the postcibal period. Phasic activity is superimposed on the tonic elevation of baseline pressure. C, Episode of pylorospasm (*) in a patient with diabetes during the postcibal period. Mixed antral and duodenal phasic activity is mixed with tonic activity (combined tonic-phasic pattern).

(From Mearin F, Camilleri M, Malagelada JR. Pyloric dysfunction in diabetics with recurrent nausea and vomiting. Gastroenterology. 1986 Jun;90(6):1919-25; used with permission.)

Figure 4.35   Pylorospasm Induced by μ-Opioid Agonist (A) in Contrast With Normal Antropyloroduodenal Coordination (B)

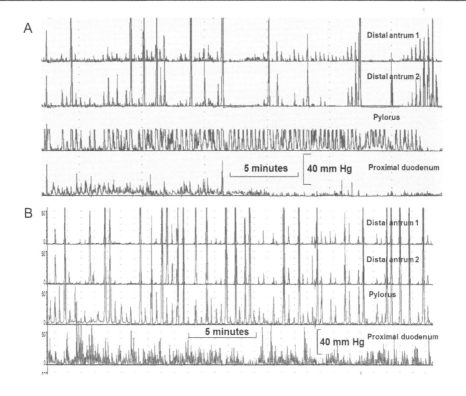

(From Camilleri M. Novel diet, drugs, and gastric interventions for gastroparesis. Clin Gastroenterol Hepatol. 2016 Aug;14(8):1072-80; used with permission.)

Aprepitant

Aprepitant (125 mg/day) is efficacious for the treatment of nausea, vomiting, and overall symptoms based on the total Gastroparesis Cardinal Symptom Index score (secondary end points in a randomized controlled trial [Pasricha 2018; see suggested reading]) (Figure 4.32) in patients with gastroparesis and related disorders. It does not retard GE, but it increases fasting and postprandial (accommodation) gastric volumes in healthy volunteers (Figure 4.33). Studies in dyspepsia or gastroparesis have not been performed.

Pyloric Interventions

Pylorospasm has been shown on manometry in patients with gastroparesis (Figure 4.34); this is suggestive of loss of inhibitory innervation and occurs in response to μ-opioid treatment (Figure 4.35).

Two randomized controlled trials (Arts 2007; Friedenberg 2008; see suggested reading) found no benefit to intrapyloric botulinum toxin type A compared with placebo. In an open-label study of intrapyloric botulinum toxin type A injection in 179 patients with gastroparesis, symptoms of gastroparesis decreased 1 to 4 months after injection in 92 patients (51.4%). Response was improved in those who received 200 U (rather than 100 U), in women, in those younger than 50 years, and in those who did not have diabetes or surgery.

Pyloroplasty, performed surgically or endoscopically (gastric peroral endoscopic myotomy or peroral pyloroplasty) (Figure 4.36), is being offered to patients who are unresponsive to other treatments, including pharmacologic approaches, enteral feeding, and gastric electrical stimulation. It is unclear whether factors such as the presence of pylorospasm, concomitant antral hypomotility, or differences in pyloric diameter or compliance (eg, as a result of scarring) affect the efficacy of pyloric interventions (Figure 4.37).

In 7 studies (Avalos 2018; see reference list for Figure 4.38) that included 130 patients with a mean duration of follow-up of 3 to 12 months, the main causes of gastroparesis were idiopathic (44.5%), diabetes (30.8%), and postgastric surgery (20.5%). Overall, the proportions of success were 87.01% (95% CI, 76.6-94.6) for clinical outcomes and 62.6% (95% CI, 49.9-74.5) for normalization of GE; adverse events occurred in 7.6% (95% CI, 1.96-16.5) of cases (Figure 4.38).

Controlled studies are required to assess the efficacy of pyloric interventions or to facilitate identification of biomarkers that predict efficacy in order to facilitate selection of patients for these interventions.

Figure 4.36   Early Human Experience With Peroral Endoscopic Pyloromyotomy in Gastroparesis

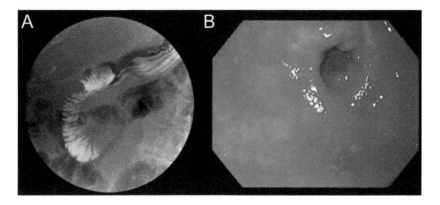

A, Upper gastrointestinal image obtained on postoperative day 1 shows free flow of contrast across the pylorus. Clips are visible at site of the mucosotomy, and there is no evidence of a leak. B, Follow-up endoscopy 3 months postoperatively shows a keyhole deformity of the pylorus at the 5–6 o'clock position corresponding to the site of the pyloromyotomy.

(From Shlomovitz E, Pescarus R, Cassera MA, Sharata AM, Reavis KM, Dunst CM, et al. Early human experience with per-oral endoscopic pyloromyotomy (POP). Surg Endosc. 2015 Mar;29(3):543-51; used with permission.)

Figure 4.37 **Algorithm Proposed for Selection of Pyloroplasty in Patients Unresponsive to Medical Treatment**

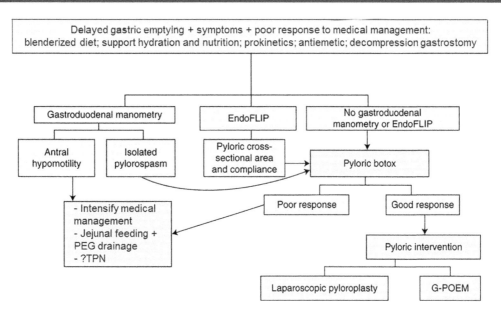

EndoFLIP indicates endoluminal functional lumen imaging probe; G-POEM, gastric peroral endoscopic myotomy; PEG, percutaneous endoscopic gastrostomy; TPN, total parenteral nutrition.

(From Lacy BE, Parkman HP, Camilleri M. Chronic nausea and vomiting: evaluation and treatment. Am J Gastroenterol. 2018 May;113(5):647-59; used with permission.)

Figure 4.38 **Results of Gastric Peroral Endoscopic Myotomy in Gastroparesis**

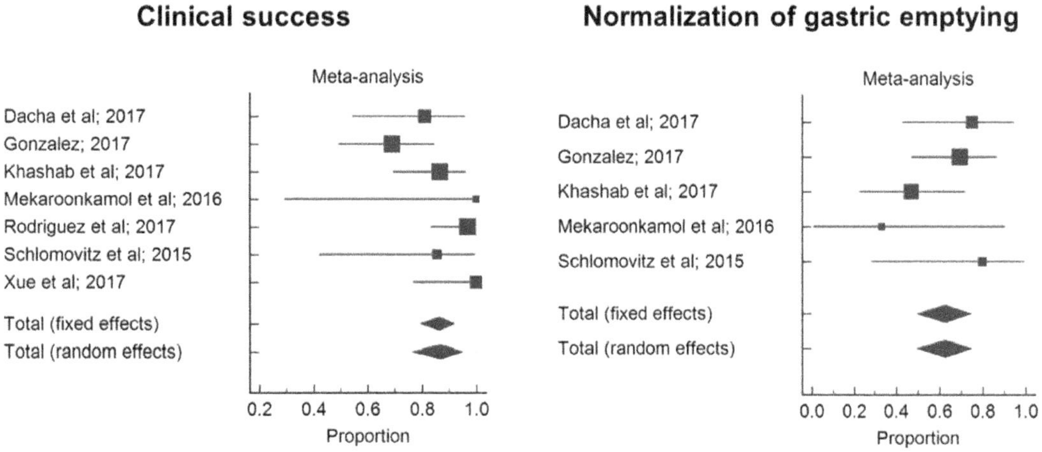

Clinical success

Normalization of gastric emptying

Meta-analysis

Dacha et al; 2017
Gonzalez; 2017
Khashab et al; 2017
Mekaroonkamol et al; 2016
Rodriguez et al; 2017
Schlomovitz et al; 2015
Xue et al; 2017

Total (fixed effects)
Total (random effects)

0.2 0.4 0.6 0.8 1.0
Proportion

Meta-analysis

Dacha et al; 2017
Gonzalez; 2017
Khashab et al; 2017
Mekaroonkamol et al; 2016
Schlomovitz et al; 2015

Total (fixed effects)
Total (random effects)

0.0 0.2 0.4 0.6 0.8 1.0
Proportion

(From Avalos DJ, Satiya J, Bashashati M, Zuckerman M, Mendoza-Ladd A, Sarosiek I, et al. Sa1584 - G-Poem improves clinical symptoms and gastric emptying in gastroparesis: a systematic review and meta-analysis [abstract]. Gastroenterology. 2018;154(6):S-320; used with permission. Full reference citations for studies listed in this figure are at the end of the chapter.)

Gastric Electrical Stimulation for Gastroparesis

Several open-label studies (reviewed in Levinthal and Bielfeldt 2017; see suggested reading) have suggested the efficacy of gastric electrical stimulation for the treatment of gastroparesis, particularly diabetic gastroparesis, and at least 2 systematic reviews and meta-analyses (O'Grady 2009; Levinthal 2017; see suggested reading) have expressed caution in recommending gastric electrical stimulation outside research studies (Figure 4.39).

Figure 4.39   Gastric Electrical Stimulation for Gastroparesis

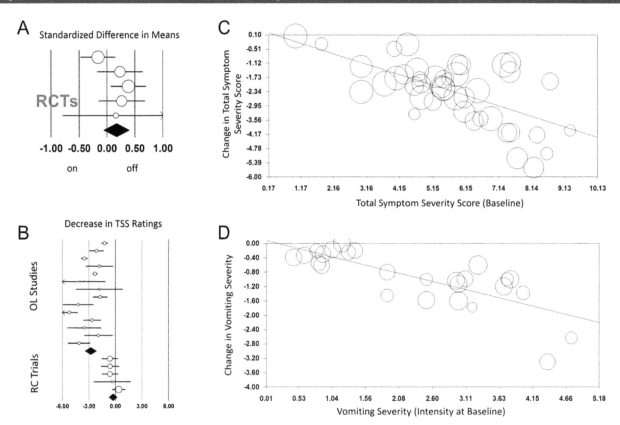

Meta-regression showing the relationship between mean changes in total symptom severity ratings and their baseline severity. Baseline symptom severity affects treatment outcome, a finding suggesting that regression to the mean likely contributes to the substantial discrepancies between the reported results of randomized controlled trials (RCTs) and open-label (OL) studies. A, Total symptom severity (TSS) scores assessed for 5 RCTs of gastric electrical stimulation comparing periods with (on) and without activation (off) of the simulator. B, Changes in total symptom severity scores for OL studies and randomized controlled (RC) trials (Q = 39.0; P<.001). C, Meta-regression showing the relationship between mean changes in TSS ratings and their baseline severity. Symbol size is proportional to the relative weight of the studies used in the analysis (slope: −0.43 [−0.59 to −0.27]; Q = 87.5; P<.01). D, Severity rating at baseline scores for vomiting. Symbol sizes are proportional to the relative weight of the studies used in the analysis (vomiting ratings: slope: −0.44 [−0.64 to −0.25]; Q = 14.8; P<.001).

(From Levinthal DJ, Bielefeldt K. Systematic review and meta-analysis: gastric electrical stimulation for gastroparesis. Auton Neurosci. 2017 Jan;202:45-55; used with permission.)

Management of Functional Dyspepsia

The diagnostic algorithm for dyspepsia in primary GI practice (Figure 4.40) suggests that upper GI endoscopy is indicated when there are alarm symptoms, such as new-onset dyspepsia at more than 55 years of age, overt GI bleeding, dysphagia (especially if progressive or associated with odynophagia), persistent vomiting, unintentional weight loss, family history of gastric or esophageal cancer, palpable abdominal or epigastric mass, abdominal adenopathy, and evidence of iron-deficiency anemia. The next consideration is to test and treat for *Helicobacter pylori*. Testing for *H pylori* is especially indicated in geographic regions where there is a high background population prevalence of *H pylori*. If such an infection is identified, *H pylori* eradication should be pursued, although the likelihood of improvement of dyspepsia in randomized controlled trials is estimated to be 10%. Alternatively, first-line

Figure 4.40   Diagnostic Algorithm for Dyspepsia in Primary Gastrointestinal Practice

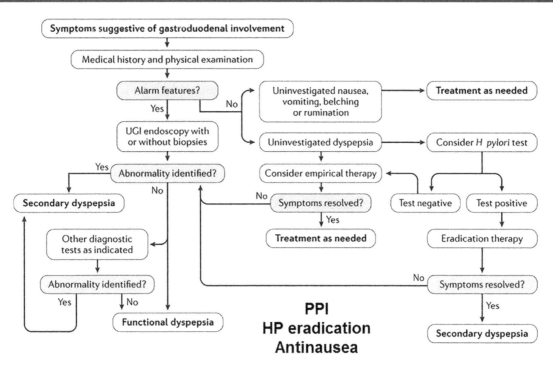

HP indicates *Helicobacter pylori*; PPI, proton pump inhibitors; UGI, upper gastrointestial.

(Modified from Stanghellini V, Chan FK, Hasler WL, Malagelada JR, Suzuki H, Tack J, et al. Gastroduodenal disorders. Gastroenterology. 2016 May;150(6):1380-92; used with permission.)

Figure 4.41   Forest Plot of Randomized Controlled Trials of the Effects of Proton Pump Inhibitors (PPI) Compared With Placebo for Functional Dyspepsia

Study or Subgroup	PPI Events	PPI Total	Placebo Events	Placebo Total	Weight	Risk Ratio M-H, Random, 95% CI
Blum 2000	272	395	170	203	9.4%	0.82 [0.75, 0.90]
Bolling-Sternevald 2002	71	100	80	97	7.1%	0.86 [0.74, 1.01]
Farup 1999	6	14	8	10	0.9%	0.54 [0.27, 1.06]
Fletcher 2011	45	70	33	35	5.9%	0.68 [0.56, 0.83]
Gerson 2005	16	21	9	19	1.4%	1.61 [0.95, 2.74]
Hengels 1998	50	131	77	138	4.2%	0.68 [0.53, 0.89]
Iwakiri 2013	194	253	71	85	8.5%	0.92 [0.82, 1.03]
Peura 2004	474	613	271	308	10.4%	0.88 [0.83, 0.93]
Suzuki 2013 (ELF)	16	23	28	30	3.8%	0.75 [0.56, 0.99]
Talley 1998 (BOND)	242	423	162	219	8.6%	0.77 [0.69, 0.87]
Talley 1998 (OPERA)	277	403	141	203	8.6%	0.99 [0.88, 1.11]
Talley 2007	653	853	84	111	8.7%	1.01 [0.90, 1.13]
Van Rensburg 2008	93	207	116	212	5.9%	0.82 [0.68, 1.00]
Van Zanten 2006	84	109	100	115	8.2%	0.89 [0.78, 1.00]
Wong 2002	231	301	107	152	8.3%	1.09 [0.97, 1.23]
Total (95% CI)		3,916		1,937	100.0%	0.87 [0.82, 0.94]
Total events	2,724		1,457			

Heterogeneity: Tau² = 0.01; Chi² = 48.93, df = 14   (*P*<.00001); I² = 71%
Test for overall effect: Z = 3.87 (*P*=.0001)

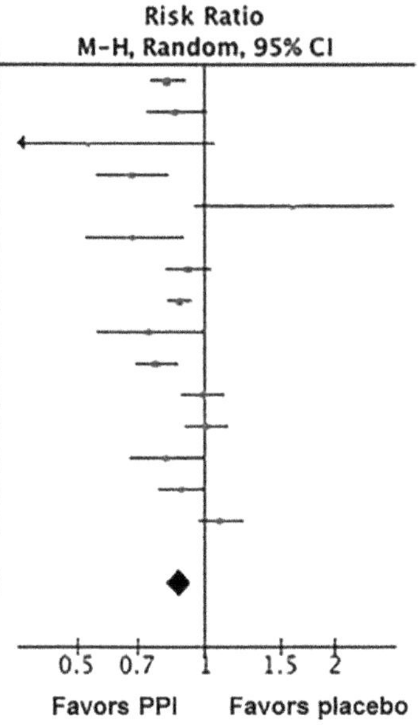

Favors PPI   Favors placebo

Note the significant heterogeneity and modest degree of efficacy. M-H indicates Mantel–Haenszel statistical test.

(From Moayyedi P, Lacy BE, Andrews CN, Enns RA, Howden CW, Vakil N. ACG and CAG clinical guideline: management of dyspepsia. Am J Gastroenterol. 2017 Jul;112(7):988-1013; used with permission. Full reference citations for studies listed in this figure can be found in the original source.)

Figure 4.42   Forest Plot of Randomized Controlled Trials Comparing *Helicobacter pylori* Eradication With Placebo Antibiotics in *Helicobacter pylori*–Infected Patients With Functional Dyspepsia

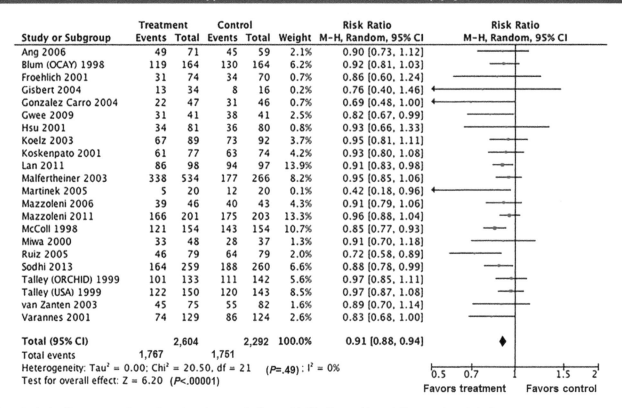

Study or Subgroup	Treatment Events	Treatment Total	Control Events	Control Total	Weight	Risk Ratio M-H, Random, 95% CI
Ang 2006	49	71	45	59	2.1%	0.90 [0.73, 1.12]
Blum (OCAY) 1998	119	164	130	164	6.2%	0.92 [0.81, 1.03]
Froehlich 2001	31	74	34	70	0.7%	0.86 [0.60, 1.24]
Gisbert 2004	13	34	8	16	0.2%	0.76 [0.40, 1.46]
Gonzalez Carro 2004	22	47	31	46	0.7%	0.69 [0.48, 1.00]
Gwee 2009	31	41	38	41	2.5%	0.82 [0.67, 0.99]
Hsu 2001	34	81	36	80	0.8%	0.93 [0.66, 1.33]
Koelz 2003	67	89	73	92	3.7%	0.95 [0.81, 1.11]
Koskenpato 2001	61	77	63	74	4.2%	0.93 [0.80, 1.08]
Lan 2011	86	98	94	97	13.9%	0.91 [0.83, 0.98]
Malfertheiner 2003	338	534	177	266	8.2%	0.95 [0.85, 1.06]
Martinek 2005	5	20	12	20	0.1%	0.42 [0.18, 0.96]
Mazzoleni 2006	39	46	40	43	4.3%	0.91 [0.79, 1.06]
Mazzoleni 2011	166	201	175	203	13.3%	0.96 [0.88, 1.04]
McColl 1998	121	154	143	154	10.7%	0.85 [0.77, 0.93]
Miwa 2000	33	48	28	37	1.3%	0.91 [0.70, 1.18]
Ruiz 2005	46	79	64	79	2.0%	0.72 [0.58, 0.89]
Sodhi 2013	164	259	188	260	6.6%	0.88 [0.78, 0.99]
Talley (ORCHID) 1999	101	133	111	142	5.6%	0.97 [0.85, 1.11]
Talley (USA) 1999	122	150	120	143	8.5%	0.97 [0.87, 1.08]
van Zanten 2003	45	75	55	82	1.6%	0.89 [0.70, 1.14]
Varannes 2001	74	129	86	124	2.6%	0.83 [0.68, 1.00]
Total (95% CI)		2,604		2,292	100.0%	0.91 [0.88, 0.94]
Total events	1,767		1,751			

Heterogeneity: Tau^2 = 0.00; Chi^2 = 20.50, df = 21   (P=.49) ; I^2 = 0%
Test for overall effect: Z = 6.20 (P<.00001)

Favors treatment   Favors control

Note the lack of heterogeneity and modest degree of efficacy. M-H indicates Mantel–Haenszel statistical test.

(From Moayyedi P, Lacy BE, Andrews CN, Enns RA, Howden CW, Vakil N. ACG and CAG clinical guideline: management of dyspepsia. Am J Gastroenterol. 2017 Jul;112(7):988-1013; used with permission. Full reference citations for studies listed in this figure can be found in the original source.)

Figure 4.43   Forest Plot of Randomized Controlled Trials of the Effects of Domperidone Compared With Placebo for Upper Gastrointestinal Symptoms

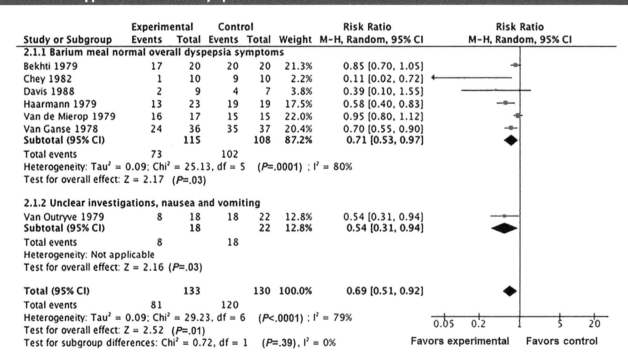

Study or Subgroup	Experimental Events	Experimental Total	Control Events	Control Total	Weight	Risk Ratio M-H, Random, 95% CI
2.1.1 Barium meal normal overall dyspepsia symptoms						
Bekhti 1979	17	20	20	20	21.3%	0.85 [0.70, 1.05]
Chey 1982	1	10	9	10	2.2%	0.11 [0.02, 0.72]
Davis 1988	2	9	4	7	3.8%	0.39 [0.10, 1.55]
Haarmann 1979	13	23	19	19	17.5%	0.58 [0.40, 0.83]
Van de Mierop 1979	16	17	15	15	22.0%	0.95 [0.80, 1.12]
Van Ganse 1978	24	36	35	37	20.4%	0.70 [0.55, 0.90]
Subtotal (95% CI)		115		108	87.2%	0.71 [0.53, 0.97]
Total events	73		102			

Heterogeneity: Tau^2 = 0.09; Chi^2 = 25.13, df = 5   (P=.0001) ; I^2 = 80%
Test for overall effect: Z = 2.17 (P=.03)

2.1.2 Unclear investigations, nausea and vomiting						
Van Outryve 1979	8	18	18	22	12.8%	0.54 [0.31, 0.94]
Subtotal (95% CI)		18		22	12.8%	0.54 [0.31, 0.94]
Total events	8		18			

Heterogeneity: Not applicable
Test for overall effect: Z = 2.16 (P=.03)

| **Total (95% CI)** | | 133 | | 130 | 100.0% | 0.69 [0.51, 0.92] |
| Total events | 81 | | 120 | | | |

Heterogeneity: Tau^2 = 0.09; Chi^2 = 29.23, df = 6   (P<.0001) ; I^2 = 79%
Test for overall effect: Z = 2.52 (P=.01)
Test for subgroup differences: Chi^2 = 0.72, df = 1   (P=.39), I^2 = 0%

Favors experimental   Favors control

Note the significant heterogeneity and modest degree of efficacy. M-H indicates Mantel–Haenszel statistical test.

(From Moayyedi P, Lacy BE, Andrews CN, Enns RA, Howden CW, Vakil N. ACG and CAG clinical guideline: management of dyspepsia. Am J Gastroenterol. 2017 Jul;112(7):988-1013; used with permission. Full reference citations for studies listed in this figure can be found in the original source.)

Figure 4.44   Treatment Algorithm in Functional Dyspepsia

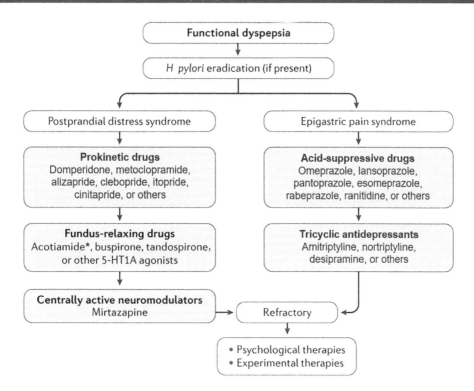

H pylori indicates *Helicobacter pylori*; 5-HT1A, serotonin 1A.

(From Enck P, Azpiroz F, Boeckxstaens G, Elsenbruch S, Feinle-Bisset C, Holtmann G, et al. Functional dyspepsia. Nat Rev Dis Primers. 2017 Nov 3;3:17081; used with permission.)

management involves treatment with proton pump inhibitors or antinausea medications (Figures 4.41 through 4.43).

Given the dominant mechanisms of GE, accommodation, hypersensitivity, and psychologic disorders, these are the main areas of management when first-line treatments for dyspepsia are ineffective. A recent systematic review (Moayyedi 2017; see suggested reading) and meta-analysis reviewed the efficacy of the different classes of drugs and the combined diagnostic and therapeutic algorithm for functional dyspepsia, as summarized in Figures 4.44 through 4.47.

Conclusions

Important advances in gastroparesis and related disorders include treating upper GI symptoms suggestive of gastroparesis on the basis of the right diagnosis, excluding iatrogenic disease, and the use of opioids. New pharmacologic agents are promising; meanwhile, off-label use of approved medications anchors current management, in addition to dietary interventions. Pyloric interventions, including endoscopic pyloroplasty, require further validation.

Figure 4.45   Forest Plot of Randomized Controlled Trials of the Effect of Serotonin 4 Prokinetic Agents With Placebo for Functional Dyspepsia

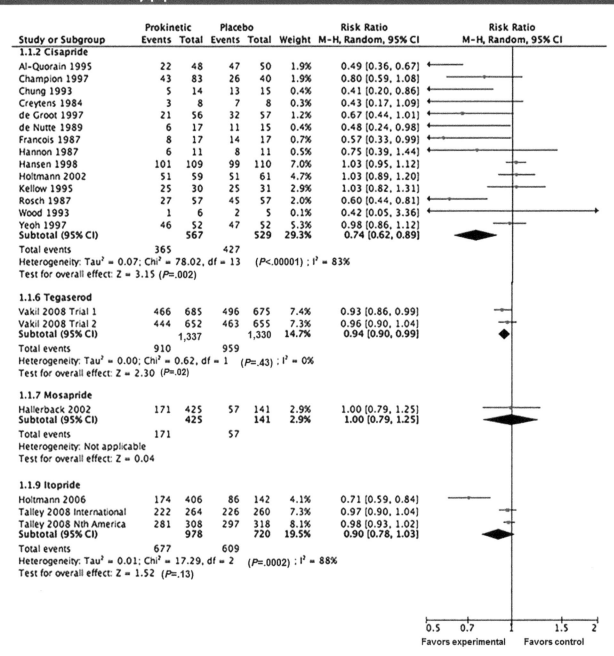

M-H indicates Mantel–Haenszel statistical test.

(From Moayyedi P, Lacy BE, Andrews CN, Enns RA, Howden CW, Vakil N. ACG and CAG clinical guideline: management of dyspepsia. Am J Gastroenterol. 2017 Jul;112(7):988-1013; used with permission. Full reference citations for studies listed in this figure can be found in the original source.)

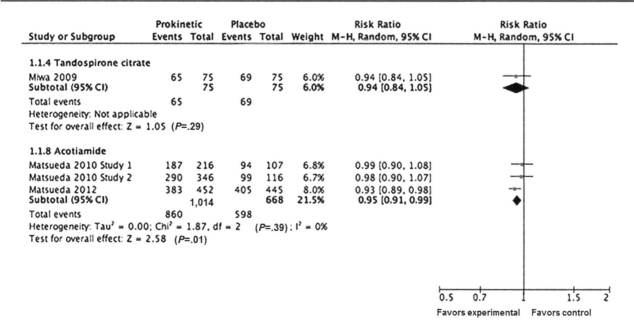

M-H indicates Mantel–Haenszel statistical test.

(From Moayyedi P, Lacy BE, Andrews CN, Enns RA, Howden CW, Vakil N. ACG and CAG clinical guideline: management of dyspepsia. Am J Gastroenterol. 2017 Jul;112(7):988-1013; used with permission. Full reference citations for studies listed in this figure can be found in the original source.)

Figure 4.47   Summary Algorithm Incorporating Diagnosis and Treatment of Functional Dyspepsia

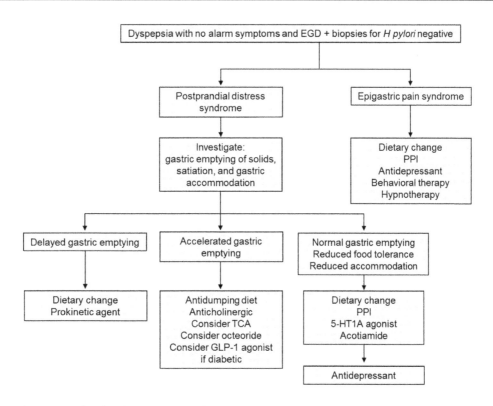

EGD indicates esophagogastroduodendoscopy; GLP-1, glucagon-like peptide-1; *H pylori, Helicobacter pylori*; PPI, proton pump inhibitor; TCA, tricyclic antidepressant; 5-HT1A, serotonin 1A.

(Modified from Camilleri M. Functional dyspepsia: mechanisms of symptom generation and appropriate management of patients. Gastroenterol Clin North Am. 2007 Sep;36(3):649-64; used with permission.)

Suggested Reading

Arts J, Holvoet L, Caenepeel P, Bisschops R, Sifrim D, Verbeke K, et al. Clinical trial: a randomized-controlled crossover study of intrapyloric injection of botulinum toxin in gastroparesis. Aliment Pharmacol Ther. 2007 Nov 1;26(9):1251–8.

Avalos DJ, Satiya J, Bashashati M, Zuckerman M, Mendoza-Ladd A, Sarosiek I, et al. Sa1584 - G-Poem improves clinical symptoms and gastric emptying in gastroparesis: a systematic review and meta-analysis [Abstract]. Gastroenterology. 2018 May;154(6 Supplement 1):S–320.

Bharucha AE, Kudva Y, Basu A, Camilleri M, Low PA, Vella A, et al. Relationship between glycemic control and gastric emptying in poorly controlled type 2 diabetes. Clin Gastroenterol Hepatol. 2015 Mar;13(3):466–76. Epub 2014 Jul 17.

Bytzer P, Talley NJ, Leemon M, Young LJ, Jones MP, Horowitz M. Prevalence of gastrointestinal symptoms associated with diabetes mellitus: a population-based survey of 15,000 adults. Arch Intern Med. 2001 Sep 10;161(16):1989–96.

Camilleri M. Clinical practice: diabetic gastroparesis. N Engl J Med. 2007 Feb 22;356(8):820–9. Epub 2007 Feb 23.

Camilleri M. Novel diet, drugs, and gastric interventions for gastroparesis. Clin Gastroenterol Hepatol. 2016 Aug;14(8):1072–80. Epub 2016 Jan 15.

Camilleri M, Chedid V, Ford AC, Haruma K, Horowitz M, Jones KL, et al. Gastroparesis. Nat Rev Dis Primers. 2018 Nov 1;4(1):41. Epub 2018 Nov 06.

Camilleri M, Parkman HP, Shafi MA, Abell TL, Gerson L; American College of Gastroenterology. Clinical guideline: management of gastroparesis. Am J Gastroenterol. 2013 Jan;108(1):18–37. Epub 2012 Nov 14.

Chedid V, Halawi H, Brandler J, Burton D, Camilleri M. Gastric accommodation measurements by single photon emission computed tomography and two-dimensional scintigraphy in diabetic patients with upper gastrointestinal symptoms. Neurogastroenterol Motil. 2019 Jun;31(6):e13581. Epub 2019 Mar 13.

Dacha S, Mekaroonkamol P, Li L, Shahnavaz N, Sakaria S, Keilin S, et al. Outcomes and quality-of-life assessment after gastric per-oral endoscopic pyloromyotomy (with video). Gastrointest Endosc. 2017 Aug;86(2):282–9. Epub 2017 Feb 1.

De Giorgio R, Cogliandro RF, Barbara G, Corinaldesi R, Stanghellini V. Chronic intestinal pseudo-obstruction: clinical features, diagnosis, and therapy. Gastroenterol Clin North Am. 2011 Dec;40(4):787–807. Epub 2011 Nov 22.

Di Nardo G, Di Lorenzo C, Lauro A, Stanghellini V, Thapar N, Karunaratne TB, et al. Chronic intestinal pseudo-obstruction in children and adults: diagnosis and therapeutic options. Neurogastroenterol Motil. 2017 Jan;29(1):e12945. Epub 2016 Sep 30.

Enck P, Azpiroz F, Boeckxstaens G, Elsenbruch S, Feinle-Bisset C, Holtmann G, et al. Functional dyspepsia. Nat Rev Dis Primers. 2017 Nov 3;3:17081. Epub 2017 Nov 04.

Friedenberg FK, Palit A, Parkman HP, Hanlon A, Nelson DB. Botulinum toxin A for the treatment of delayed gastric emptying. Am J Gastroenterol. 2008 Feb;103(2):416–23. Epub 2007 Dec 5.

Ganzini L, Casey DE, Hoffman WF, McCall AL. The prevalence of metoclopramide-induced tardive dyskinesia and acute extrapyramidal movement disorders. Arch Intern Med. 1993 Jun 28;153(12):1469–75.

Gonzalez JM, Benezech A, Vitton V, Barthet M. G-POEM with antro-pyloromyotomy for the treatment of refractory gastroparesis: mid-term follow-up and factors predicting outcome. Aliment Pharmacol Ther. 2017 Aug;46(3):364–70. Epub 2017 May 15.

Homko CJ, Duffy F, Friedenberg FK, Boden G, Parkman HP. Effect of dietary fat and food consistency on gastroparesis symptoms in patients with gastroparesis. Neurogastroenterol Motil. 2015 Apr;27(4):501–8. Epub 2015 Jan 19.

Jehangir A, Parkman HP. Chronic opioids in gastroparesis: relationship with gastrointestinal symptoms, healthcare utilization and employment. World J Gastroenterol. 2017 Oct 28;23(40):7310–20.

Keller J, Bassotti G, Clarke J, Dinning P, Fox M, Grover M, et al. Expert consensus document: advances in the diagnosis and classification of gastric and intestinal motility disorders. Nat Rev Gastroenterol Hepatol. 2018 May;15(5):291–308. Epub 2018 Apr 07.

Khashab MA, Ngamruengphong S, Carr-Locke D, Bapaye A, Benias PC, Serouya S, et al. Gastric per-oral endoscopic myotomy for refractory gastroparesis: results from the first multicenter study on endoscopic pyloromyotomy (with video). Gastrointest Endosc. 2017 Jan;85(1):123–8. Epub 2016 Jun 25.

Lacy BE, Parkman HP, Camilleri M. Chronic nausea and vomiting: evaluation and treatment. Am J Gastroenterol. 2018 May;113(5):647–59. Epub 2018 Mar 17.

Levinthal DJ, Bielefeldt K. Systematic review and meta-analysis: gastric electrical stimulation for gastroparesis. Auton Neurosci. 2017 Jan;202:45–55. Epub 2016 Apr 11.

Mekaroonkamol P, Dacha S, Wang L, Li X, Jiang Y, Li L, et al. Gastric peroral endoscopic pyloromyotomy reduces symptoms, increases quality of life, and reduces health care use for patients with gastroparesis. Clin Gastroenterol Hepatol. 2019 Jan;17(1):82–9. Epub 2018 Apr 13.

Moayyedi PM, Lacy BE, Andrews CN, Enns RA, Howden CW, Vakil N. ACG and CAG clinical guideline: management of dyspepsia. Am J Gastroenterol. 2017 Jul;112(7):988–1013. Epub 2017 Jun 21.

O'Grady G, Egbuji JU, Du P, Cheng LK, Pullan AJ, Windsor JA. High-frequency gastric electrical stimulation for the treatment of gastroparesis: a meta-analysis. World J Surg. 2009 Aug;33(8):1693–701.

Olausson EA, Storsrud S, Grundin H, Isaksson M, Attvall S, Simren M. A small particle size diet reduces upper gastrointestinal symptoms in patients with diabetic gastroparesis: a randomized controlled trial. Am J Gastroenterol. 2014 Mar;109(3):375–85. Epub 2014 Jan 14.

Park SY, Acosta A, Camilleri M, Burton D, Harmsen WS, Fox J, et al. Gastric motor dysfunction in patients with functional gastroduodenal symptoms. Am J Gastroenterol. 2017 Nov;112(11):1689–99. Epub 2017 Sep 13.

Parkman HP, Hallinan EK, Hasler WL, Farrugia G, Koch KL, Nguyen L, et al; NIDDK Gastroparesis Clinical Research Consortium (GpCRC). Early satiety and postprandial fullness in gastroparesis correlate with gastroparesis severity, gastric emptying, and water load testing. Neurogastroenterol Motil. 2017 Apr;29(4):e12981. Epub 2016 Oct 25.

Parkman HP, Yates K, Hasler WL, Nguyen L, Pasricha PJ, Snape WJ, et al; National Institute of Diabetes and Digestive and Kidney Diseases Gastroparesis Clinical Research Consortium. Clinical features of idiopathic gastroparesis vary with sex, body mass, symptom onset, delay in gastric emptying, and gastroparesis severity. Gastroenterology. 2011 Jan;140(1):101–15. Epub 2010 Oct 20.

Pasricha PJ, Parkman HP. Gastroparesis: definitions and diagnosis. Gastroenterol Clin North Am. 2015 Mar;44(1):1–7. Epub 2015 Feb 11.

Pasricha PJ, Yates KP, Sarosiek I, McCallum RW, Abell TL, Koch KL, et al; NIDDK Gastroparesis Clinical Research Consortium (GpCRC). Aprepitant has mixed effects on nausea and reduces other symptoms in patients with gastroparesis and related disorders. Gastroenterology. 2018 Jan;154(1):65–76.

Rodriguez JH, Haskins IN, Strong AT, Plescia RL, Allemang MT, Butler RS, et al. Per oral endoscopic pyloromyotomy for refractory gastroparesis: initial results from a single institution. Surg Endosc. 2017 Dec;31(12):5381–8. Epub 2017 May 31.

Shlomovitz E, Pescarus R, Cassera MA, Sharata AM, Reavis KM, Dunst CM, et al. Early human experience with per-oral endoscopic pyloromyotomy (POP). Surg Endosc. 2015 Mar;29(3):543–51. Epub 2014 Aug 9.

Soykan I, Sivri B, Sarosiek I, Kiernan B, McCallum RW. Demography, clinical characteristics, psychological and abuse profiles, treatment, and long-term follow-up of patients with gastroparesis. Dig Dis Sci. 1998 Nov;43(11):2398–404.

Talley NJ, Locke GR, Saito YA, Almazar AE, Bouras EP, Howden CW, et al. Effect of amitriptyline and escitalopram on functional dyspepsia: a multicenter, randomized controlled study. Gastroenterology. 2015 Aug;149(2):340–9. Epub 2015 Apr 25.

Xue HB, Fan HZ, Meng XM, Cristofaro S, Mekaroonkamol P, Dacha S, et al. Fluoroscopy-guided gastric peroral endoscopic pyloromyotomy (G-POEM): a more reliable and efficient method for treatment of refractory gastroparesis. Surg Endosc. 2017 Nov;31(11):4617–24. Epub 2017 Apr 13.

References Listed in Figure 4.39

Dacha S, Mekaroonkamol P, Li L, Shahnavaz N, Sakaria S, Keilin S, et al. Outcomes and quality-of-life assessment after gastric per-oral endoscopic pyloromyotomy (with video). Gastrointest Endosc. 2017 Aug;86(2):282–9. Epub 2017 Feb 1.

Gonzalez JM, Benezech A, Vitton V, Barthet M. G-POEM with antro-pyloromyotomy for the treatment of refractory gastroparesis: mid-term follow-up and factors predicting outcome. Aliment Pharmacol Ther. 2017 Aug;46(3):364–70. Epub 2017 May 15.

Khashab MA, Ngamruengphong S, Carr-Locke D, Bapaye A, Benias PC, Serouya S, et al. Gastric per-oral endoscopic myotomy for refractory gastroparesis: results from the first multicenter study on endoscopic pyloromyotomy (with video). Gastrointest Endosc. 2017 Jan;85(1):123–8. Epub 2016 Jun 25.

Mekaroonkamol P, Dacha S, Wang L, Li X, Jiang Y, Li L, et al. Gastric peroral endoscopic pyloromyotomy reduces symptoms, increases quality of life, and reduces health care use for patients with gastroparesis. Clin Gastroenterol Hepatol. 2019 Jan;17(1):82–9. Epub 2018 Apr 13.

Rodriguez JH, Haskins IN, Strong AT, Plescia RL, Allemang MT, Butler RS, et al. Per oral endoscopic pyloromyotomy for refractory gastroparesis: initial results from a single institution. Surg Endosc. 2017 Dec;31(12):5381–8. Epub 2017 May 31.

Shlomovitz E, Pescarus R, Cassera MA, Sharata AM, Reavis KM, Dunst CM, et al. Early human experience with per-oral endoscopic pyloromyotomy (POP). Surg Endosc. 2015 Mar;29(3):543–51. Epub 2014 Aug 9.

Xue HB, Fan HZ, Meng XM, Cristofaro S, Mekaroonkamol P, Dacha S, et al. Fluoroscopy-guided gastric peroral endoscopic pyloromyotomy (G-POEM): a more reliable and efficient method for treatment of refractory gastroparesis. Surg Endosc. 2017 Nov;31(11):4617–24. Epub 2017 Apr 13.

Introduction

The gastrointestinal causes of nausea and vomiting include delayed gastric emptying (GE), such as chronic gastroparesis and chronic intestinal pseudo-obstruction; impaired gastric accommodation; rumination syndrome; colonic motor dysfunction or rectal evacuation disorder manifesting as associated constipation; and, extremely rarely, brainstem tumor.

For the evaluation of patients, there are critically important requirements. First, there should be an understanding of what patients really mean when they report nausea or vomiting (Figure 5.1), which may be mistaken for early postprandial fullness and effortless food regurgitation.

Figure 5.1 Patient Complaint: Nausea and Vomiting

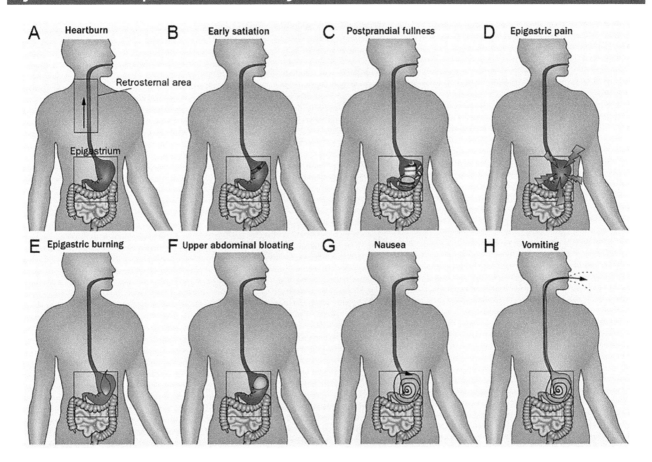

Patients may confuse nausea with upper gastrointestinal symptoms (A-H).

(From Tack J, Talley NJ. Functional dyspepsia: symptoms, definitions and validity of the Rome III criteria. Nat Rev Gastroenterol Hepatol. 2013;10(3):134-41; used with permission.)

Second, iatrogenic factors should always be excluded, particularly concomitant medications, including opioids, cannabinoids, and glucagon-like peptide 1 or amylin analogs in patients with diabetes mellitus.

Third, gastroparesis should be confirmed or excluded with an accurate GE test (Figure 5.2). National organizations (American Neurogastroenterology and Motility Society, Society of Nuclear Medicine) have recommended the scintigraphic GE test (meal of 300 kcal, 2% fat), for which the result is abnormal if more than 10% of the meal is retained at 4 hours.

Other approved tests are the well-validated GE test at Mayo Clinic (meal of 320 kcal, 32% fat, scintigraphy), for which GE is considered delayed if more than 25% of the meal is retained at 4 hours; the wireless motility capsule test (retention at 5 hours); and the stable isotope GE test. GE rates differ according to meal consistency, calories, and fat content (Chapter 4, "Gastroparesis, Chronic Intestinal Pseudo-Obstruction, and Functional Dyspepsia"). The normal values for the Mayo Clinic GE test are listed in Table 5.1.

Figure 5.2   Exclusion of Gastroparesis With an Accurate Gastric Emptying (GE) Test (Duration, at Least 3 Hours)

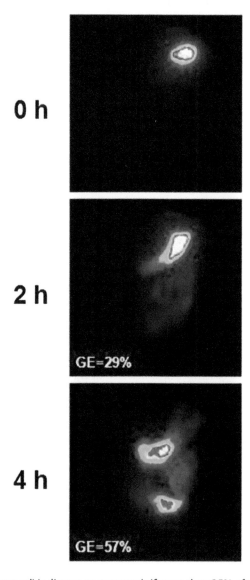

Mayo Clinic GE test (320 kcal, 30% fat egg meal) indicates gastroparesis if more than 25% of meal is retained in stomach at 4 hours.

(Modified from Shin A, Camilleri M, Busciglio I, Burton D, Smith SA, Vella A, et al. The ghrelin agonist RM-131 accelerates gastric emptying of solids and reduces symptoms in patients with type 1 diabetes mellitus. Clin Gastroenterol Hepatol. 2013 Nov;11(11):1453-9; used with permission.)

Table 5.1	Normal Values of Mayo Clinic Gastric Emptying (GE) Test at Different Times and Inter-individual Variation				
Group	GE $t_{1/2}$, min	GE at 1 h,%	GE at 2 h,%	GE at 3 h,%	GE at 4 h,%
All participants					
Mean (SD)	121.7 (29.8)	18.1 (9.5)	51.4 (15.7)	78.1 (14.5)	93.2 (8.9)
Median (5th, 95th %)	120 (78.4, 174.0)	17 (4.4, 35.0)	50 (25.0, 78.5)	80 (52.0, 98.0)	96 (76.2, 100.0)
No.	319	319	319	314	315
COV$_{inter}$, %	24.5	52.7	30.6	18.6	9.6
Women					
Mean (SD)	127.7 (28.7)	16.5 (8.3)	47.8 (14.3)	75.3 (14.2)	92.1 (9.4)
Median (5th, 95th %)	125 (89.0, 180.0)	16 (4.3, 31.4)	47.2 (25.0, 71.0)	76 (50.0, 95.9)	94.8 (76.2, 100.0)
No.	214	214	214	211	211
COV$_{inter}$, %	22.5	50.5	29.9	18.8	10.2
Men					
Mean (SD)	109.9 (28.6)	21.3 (10.9)	58.6 (15.1)	83.8 (13.6)	92.1 (9.4)
Median (5th, 95th %)	105 (73.2, 165.0)	19 (4.7, 40.0)	60 (28.4, 82.0)	88 (55.0, 100.0)	98.3 (77.0, 100.0)
No.	105	105	105	103	104
COV$_{inter}$, %	26.0	51.3	27.5	16.2	7.7

Abbreviation: COV$_{inter}$, intersubject coefficient of variation.

From Camilleri M, Iturrino J, Bharucha AE, Burton D, Shin A, Jeong ID, et al. Performance characteristics of scintigraphic measurement of gastric emptying of solids in healthy participants. Neurogastroenterol Motil. 2012 Dec;24(12):1076-e562; used with permission.

Case Examples

Case 1

A 72-year-old man presented with weight loss, food intolerance, and stool incontinence; he had never smoked. He complained of back pain (was known to have back degenerative joint disease) and was unable to walk, presenting with peripheral weakness of his legs and feet. Test results were as follows: His erythrocyte sedimentation rate was 23 mm in the first hour, and he had macrocytic anemia with normal vitamin B$_{12}$ and ferritin levels. There were minor abnormalities of the following tests: serum albumin, 3.1 g/dL; creatinine, 1.8 mg/dL; sensitive thyroid-stimulating hormone, 6.5 mIU/L; glucose, 118 mg/dL; and urine protein, 236 mg/24 hours. Special serum protein studies with electrophoresis, including immunofixation, had negative results. Other serologic tests, including paraneoplastic screen serology and tests for syphilis and urine heavy metals, had negative results, as did chest radiography and bone survey for myeloma.

The patient had delayed GE (Figure 5.3), abnormal sweating (Figure 5.4), and a widespread autonomic (cardiovagal, cardiovascular, adrenergic, and post-ganglionic sympathetic sudomotor) (Figure 5.5) and a length-dependent peripheral neuropathy documented on electromyography and nerve conduction studies: a length-dependent axonal sensorimotor neuropathy. In addition, in view of the fecal incontinence, anal sphincter pressure was measured. The resting pressure of 54 mm Hg and the squeeze pressure of 83 mm Hg were suggestive of external anal sphincter denervation due to pudendal nerve dysfunction.

Further examination by a neurologist identified macroglossia and dysgeusia, and special urine protein studies showed a small monoclonal κ light chain, all suggestive of amyloidosis, which was confirmed by Congo red staining on a fat aspirate. Echocardiography showed left ventricular wall thickness, diastolic dysfunction, and biatrial enlargement, and bone marrow examination showed systemic amyloidosis, AL type, comprised of κ immunoglobulin light chains.

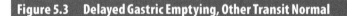

Figure 5.3   Delayed Gastric Emptying, Other Transit Normal

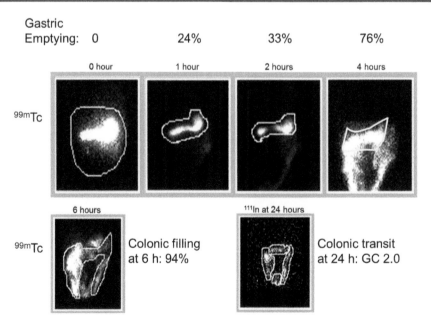

GC indicates geometric center, the weighted average location of colonic isotope (0=ileocecal valve, 5=stool); ^{111}In, indium In 111; ^{99m}Tc, technetium Tc 99m. Area outlined in yellow on 4-hour result indicates gastric region of interest with background of ^{99m}Tc in small bowel.

Figure 5.4   Thermoregulatory Sweat Test Showing Anhidrosis

Indication: GI motility disorder; peripheral & truncal neuropathy

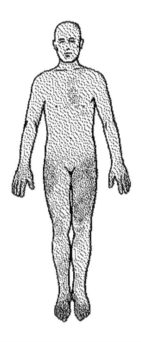

RESULTS:
Sweating in shaded areas
Oral temperature: **36.7°C** before, **38.0°C** after
Body surface anhidrosis: **91%**
Distribution: **global**

IMPRESSION:
The patient was essentially anhidrotic, with relative sparing of he hands, thighs, and distal aspects of feet. Such pattern can occur in widespread autonomic neuropathies or central autonomic disorder.

Figure 5.5   Results on Autonomic Reflex Screen

Heart rate responses

Test	Parameter	Result	[Normal range for age, sex]
Valsalva maneuver	Valsalva ratio	1.14	[> 1.29]
Deep breathing	Heart rate range (bpm)	1.3	[> 7]

Blood pressure and heart rate responses to tilt

		Values with patient to 70° tilt up		
	Supine	1 min	5 min	7 min
BP (mm Hg)	134/78	108/64	80/54	80/60
Pulse (bpm)	74	78	83	81

Quantitative sudomotor axon reflex test (QSART)

Site	Current (mA)	Test duration (min)	Sweat output (μL/cm²)	Normal values (μL/cm²)
L Forearm	2	10	4.76	[M 0.84-5.42;F 0.12-4.39]
L Proximal leg	2	10	2.11	[M 0.76-3.91;F 0.20-2.36]
L Distal leg	2	10	0.19	[M 0.93-4.98;F 0.20-2.98]
L Foot	2	10	0.50	[M 0.70-5.39;F 0.16-3.03]

Reduced heart period responses to deep breathing suggest cardiovagal dysfunction (top red box outlines abnormal heart period responses to deep breathing and Valsalva ratio), postural drop in systolic blood pressure and modest pulse rate increase (outlined in middle red box) suggest sympathetic adrenergic denervation, and reduced sweat output in lower limbs (outlined in bottom red box) is consistent with sympathetic cholinergic denervation. Sympathetic cholinergic denervation is not generalized and may be indicative of peripheral neuropathy rather than pan-autonomic neuropathy. BP indicates blood pressure; bpm, beats per minute; F, female; L, left; M, male.

Case 2

A 29-year-old woman presented with a 25-year history of insulin-dependent, ketosis-prone diabetes mellitus with recurrent hypoglycemic episodes. Her glycosylated hemoglobin value was 7.9%, and her fasting blood glucose concentration was often more than 200 mg/dL. She was also known to have well-controlled hypothyroidism while receiving replacement thyroxine. On physical examination, autonomic neuropathy with involvement of both cholinergic and adrenergic nerves was suggested, there was a pupillary abnormality (minimal response to light, normal response to accommodation), and blood pressure was 117/77 mm Hg prone and 110/60 standing (delta diastolic blood pressure >15 mm Hg). Her fasting blood glucose value was 278 mg/dL. On a 4-hour GE test, 15% of the meal emptied at 1 hour, 25% at 2 hours, and 73% at 4 hours; at 6 hours, 30% of the activity had reached the colon. The patient was prescribed a blenderized diet and prokinetics (metoclopramide); her nutrition and diabetes control were to be reviewed in a month and the plan revised as needed.

Diabetic autonomic neuropathy affecting motility is often not limited to the stomach. Therefore, treating only the stomach may not be enough. This patient had a second problem: constipation. On examination, there was no succussion splash in the abdomen, the right and left lower quadrants had palpable masses consistent with stool, and there was tenderness in the left lower quadrant over palpable stool. Rectal examination showed minimal perineal descent with anterior traction of the anal verge. Palpation of the puborectalis caused exquisite tenderness and, with the finger in the rectum, there was descent of about 1 or 1.5 cm during attempts to expel the examining finger. Rectal mucosa was normal to palpation.

Figure 5.6   Abdominal Radiograph Showing Volume of Retained Gas in Pelvis Above the Level of the Pelvic Floor and Below the Lower Margin of the Sacroiliac Joints

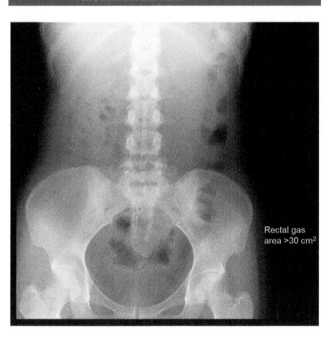

Rectal gas area >30 cm^2

A gas area more than 9 cm^2 is approximately 75% predictive of rectal evacuation disorder.

Other investigations showed borderline slow colonic transit, geometric center at 24 hours, 1.7; anal resting pressure, 81.6 mm Hg; anal squeeze pressure, 123.57 mm Hg; and balloon expulsion requirement more than 586 grams. Abdominal radiography showed retained gas in the pelvis (Figure 5.6), suggestive of a rectal evacuation disorder.

The overall diagnoses were diabetic gastroparesis, autonomic neuropathy, and rectal evacuation disorder. The treatment was biofeedback retraining of the pelvic floor and symptomatic and pharmacologic treatment of the gastroparesis.

Case 3

In a 42-year-old man with diabetes mellitus, cyclical vomiting syndrome was diagnosed 5 years previously, at which time results of transit measurement, gastric accommodation testing, and brain magnetic resonance imaging were all normal. He now presents with a total symptom duration of 7 years, dominated by nausea and vomiting in the morning. He reports acute attacks occurring approximately once every month for the past 6 years that required multiple hospital admissions for 24 to 48 hours after presentation to the emergency department. He experiences excessive heat and sweating during episodes of acute emesis. In the past year, he has required intramuscular promethazine and midazolam to abort the episodes of severe nausea and vomiting.

The patient denies a history of retinopathy, neuropathy, or nephropathy in association with diabetes, and the onset of the nausea and vomiting was very soon after the onset of the diabetes. Current medications are metformin, 500 mg twice daily, and exenatide, 5 µg daily. He acknowledges that he may use marijuana to control the nausea and that, if this is available, he would even use it on a daily basis. He also acknowledges exposure to marijuana in his late teens.

Scintigraphic GE at 1 hour was 22% (normal, 4%-35%); at 2 hours, 56% (normal, 25%-78.5%), and at 4 hours, 87% (normal, 76.2%-100%). Gastric accommodation (postprandial minus fasting volume) was 432 mL (normal, >428 mL).

The diagnosis was cannabinoid hyperemesis, and the patient was referred to psychiatry for withdrawal from cannabinoids.

Case 4

A 56-year-old woman presented with a history of type 1 diabetes mellitus since age 19 years. She had previously had 2 pancreas transplants that failed. She presents with daily postprandial fullness and major episodes of nausea and vomiting that occur once per month on average. She experiences frequent postprandial hypoglycemia (commonly a glucose level of approximately 20 mg/dL), during which she requires administration of glucagon to reverse the hypoglycemia. She also complains of constipation; she passes bowel movements once every 5 days with excessive straining and abdominal bloating and requires polyethylene glycol regularly to relieve the constipation. She also has performed anal canal digitation to assist stool evacuation, but she denies vaginal pressure or splinting to evacuate stool. She has no difficulty urinating or does not have recurrent urinary tract infections. She has not had any vaginal deliveries. She has several complications of diabetes: proliferative retinopathy, peripheral neuropathy, stocking paresthesias, postural dizziness, and eye discomfort when moving from a dark to a bright environment. She has normal sweating.

On physical examination, blood pressure was 106/64 mm Hg, the right pupil was 3 mm in diameter and nonreactive to light, and the left pupil was distorted after a prior iridectomy. Abdominal examination showed multiple scars, subcutaneous injury from insulin injections, no succussion splash, quiet bowel sounds, and no organomegaly, bruit, or masses. Rectal examination showed normal perianal sensation, no spasticity of the puborectalis, low-normal anal resting tone, and reduced anal squeeze pressure. Results of other investigations were as follows: blood glucose, 48 mg/dL; hemoglobin A_{1c}, 7.2%; and anorectal manometry, normal. GE was delayed (Figure 5.7), as was colonic transit (Figure 5.8). An electrocardiogram showed absence of sinus arrhythmia, consistent with vagal neuropathy (Figure 5.9).

Figure 5.7   Gastric Emptying

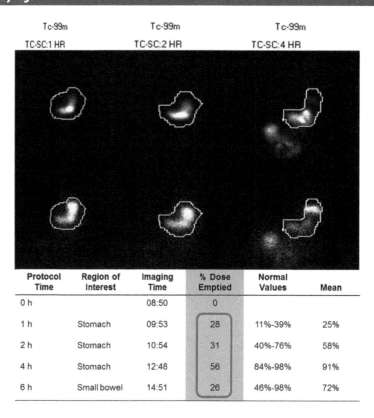

Protocol Time	Region of Interest	Imaging Time	% Dose Emptied	Normal Values	Mean
0 h		08:50	0		
1 h	Stomach	09:53	28	11%-39%	25%
2 h	Stomach	10:54	31	40%-76%	58%
4 h	Stomach	12:48	56	84%-98%	91%
6 h	Small bowel	14:51	26	46%-98%	72%

Emptying was delayed at 2 hours (31% emptied) and 4 hours (56% emptied). Tc-99m indicates technetium Tc 99m; TC-SC, technetium sulfur colloid. Red box outlines the abnormal gastric emptying and reduced colonic filling results, probably due to the delayed gastric emptying.

Figure 5.8   Colonic Transit

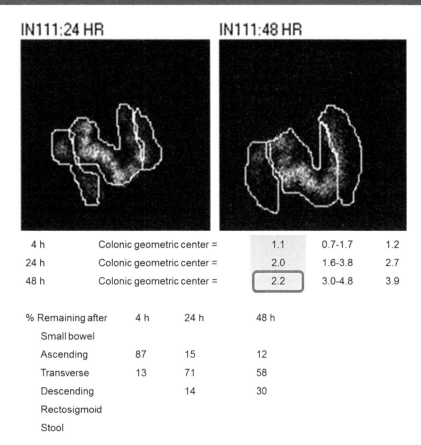

IN111:24 HR   IN111:48 HR

4 h	Colonic geometric center =		1.1	0.7-1.7	1.2
24 h	Colonic geometric center =		2.0	1.6-3.8	2.7
48 h	Colonic geometric center =		2.2	3.0-4.8	3.9

% Remaining after	4 h	24 h	48 h
Small bowel			
Ascending	87	15	12
Transverse	13	71	58
Descending		14	30
Rectosigmoid			
Stool			

Predominant retention is in the transverse colon, 71% at 24 hours and 58% at 48 hours. In111 indicates indium In 111. Red box outlines the 48-hour geometric center, which indicates slow colonic transit. The change from 24 to 48 hours is below the lower limit of normal (for males >0.290, for females >0.380).

Figure 5.9   Electrocardiogram Showing Absence of Sinus Arrhythmia

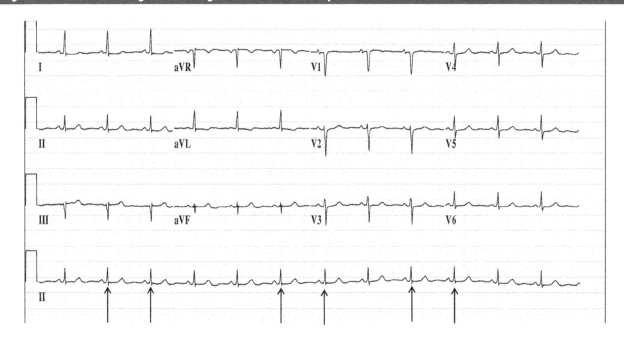

This finding, shown by the consistent R-R interval (arrows), suggests cardiovagal neuropathy.

Figure 5.10   Delayed Colonic Transit at 24 Hours in Patients With Diabetes Mellitus and Autonomic Neuropathy

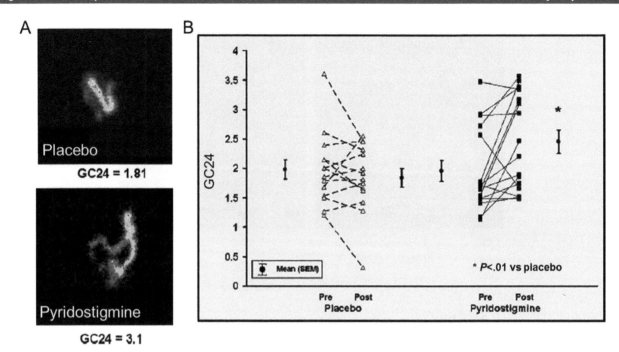

A, Retention was predominantly in transverse colon; isotope progressed to distal colon with pyridostigmine. B, Placebo had no overall effect, in contrast to the increase in geometric center at 24 hours after pyridostigmine (GC24), a finding indicating accelerated colonic transit.

(Modified from Bharucha AE, Low P, Camilleri M, Veil E, Burton D, Kudva Y, et al. A randomised controlled study of the effect of cholinesterase inhibition on colon function in patients with diabetes mellitus and constipation. Gut. 2013 May;62(5):708-15; used with permission.)

The diagnoses were diabetic vagal neuropathy with gastroparesis; slow-transit constipation, probably due to the type 1 diabetes mellitus; and autonomic neuropathy. Treatment options included the acetylcholinesterase inhibitor pyridostigmine, 60 mg 3 times daily. Clinical research studies have found acceleration of colonic transit and amelioration of bowel function with this agent (Figures 5.10 and 5.11).

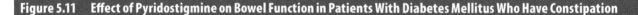

Figure 5.11   Effect of Pyridostigmine on Bowel Function in Patients With Diabetes Mellitus Who Have Constipation

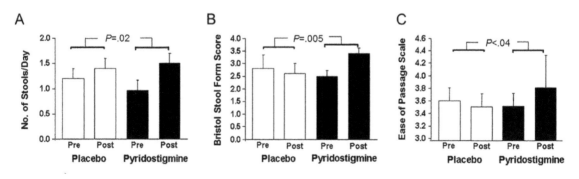

A, Stool frequency. B, Stool form. C, Ease of passage.

(From Bharucha AE, Low P, Camilleri M, Veil E, Burton D, Kudva Y, et al. A randomised controlled study of the effect of cholinesterase inhibition on colon function in patients with diabetes mellitus and constipation. Gut. 2013 May;62(5):708-15; used with permission.)

Case 5

A 43-year-old woman with a recent history of breast cancer (will require chemotherapy and radiotherapy) presented with a 3-year history of chronic vomiting. She was extensively evaluated elsewhere, including upper gastrointestinal endoscopy, gastroduodenal manometry, esophageal manometry and impedance, and reflux pH testing, results of which were negative. She had undergone cholecystectomy for a small stone in the gallbladder.

The patient experienced daily, effortless vomiting occurring after every meal, starting within 1 hour of eating, typically immediately after breakfast. The patient reported the food tasted just like the food she had just eaten as it regurgitated to the throat. Sometimes she had acid or a burning sensation with food coming back into her throat. She did not reswallow the food but expelled it from the throat and mouth.

The patient has rumination syndrome, which is characterized by repetitive regurgitation of gastric contents, occurring within minutes after a meal; the episodes often persist for 1 to 2 hours; the regurgitant consists, at least partially, of recognizable food; and regurgitation is effortless or preceded by a sensation of belching immediately before arrival of food in the pharynx. Typically, no retching or nausea precedes the regurgitation. The patient then makes a conscious decision: swallow or spit the regurgitated material, and this is often determined by the volume of the regurgitated material. This regurgitation happens every day, with every meal: a "meal in, meal out, day in, day out" behavior. The patient insisted on undergoing more tests, which showed modestly delayed GE (Figure 5.12) and normal gastric accommodation (432 mL, normal >428 mL).

Rumination syndrome is characterized by involuntary abdominal contractions that result in food

Figure 5.12   Gastric Emptying May Be Modestly Delayed in Rumination Syndrome as Food Moves Back and Forth in the Stomach

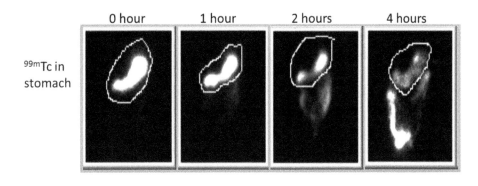

Time (h)	Region	% Emptied	Normal Mean (%)	Normal Range (%)
0	Stomach	0	0	
1	Stomach	13	25	11%-39%
2	Stomach	44	58	40%-76%
4	Stomach	82	91	84%-98%

99mTc indicates technetium Tc 99m. Red box outlines borderline gastric emptying at 2 hours, which may reflect movement of meal back and forth in stomach regions as part of rumination syndrome.

Figure 5.13   Proposed Pathophysiology of Rumination Syndrome

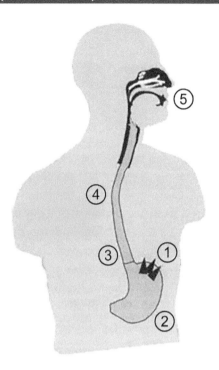

Gastric distention occurs with food (1); abdomen compresses (2); lower esophageal sphincter relaxes (3); gastric contents are regurgitated (4); and food is expelled or reswallowed, depending on social circumstances (5).

(Modified from Malcolm A, Thumshirn MB, Camilleri M, Williams DE. Rumination syndrome. Mayo Clin Proc. 1997;72(7):646-52; used with permission.)

regurgitation; there is evidence that lower fundic pressures are required to induce lower esophageal sphincter relaxation (Figure 5.13). Prolonged pH monitoring studies show early postprandial acidification in the esophagus with no such reflux episodes in the supine position (Figure 5.14), in contrast to the usual preponderance of reflux at night, when patients are supine, in classic gastroesophageal reflux disease.

Figure 5.14   Meal-related "Reflux" With No Pain and No Supine pH Drops in Rumination Syndrome (A), in Contrast to True Reflux, Which Occurs Postprandially and Is Aggravated in Supine Position (B)

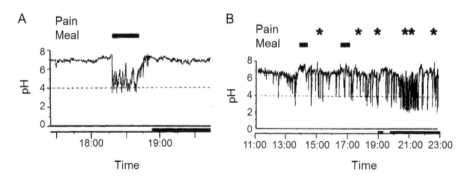

Asterisks indicate patient report of pain; bars on time axis indicate when patient was supine.

(From Malcolm A, Thumshirn MB, Camilleri M, Williams DE. Rumination syndrome. Mayo Clin Proc. 1997;72(7):646-52; used with permission.)

Figure 5.15   High-Resolution Manometry (A) With Impedance Measurement (B) Showing Flow

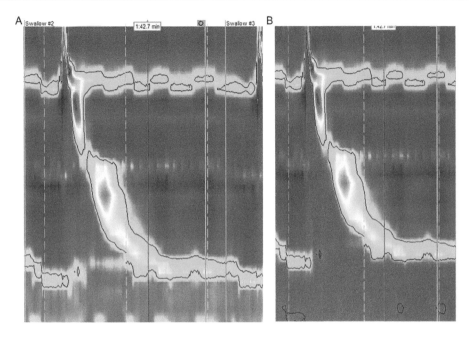

Purple areas indicate presence of fluid in the esophagus, measured as impedance.

(Courtesy of M. Halland, MD, Mayo Clinic, Rochester, Minnesota; used with permission.)

Specialized high-resolution manometry, with impedance (flow) measurements, shows the retrograde flow during episodes of rumination (Figures 5.15 and 5.16). This can be corrected by behavioral intervention with diaphragmatic breathing (Figures 5.17 and 5.18), which this patient underwent.

Figure 5.16   High-Resolution Manometry (A) With Impedance Measurement (B) Showing Flow

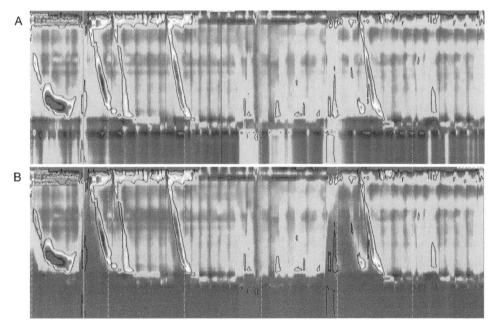

Rumination with retrograde flow followed by normal swallows.

Figure 5.17   Behavioral Intervention for the Treatment of Rumination

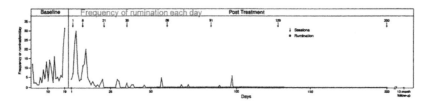

This is the record of the first patient treated with diaphragmatic breathing behavioral modification at Mayo Clinic. Arrows indicate treatment sessions; numbers above arrows, day on which treatment occurred. Duration of each treatment was about 45 minutes.

(From Wagaman JR, Williams DE, Camilleri M. Behavioral intervention for the treatment of rumination. J Pediatr Gastroenterol Nutr. 1998;27(5):596-8; used with permission.)

Figure 5.18   High-Resolution Manometry With Impedance Measurement During Diaphragmatic Breathing

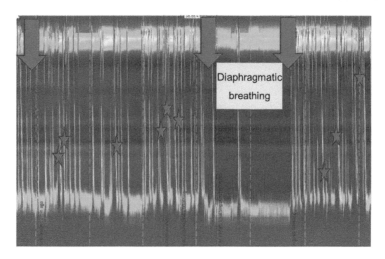

Red arrows indicate diaphragmatic breathing; red stars, aborted episodes of rumination.

Case 6

A 21-year-old woman presented with a 5-year history of her "stomach not allowing food to digest." She reported effortless food regurgitation daily, immediately after every meal, which might persist for several hours, affecting both solids and liquids. Initially the regurgitated material did not taste like acid and she would reswallow it, but later it tasted like acid or was bitter and she would then not reswallow the regurgitant. She reported other symptoms of abdominal bloating, nausea with no vomiting, weight fluctuation, burning retrosternal sensation, and constipation.

Her past medical history included anorexia nervosa, bulimia, bipolar disorder, attention-deficit/hyperactivity disorder, esophagogastroduodenoscopy showing grade C esophagitis (Los Angeles classification), abnormal gastroesophageal junction, and hypotensive lower esophageal sphincter on esophageal manometry that led to laparoscopic Nissen fundoplication. Unfortunately, this procedure was complicated by a leak, leading to localized gastric resection and requiring gastrostomy tube feeding for 3 months.

On physical examination, her body mass index was 18.3 kg/m^2 and the abdomen showed multiple scars, normal bowel sounds, and no succussion splash, organomegaly, or mass. Rectal examination showed no signs of evacuation disorder. GE testing showed marked retention of solids, gastric accommodation was reduced, and there was evidence of vagal dysfunction based on the pancreatic polypeptide response to modified sham feeding (Figures 5.19 through 5.21).

The patient underwent treatment with diaphragmatic breathing for rumination syndrome; homogenized solids and liquid-formula metoclopramide, 5 mg

Figure 5.19   Gastric Emptying of Solids

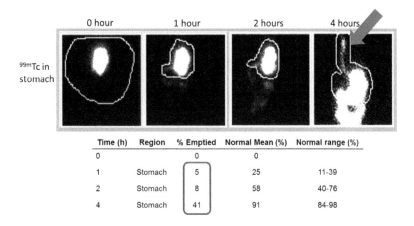

Time (h)	Region	% Emptied	Normal Mean (%)	Normal range (%)
0		0	0	
1	Stomach	5	25	11-39
2	Stomach	8	58	40-76
4	Stomach	41	91	84-98

Emptying is markedly delayed: 5% emptied at 1 hour; 8% emptied at 2 hours; 41% emptied at 4 hours (outlined in red box). Esophagus contains regurgitated material 4 hours after meal ingestion (arrow). ^{99m}Tc indicates technetium Tc 99m.

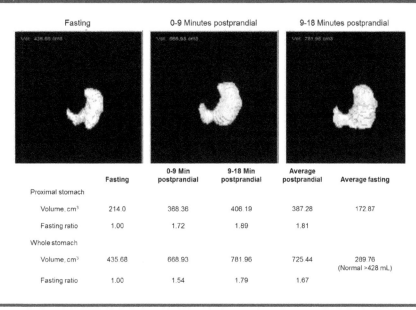

	Fasting	0-9 Min postprandial	9-18 Min postprandial	Average postprandial	Average fasting
Proximal stomach					
Volume, cm³	214.0	368.36	406.19	387.28	172.87
Fasting ratio	1.00	1.72	1.89	1.81	
Whole stomach					
Volume, cm³	435.68	668.93	781.96	725.44	289.76 (Normal >428 mL)
Fasting ratio	1.00	1.54	1.79	1.67	

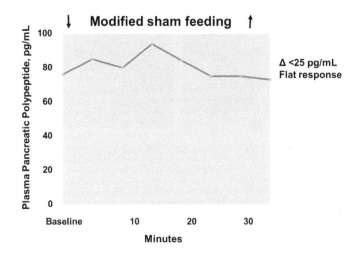

The increase in plasma pancreatic polypeptide is less than 25 pg/mL relative to baseline in samples obtained during sham feeding. This finding is consistent with abdominal vagal dysfunction, but it does not differentiate reversible dysfunction from complete denervation.

4 times a day, for severe gastroparesis; buspirone, 5 mg twice a day, for poor accommodation and anxiety; and a slurry containing aluminum and magnesium salts, 30 mL 3 times a day, for bile acid reflux.

Case 7

An 18-year-old woman presented with a 10-year history of abdominal pain. The pain was sharp, located in the epigastrium, without radiation, and relieved by lying down, curling up in bed, or stooping forward. She experienced vomiting that was worse with fast foods, red sauces, and anxiety and was associated with nausea and loss of appetite. Food would regurgitate in an effortless manner, almost on its own, without any straining, retching, or contraction of the abdominal muscles. The regurgitated food consisted of material that contained unchanged food, but, when regurgitation occurred repeatedly, the regurgitant was bitter or acidic to taste. Three esophagogastroduodenoscopies and colonoscopy elsewhere had negative results. She had been given domperidone, 1 to 2 10-mg tablets, to be taken immediately after waking in the morning.

On examination, there was palpable stool in the lower right and left quadrants of the abdomen and, on rectal examination, 2 of 4 maneuvers to evacuate the examining finger were associated with paradoxic contraction of the puborectalis and anal sphincter.

Gastric and small bowel transit were unremarkable. Physiologic tests showed reduced gastric accommodation (290 mL; normal, >428 mL) and retardation of colonic transit with predominant retention in the left colon (Figures 5.22 and 5.23).

On anorectal manometry, resting anal pressure was 160 mm Hg, squeeze anal pressure was 289 mm Hg, and rectoanal pressure differential was −30.6 mm Hg. Balloon expulsion was achieved with addition of 94 g.

The diagnoses were rumination syndrome plus rectal evacuation disorder, delayed GE, and reduced gastric accommodation.

Among 438 patients evaluated for rectal evacuation disorder at Mayo Clinic over a 19-year period, 57 (13%) had concomitant rumination syndrome: 95% females, 89% white, mean age (SD) 30.3 (1.6) years (8 being <18 years old), and body mass index (SD) 20.8 (0.5) kg/m^2 (15 having body mass index <18.5 kg/m^2) (Table 5.2).

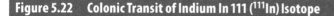

Figure 5.22   Colonic Transit of Indium In 111 (^{111}In) Isotope

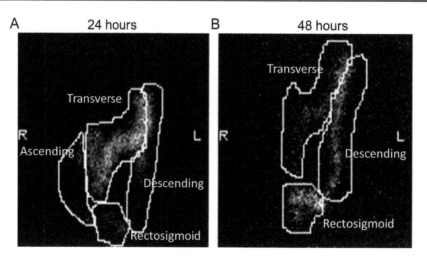

Time (h)	Colonic GC	Normal Range (%)
24	2.3	1.3-4.4
48	3.2	1.9-5.0

A and B, Predominant retention in the left colon, especially the rectosigmoid region at 48 hours (B). Overall numerical values for colonic transit are normal. GC indicates geometric center; L, left; R, right.

Figure 5.23   Slow Gastrointestinal and Colonic Transit

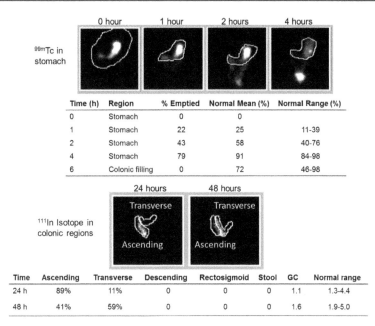

Time (h)	Region	% Emptied	Normal Mean (%)	Normal Range (%)
0	Stomach	0	0	
1	Stomach	22	25	11-39
2	Stomach	43	58	40-76
4	Stomach	79	91	84-98
6	Colonic filling	0	72	46-98

Time	Ascending	Transverse	Descending	Rectosigmoid	Stool	GC	Normal range
24 h	89%	11%	0	0	0	1.1	1.3-4.4
48 h	41%	59%	0	0	0	1.6	1.9-5.0

The most common cause of slow small bowel transit (low colonic filling at 6 hours) is slow colonic transit. GC indicates geometric center; ^{111}In, indium In 111; ^{99m}Tc, technetium Tc 99m.

Table 5.2   Anorectal Dysfunction in 57 Patients With Rumination Syndrome and Rectal Evacuation Disorder

Clinical Feature	Feature Present/Feature Documented in Medical Record, No. of Patients	% of Patients
Rectal evacuation disorder history		
Support perineum	2/26	8
Anal digitation	7/35	20
Vaginal digitation	0/28	0
Excessive strain	32/40	80
Incomplete rectal evacuation	15/22	68
Digital rectal examination		
Decreased perianal sensation	0/38	0
Decreased perineal descent (≤1 cm)	43/53	81
Resting anal sphincter pressure	26/52	50
Paradoxical contractions	24/37	65
Puborectalis tenderness	28/39	72
Rectal examination combinations		
All	9/56	16
3	12/56	21
2	17/56	30
1	15/56	27
None	3/56	5

From Vijayvargiya P, Iturrino J, Camilleri M, Shin A, Vazquez-Roque M, Katzka DA, et al. Novel association of rectal evacuation disorder and rumination syndrome: diagnosis, co-morbidities and treatment. United European Gastroenterol J. 2014 Feb 1;2(1):38-46; used with permission.

Case 8

A 50-year-old woman presented with a 2-year history of constant epigastric pain, nausea, and malaise. She had a history of "gastroparesis" not responding to treatment,; she also had an antecedent history of food poisoning, starting with vomiting and diarrhea, during a visit to the Dominican Republic, suggesting a possible post-viral cause. In relation to her other complaint of constipation, she had 4 biological children born by vaginal delivery, and she had features suggesting descending perineum syndrome: excessive straining, vaginal splinting, and anal digitation to evacuate. Anorectal manometry showed a resting anal sphincter pressure of 39 mm Hg and squeeze anal sphincter pressure of 91 mm Hg, and balloon expulsion was achieved with no weight added. Gastrointestinal and colonic transit were slow, and colonic tone was essentially reduced, but the compliance measurement was normal, and this finding excluded megacolon (Figure 5.24).

The diagnosis was colonic inertia and descending perineum syndrome. Management was strengthening of anal sphincters first, followed by laparoscopic colectomy with ileorectal anastomosis.

Figure 5.24   Colonic Tone at 14 mm Hg Baseline Operating Pressure

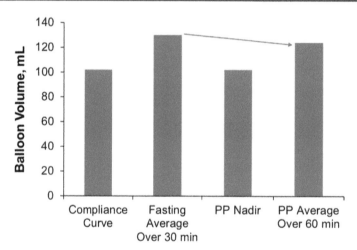

The minimal tone increase after the meal was consistent with colonic inertia. The volume of the 10-cm balloon at 14 mm Hg distention during measurement of compliance was approximately 100 mL, a finding excluding megacolon as the cause of the colonic inertia. PP indicates postprandial.

Conclusion

Several options can be followed when a patient presents with nausea and vomiting:

- Inquire whether the patient has constipation and/or rumination

- Examine the whole patient (especially pupils, rectum)

- Consider iatrogenic disease

- Measure whole gastrointestinal and colonic transit, not just GE

- Have a low threshold to evaluate rectal emptying

- Occam's razor (aka, law of economy or law of parsimony), "Among competing hypotheses, the hypothesis with the fewest assumptions should be selected," does not work in many patients presenting with nausea and vomiting, and there may be more than 1 cause of a patient's symptoms.

Pathophysiologic Mechanisms of Appetite, Obesity, and Gut Hormones[a]

Introduction

Multiple peripheral mechanisms regulate appetite, including the rate of gastric emptying (GE) and fasting and accommodation gastric volumes. The stomach is one of the organs that convey symptoms of satiation to the brain. Several peripherally released peptides and hormones originating from the stomach, small bowel, and pancreas provide feedback on arrival of nutrients in different regions of the gut. The release of these chemicals (paracrine, endocrine, or neurocrine messengers) exerts effects on satiation centers in the brainstem or hypothalamus or regulates metabolism (particularly glucose) through their incretin effects. Ultimately, input to the highly organized hypothalamic circuits and vagal complex of nuclei leads to cessation of energy intake during meal ingestion. Conversely, when the levels of these peptides and hormones are reduced during the interdigestive period, appetite and hunger return over time. In the overall control of appetite, one cannot underestimate the important roles of motivation and behavioral aspects of feeding, the interaction with input of hypothalamic peptidergic circuits to vagal nuclei, and hormones derived from adipose tissue (Figures 6.1 and 6.2).

An understanding of the neural and hormonal mechanisms (Figure 6.3 and see Figure 3.3) and the functions of the stomach is essential to physiologic control of feeding, as is an understanding of the derangements that occur in obesity and their restoration with treatment (as demonstrated by the effects of bariatric surgery) and of the scientific rationale for the potential for novel therapeutic approaches for anorexia, cachexia, and obesity.

Definitions of Satiation and Satiety

Satiation is the pleasant postprandial feeling of fullness; increased satiation may be associated with discomfort and other symptoms such as nausea or bloating. Practical measurements of satiation are the volume to comfortable fullness, the maximum tolerated volume of a liquid nutrient meal, and the intraprandial and postprandial symptoms experienced with the nutrient drink test, as discussed in Chapter 2 ("Measurement of Gastrointestinal and Colonic Motility in Clinical Practice") and shown in Figure 6.4. Normal values for adults and adolescents have been published (Figure 6.5). Volume to feeling comfortably full is indicated by grade 3 on the satiation scale.

Satiety is the appetite to ingest meals after a period of fasting, and it may be operationally defined by the kilocalories ingested at an ad libitum buffet meal after

---

[a] Portions previously published in Camilleri M. Peripheral Mechanisms in Appetite Regulation. Gastroenterology. 2015;148(6):1219-33; used with permission.

Figure 6.1   Complex Motivational Behavior in Feeding

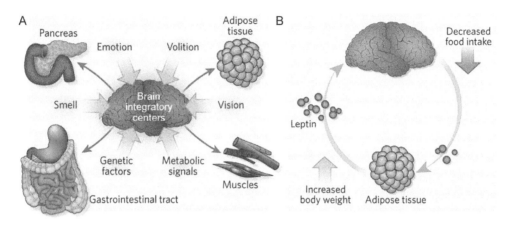

A, Feeding is a complex motivational behavior. Several behavioral, genetic, and metabolic signals regulate feeding through signals that travel from distinct peripheral tissues to integratory centers in the brain. After processing these signals, the brain modifies feeding and also sends appropriate commands to specific peripheral tissues to regulate metabolism. B, Leptin and the control of body fat. With increased body weight, adipose tissue secretes higher levels of leptin. This hormone then travels to the brain, where it binds to leptin receptors in various regions, including the hypothalamus. The result is a sensation of satiety and thus a decrease in food intake. Conversely, a reduction in body weight lowers leptin levels and increases food intake. Thus, relative constancy of weight can be maintained.

(From Friedman JM. Obesity: Causes and control of excess body fat. Nature. 2009 May 21;459(7245):340-2; used with permission.)

a specified time from a prior standard meal, typically ingested 4 hours previously (eg, a 300-kcal meal).

There is a significant relationship between satiation (volume to comfortable fullness) during a nutrient drink test and satiety at a buffet meal (Figure 6.6), and both are also inversely correlated with the rate of GE. Thus, slow emptying characterized by a longer GE of half the radioactivity in a test meal is associated with lower calorie intake.

Postprandial satiation and satiety are critically relevant to the development of obesity (Figure 6.7) because they determine the total energy consumed daily and, therefore, affect the balance between energy consumed and expended.

Phases of Digestion

Gastric motility is critically involved in the cephalic, gastric, and enteric phases of digestion; these functions are integrated.

Taste and other visceral sensations project along vagal afferents into the nucleus of the solitary tract, which is the vagal sensory complex. This tract is linked to the dorsal motor nucleus of the vagus in the brainstem to activate the processes of digestion. The dorsal motor nucleus of the vagus is the nucleus from which efferents from the vagus control diverse functions of the foregut and midgut, including the cephalic phase of gastric motility and digestion. The nucleus of the solitary tract and the dorsal motor nucleus of the vagus are linked through neurons secreting acetylcholine, neuropeptide Y, and thyrotrophin-releasing hormone. The vagus nerve's main neurotransmitter is acetylcholine. A coordinated digestive response, including gastric acid and pepsin secretion, gastric motility and emptying, and integrated pancreaticobiliary secretion, involves other modulators, specifically cholecystokinin (CCK) and gastrin. Descending projections from higher senses in the forebrain, as well as centers of olfaction and vision, modulate these brainstem (predominantly vagal) reflexes.

Motor and secretory functions of the upper gut and midgut that are stimulated by cephalic mechanisms contribute to more than half of the overall postprandial response. Food ingestion results in release of several hormones from the upper gut (gastrin, CCK,

Figure 6.2   Hormonal and Neural Pathways Regulate Food Intake

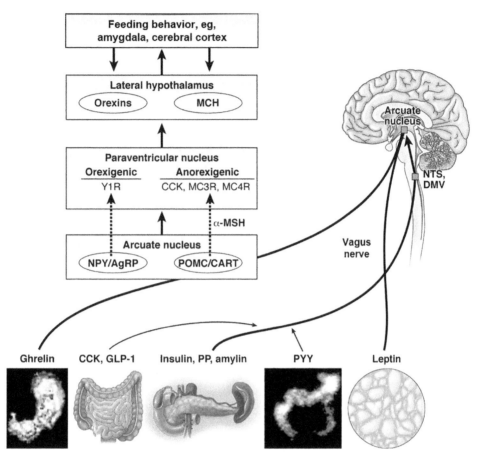

Peripheral and central factors modulating appetite centers in the brain are shown. Gastrointestinal and fat-derived hormones stimulate specific areas of the hypothalamus and brainstem that sense nutrients and coordinate the response to hunger and the intake of food. The arcuate nucleus in the hypothalamus receives input from brainstem (eg, vagal) nuclei and direct stimulation by circulating hormones through an incomplete blood-brain barrier. Neurons in the arcuate nucleus are either orexigenic (eg, contain neuropeptide Y [NPY] through Y1 receptors [Y1R] or agouti-related peptide [AgRP]) or anorexigenic (eg, contain pro-opiomelanocortin [POMC], cocaine- and amphetamine-related transcript [CART]). POMC is a precursor of α-melanocyte stimulating hormone (α-MSH). Ultimately, other regions of the hypothalamus (the paraventricular nucleus and lateral hypothalamus) and higher centers (such as amygdala, limbic system, and cerebral cortex) are stimulated to change feeding behavior by influencing the functions of the same hypothalamic nuclei. CCK indicates cholecystokinin; DMV, dorsal motor nucleus of the vagus nerve; GLP-1, glucagon-like peptide-1; MC4R, melanocortin-4 receptor; MCH, melanin-concentrating hormone; MC3R, melanocortin-3 receptor; NTS, nucleus of the tractus solitarius; PP, pancreatic polypeptide; PYY, peptide tyrosine-tyrosine.

(From Camilleri M. Peripheral mechanisms in appetite regulation. Gastroenterology. 2015 May;148(6):1219-33 as redrawn from Camilleri M, Grudell AB. Appetite and obesity: a gastroenterologist's perspective. Neurogastroenterol Motil. 2007 May;19(5):333-41; used with permission; with data from Kopelman PG, Grace C. New thoughts on managing obesity. Gut. 2004 Jul;53(7):1044-53 and Huda MS, Wilding JP, Pinkney JH. Gut peptides and the regulation of appetite. Obes Rev. 2006 May;7(2):163-82.)

glucose-dependent insulinotropic peptide [GIP], ghrelin, gastric leptin, and pancreatic polypeptide) that activate gastrointestinal (GI) motility, gastric and pancreaticobiliary secretion, digestion, and absorption. Incretins such as glucagon-like peptide (GLP)-1, peptide YY, and oxyntomodulin secreted from the proximal and distal small bowel counter postprandial glycemia, inhibit the cephalic phase mediated through the vagus nerve, and reduce appetite. Hormones such as CCK and GIP, released from the duodenum and most proximal small bowel, inhibit gastric motility, relax the gastric fundus, inhibit antral contractions or stimulate pyloric contraction to inhibit GE, slow meal digestion, and induce satiation.

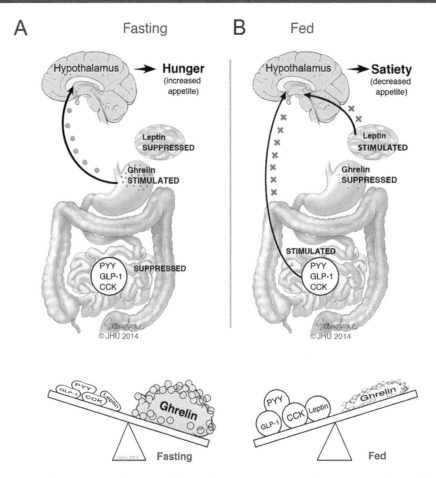

A, During the fasting/preprandial state, ghrelin released from the stomach acts on the arcuate nucleus of the hypothalamus and vagus nucleus in the brainstem to stimulate hunger. B, In the postprandial state, anorectic hormones (peptide tyrosine tyrosine [PYY], glucagon-like peptide [GLP]-1, oxyntomodulin, and pancreatic polypeptide) released from the intestine act on the arcuate nucleus, brainstem, and vagus nerve to cause satiation. CCK indicates cholecystokinin.

(From Weiss CR, Gunn AJ, Kim CY, Paxton BE, Kraitchman DL, Arepally A. Bariatric embolization of the gastric arteries for the treatment of obesity. J Vasc Interv Radiol. 2015 May;26(5):613-24; used with permission of John Hopkins University.)

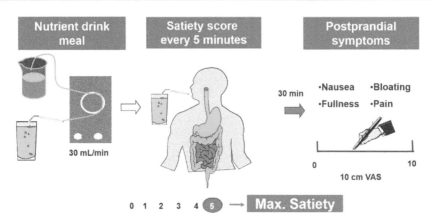

Max indicates maximum; VAS, visual analog scale.

(Modified from Delgado-Aros S, Kim DY, Burton DD, Thomforde GM, Stephens D, Brinkmann BH, et al. Effect of GLP-1 on gastric volume, emptying, maximum volume ingested, and postprandial symptoms in humans. Am J Physiol Gastrointest Liver Physiol. 2002 Mar;282(3):G424-31.)

Figure 6.5   Satiation: Adult and Adolescent Normal Values

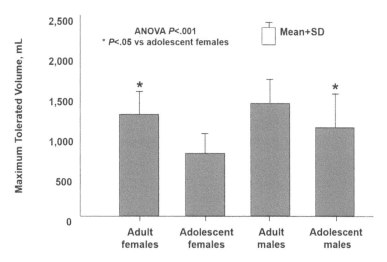

Liquid nutrient drink at 30 mL/min. ANOVA indicates analysis of variance.

(Data from Chial HJ, Camilleri C, Delgado-Aros S, Burton D, Thomforde G, Ferber I, et al. A nutrient drink test to assess maximum tolerated volume and postprandial symptoms: effects of gender, body mass index and age in health. Neurogastroenterol Motil. 2002 Jun;14(3):249-53.)

Figure 6.6   Satiation and Satiety

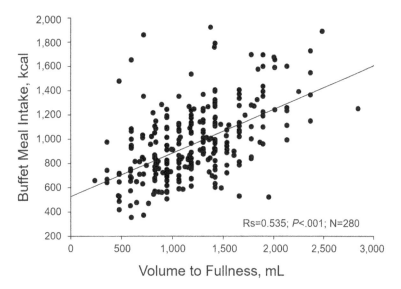

There is a significant relationship between satiation (volume to comfortable fullness) during nutrient drink test and satiety at a buffet meal. Rs indicates Spearman rank correlation coefficient.

(From Halawi H, Camilleri M, Acosta A, Vazquez-Roque M, Oduyebo I, Burton D, et al. Relationship of gastric emptying or accommodation with satiation, satiety, and post-prandial symptoms in health. Am J Physiol Gastrointest Liver Physiol. 2017 Nov 1;313(5):G442-7.)

Figure 6.7   Is Obesity a Problem of the Brain-Gut Axis?

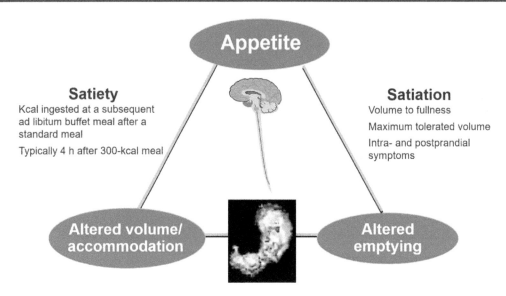

Obesity is related to appetite, satiation (operationally measured as volume to fullness or maximum tolerated volume), and satiety (operationally measured as kcal intake at an ad libitum meal). All functions are influenced by gastric volume, accommodation, and emptying.

Role of Gastric Motor Functions in Postprandial Symptoms, Satiation, and Satiety

In patients with dyspepsia, gastric motor functions (such as emptying and accommodation) and gastric sensation induce symptoms during and after a meal. Moreover, fats with at least a 12-carbon chain length influence satiation in health and dyspepsia.

In obese persons, postprandial symptoms such as fullness are affected by small fasting gastric volume, accelerated GE at 1 hour, delayed GE at 4 hours, waist circumference, and behavioral (psychologic) traits; age and sex are statistically significant covariates of the effect of body mass index (BMI) on these functions.

Dysregulation of Gastric Function, Satiety, and Satiation Mechanisms in Obesity

GE may be rapid, normal, or slow in obese persons. Similarly, there is wide variation in stomach size, with no statistically significant or meaningful relationship to body weight except in binge eating disorder which is associated with larger stomach volume (measured using intragastric latex balloon). Obese persons consume more food per minute than nonobese persons. In

relatively small studies (<40 participants), binge eaters choose small, immediate rewards over larger, delayed rewards, a behavior suggesting motor impulsivity and a tendency to respond rapidly without forethought or attention to consequences.

In a prospective study of 328 participants with BMI ranging from normal to class III obesity, obesity was associated with 1 or more phenotypes: higher fasting gastric volume, accelerated GE of solids and liquids, lower postprandial levels of the satiety hormone peptide tyrosine tyrosine (PYY), and higher postprandial GLP-1 levels (which may be the result of accelerated GE of nutrients). Obesity was also associated with reduced satiation (larger maximum tolerated volume). The total calorie intake at an ad libitum meal was not appreciably related to BMI, but it was greater in persons with higher waist circumference.

In a principal components analysis of approximately 500 obese or normal-weight participants, latent dimensions together accounted for approximately 81% of the variance in obesity: satiety/satiation (21%), gastric motility (14%), psychologic (13%), and gastric sensorimotor (11%). Thus, measurements of these quantitative traits associated with obesity (Figures 6.8 through 6.10) may provide the rationale for individualized treatment.

GE of solids and liquids is accelerated in obesity (Figure 6.11); GE of solids is notably associated with

Figure 6.8   Relationship Between Satiation and Obesity

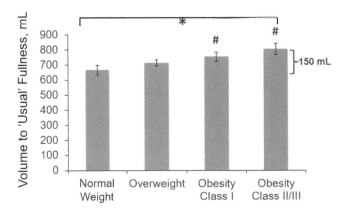

* ANOVA P value <.05;
# P value <.05 compared with normal weight
(Dunnett test)

Volume to fullness is greater in obesity class I or II/III. ANOVA indicates analysis of variance.

(Data from Acosta A, Camilleri M, Shin A, Vazquez-Roque MI, Iturrino J, Burton D, et al. Quantitative gastrointestinal and psychological traits associated with obesity and response to weight-loss therapy. Gastroenterology. 2015 Mar;148(3):537-46.)

calorie intake at nutrient drink test and ad libitum buffet meal, and faster emptying is associated with increased calorie intake (Figure 6.12). The relevance of these factors is also demonstrated by effects of sleeve gastrectomy on appetite and weight loss (discussed below).

Principal Sites of Synthesis of GI Peptides Implicated in Regulation of Food Intake

The principal sites of synthesis of GI peptides or amines implicated in the regulation of food intake are illustrated in Figure 6.13.

The GI hormones released from the foregut, midgut, and hindgut affect hunger and satiety by effects mediated through behavioral brain effects (Table 6.1), although several also have feedback effects inhibiting gastric functions that may also result in satiation.

For example, CCK, GLP-1, and PYY retard GE. In obesity, there is a reduction in peak postprandial PYY levels (Figure 6.14), and this decrease may be a factor

Figure 6.9   Gastric Volume and Accommodation Measured by Single-Photon Emission Computed Tomography (SPECT)

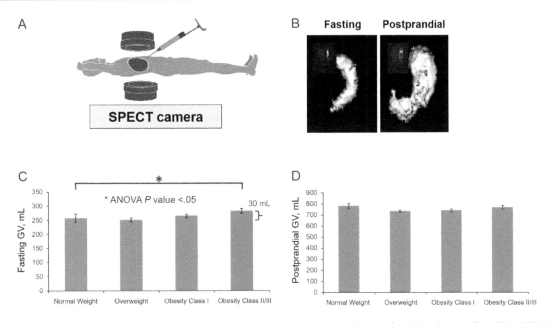

(A through D) SPECT shows higher fasting but normal postprandial gastric volume (GV) in class II/III obesity (C and D). ANOVA indicates analysis of variance.

(Modified from Delgado-Aros S, Kim DY, Burton DD, Thomforde GM, Stephens D, Brinkmann BH, et al. Effect of GLP-1 on gastric volume, emptying, maximum volume ingested, and postprandial symptoms in humans. Am J Physiol Gastrointest Liver Physiol. 2002 Mar;282(3):G424-31; Data from Acosta A, Camilleri M, Shin A, Vazquez-Roque MI, Iturrino J, Burton D, et al. Quantitative gastrointestinal and psychological traits associated with obesity and response to weight-loss therapy. Gastroenterology. 2015 Mar;148(3):537-46.)

Figure 6.10 Satiety Test: Ad Libitum Buffet Meal 4 Hours After Standard 300 kcal Liquid Breakfast

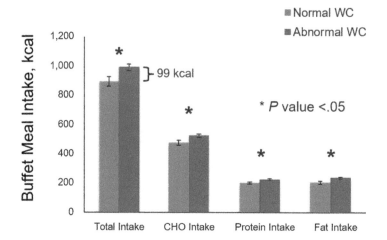

Central obesity associated with larger waist circumference (WC) is associated with 50 to 100 kcal more ingested during meal; increased calorie intake over time would lead to obesity. CHO indicates carbohydrate; World Health Organization WC classification: normal women, <88 cm; normal men, <102 cm.

(Data from Acosta A, Camilleri M, Shin A, Vazquez-Roque MI, Iturrino J, Burton D, et al. Quantitative gastrointestinal and psychological traits associated with obesity and response to weight-loss therapy. Gastroenterology. 2015 Mar;148(3):537-46.)

Figure 6.11 Association of Altered Gastric Emptying and Body Mass Index

A

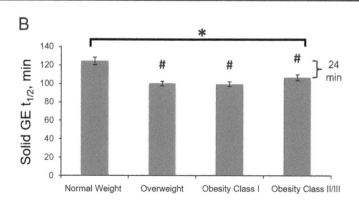

* ANOVA *P*<.05
# *P*<.05 compared with normal
weight (Dunnett test)

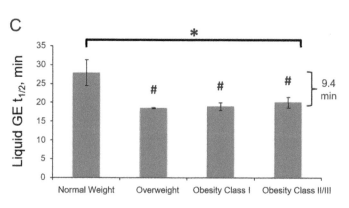

A, External gamma camera imaging of radioisotopically labeled gastric content. Gastric emptying time for half of radioactive meal (GE $t_{1/2}$) of solids (B) and liquids (C) in normal-weight persons compared with that in overweight and obese persons. ANOVA indicates analysis of variance.

(Data from Acosta A, Camilleri M, Shin A, Vazquez-Roque MI, Iturrino J, Burton D, et al. Quantitative gastrointestinal and psychological traits associated with obesity and response to weight-loss therapy. Gastroenterology. 2015 Mar;148(3):537-46.)

Figure 6.12   Relationship of Gastric Emptying (Measured With Scintigraphy) With Satiation (Nutrient Drink Test) and With Satiety (Buffet Meal kcal Intake) Measurements

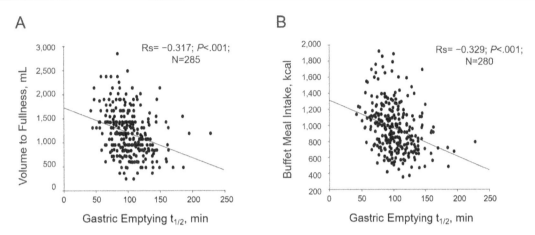

The kcal intake is lower with both nutrient drink (1 mL = 1 kcal) ingested at 30 mL/min (A) and ad libitum buffet meal (B) with slower gastric emptying time for half of radioactive meal (GE $t_{1/2}$). Rs indicates Spearman rank correlation coefficient.

(From Halawi H, Camilleri M, Acosta A, Vazquez-Roque M, Oduyebo I, Burton D, et al. Relationship of gastric emptying or accommodation with satiation, satiety, and post-prandial symptoms in health. Am J Physiol Gastrointest Liver Physiol. 2017 Nov 1;313(5):G442-7.)

Figure 6.13   Principal Sites of Synthesis of Gastrointestinal Peptides Involved in the Regulation of Food Intake

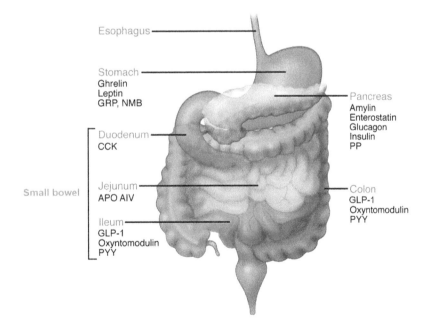

APO AIV indicates apolipoprotein A-IV; CCK, cholecystokinin; GLP-1, glucagon-like peptide-1; GRP, gastrin-releasing peptide; NMB, neuromedin B; PP, pancreatic polypeptide; PYY, peptide YY.

(From Cummings DE, Overduin J. Gastrointestinal regulation of food intake. J Clin Invest. 2007 Jan;117(1):13-23; used with permission.)

Table 6.1   Gastrointestinal Hormones Affecting Hunger and Satiety

Gastrointestinal Hormone	Amino Acid Number	Embryonic Site of Origin	Behavioral Brain Effects	
			Hunger	Satiety
Ghrelin	28	Stomach (upper foregut)	Increased	Decreased
Obestatin	23	Stomach (upper foregut)	Effect unknown	Effect unknown
Pancreatic polypeptide	36	Foregut and midgut	Decreased	Effect unknown
Cholecystokinin	Several	Foregut and midgut	Decreased	Increased
Gastric inhibitory polypeptide	42	Hindgut	Effect unknown	Effect unknown
Glucagon-like peptide-1	30	Hindgut	Decreased	Increased
Oxyntomodulin	37	Hindgut	Decreased	Increased
Peptide YY	36	Hindgut	Decreased	Increased

Modified from Camilleri M. Peripheral mechanisms in the control of appetite and related experimental therapies in obesity. Regul Pept. 2009;156(1–3):24-7; used with permission.

in reducing postprandial satiation and increased food intake.

On the basis of these observations, a principal component analysis in 500 humans at all ranges of the BMI spectrum (Acosta 2015; see suggested reading) identified several latent dimensions in obesity, that is, discrete phenotypic characteristics and behavioral traits (Figure 6.15) that could be considered biomarkers or targets for treatment of obesity based on the principal component analysis: satiety/satiation (21%), psychological/behavioral overeating (19%), gastric sensorimotor function (17%), gastric capacity (14%), peak postprandial hormone levels (9%), and unspecified (20%).

The potential of these biomarkers is shown by the weight loss predictors for phentermine-topiramate

Figure 6.14   Peak Postprandial Polypeptide YY (PYY) Concentration in Obesity

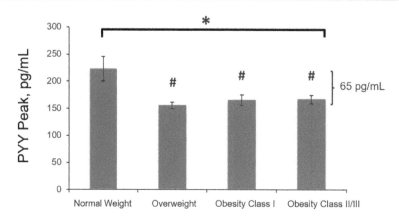

* ANOVA $P<.05$
# $P<.05$ compared with normal weight (Dunnett test)

ANOVA indicates analysis of variance.

(Data from Acosta A, Camilleri M, Shin A, Vazquez-Roque MI, Iturrino J, Burton D, et al. Quantitative gastrointestinal and psychological traits associated with obesity and response to weight-loss therapy. Gastroenterology. 2015 Mar;148(3):537-46.)

Figure 6.15   Behavioral Traits

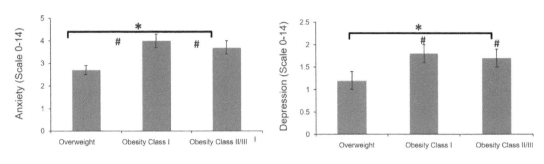

* ANOVA *P*<.05
# *P*<.05 compared with overweight (Dunnett test)

Anxiety and depression are more frequent in obesity, although it is unclear which is the cause and which is the consequence. ANOVA indicates analysis of variance.

(Data from Acosta A, Camilleri M, Shin A, Vazquez-Roque MI, Iturrino J, Burton D, et al. Quantitative gastrointestinal and psychological traits associated with obesity and response to weight-loss therapy. Gastroenterology. 2015 Mar;148(3):537-46.)

extended release (Figure 6.16). Weight loss was predicted by calorie intake at a buffet meal, but it was unrelated to other GI traits (satiation, GE, fasting gastric volume, and postprandial peak PYY).

These data support the notion that gastric motor functions are important predictors of the sensation of fullness or satiation and may determine a person's choice to stop ingesting food.

Figure 6.16   Weight Loss Predictors for Treatment With Phentermine-Topiramate Extended Release (Phen-Top ER)

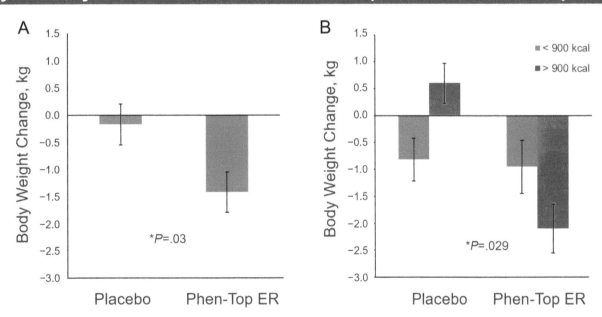

A, Body weight change after 2 weeks of treatment. B, Body weight change after 2 weeks of treatment according to calorie intake in a prior satiety test. The degree of weight loss was substantially greater in obese patients who ingested more than 900 kcal at ad libitum meal. Other gastrointestinal traits (satiation, gastric emptying, fasting gastric volume, and postprandial peak peptide tyrosine tyrosine) were not significant predictors of weight loss.

(Data from Acosta A, Camilleri M, Shin A, Vazquez-Roque MI, Iturrino J, Burton D, et al. Quantitative gastrointestinal and psychological traits associated with obesity and response to weight-loss therapy. Gastroenterology. 2015 Mar;148(3):537-46.)

Gut-Brain Communication

The vagal nuclei and the vagus nerve provide the extrinsic neural control of the sections of the GI tract involved in energy intake, satiation, and digestion. As a result of change in viscus tension by food, or later chyme, and of response to chemical stimuli activating taste receptors (see below) resulting in the release of peptides or amines from mucosal enteroendocrine cells, the vagal afferents are stimulated to either increase appetite (an orexigenic effect, eg, ghrelin) or induce satiety (eg, gastric leptin, CCK, GLP-1, or PYY).

After absorption from the digestive tract, circulating nutrients can be sensed in the area postrema in the floor of the fourth ventricle, where there is a thin blood-brain barrier. In response, the brainstem affects upper gut functions through the vagus nerve, which modulates the enteric nervous system. Through direct vagal connections to the hypothalamic circuits, calorie intake is reduced when nutrients are sensed by the area postrema. Conversely, interfering with vagal function induces early satiety and weight loss, possibly by reducing GE and inducing satiation. Methods that are used for this purpose include, for example, partial vagotomy, total subdiaphragmatic vagotomy, or intermittent vagal nerve electrical stimulation with a US Food and Drug Administration–approved device for obesity treatment.

Mechanisms Regulating Appetite

Several interacting control mechanisms (Figures 6.1 and 6.2) that involve hormonal and neural pathways result in regulation of food intake by the peripheral and central factors that modulate appetite centers in the brain.

Hypothalamic and Brainstem Mechanisms

Hypothalamic circuits that control appetite and food intake involve several peptide receptors or their ligands: cannabinoid molecules, neuropeptide Y, pro-opiomelanocortin, melanin-concentrating hormone, α-melanocyte stimulating hormone, agouti-related peptide, cocaine- and amphetamine-regulated transcript, CCK, and GLP-1. The nuclei in the hypothalamus and brainstem may also be affected by GI hormones, including leptin, cholecystokinin, PYY, oxyntomodulin, and GLP-1; the passage of such hormones from the peripheral circulation into the brain regions occurs where the blood-brain barrier allows direct interaction between these hormones with the nuclei, as occurs with nutrients. Thus, circulating peptides inhibit the agouti-related peptide/neuropeptide Y pathway in the arcuate nucleus of the hypothalamus, thereby reducing appetite, and stimulate the pro-opiomelanocortin/α-melanocyte stimulating hormone pathway, indirectly reducing appetite.

Bidirectional pathways link the nuclei of the hypothalamus to higher centers (reward involving neuropeptide Y and dopaminergic receptors or well-being) and to the brainstem nuclei such as the nucleus of the solitary tract (the nucleus receiving most sensory input from vagal afferents) and dorsal motor nucleus of the vagus (the predominant efferent vagal nucleus). For example, activation of the hypothalamus by intake of food and induction of satiation can result in slow GE by stimulating vagal fibers that activate gastric inhibitory (eg, nitrergic) neurons to decrease gastric motility and, as a consequence, decrease calorie consumption.

The hypothalamus and other brain regions in humans seem to respond differently to the monosaccharides fructose and glucose. Thus, after glucose ingestion, compared with fructose, there is appreciably greater reduction in cerebral blood flow in the hypothalamus and in cerebral cortical areas. There are also differences in connectivity of brain centers in response to these different monosaccharides.

Taste Receptors for Sweet or Amino Acids (Umami)

There are chemosensory molecular mechanisms in neuroepithelial taste receptor cells of the tongue and in gut enteroendocrine cells. This sensing controls digestion and initiates hormonal or afferent (predominantly vagal) pathways leading to regulation of calorie intake, pancreatic insulin secretion, and changes in metabolism (eg, glycemic control). Intestinal mucosal vagal afferent nerve terminals express receptors for several regulatory peptides and neurotransmitters (eg, GLP-1, GLP-2, serotonin).

There are 3 distinct subunits of the G protein–coupled taste receptors (T1Rs) that can be activated by natural sugars, sweet proteins, and artificial sweeteners. These form heterodimers that sense either sweet (T1R2 and T1R3) or amino acids (umami, T1R1 and T1R3). The subunits of T1R2 and T1R3 interact with Gα-gustducin, expressed in intestinal enteroendocrine cells that express PYY in the colon or GLP-1 and serotonin in the small bowel. T1Rs upregulate the sodium-coupled transporter SGLT-1 (sodium-glucose linked transporter 1) and GLUT2 (glucose transporter 2, which is independent of sodium cotransport) in the intestinal epithelium in response to glucose, and T1Rs also regulate GLP-1 secretion. Gut endocrine cells may also detect microbiota because they also express toll-like receptor molecules that recognize bacterial breakdown products.

Gut Peptidergic and Hormonal Control of Response to Feeding and Satiation

Through mechanical, chemical, and osmotic effects, nutrients and their digestion products result in signals (through gastric and duodenal vagal afferents) that initiate digestion and absorption and a feeling of satiation through direct effects on gastric functions or indirectly through stimulation of satiation hormones and transmitters leading to meal termination.

Function of GI Hormones and Incretins on Appetite-Related Mechanisms

The following is a summary of the main effects of the predominant hormones or peptides on food intake or appetite. Ghrelin is an orexigen important in short-term food intake; in contrast, leptin (gastric), a minor orexigen, and obestatin, a peptide encoded by the ghrelin gene, oppose ghrelin's effects on food intake, delay GE, and inhibit jejunal motility. Table 6.2 reviews in greater detail the role of GI peptides and

Table 6.2	**Peptides, Hormones, and Receptors Involved in the Peripheral Control of Upper Gastrointestinal Functions Associated With Satiation and Appetite**	
Peptide/Hormone/ Receptor[a]	**Predominant Site of Synthesis/ Release**	**Main Functions**
Gastrins	17-AA peptide hormone from gastric mucosa	Blood-borne regulator of gastric acid secretion, interacting with somatostatin and EC cells Regulates gastric epithelial organization, proliferation, and function
Motilin	22-AA peptide from duodenal mucosa	Stimulates contractility of gastrointestinal smooth muscle directly and via release of acetylcholine from enteric nerves Plasma motilin fluctuates with changes in phase of MMC in the stomach and small bowel, peaking at end phase II Peaking corresponds with increase in hunger but reduces gastric accommodation and food intake
CCK	Peptide from I cells in duodenal mucosa, particularly >12 carbon fatty acids; molecular forms, eg, CCK 8, 33	Activates vagal afferents directly and modifies the response of vagal mechanosensitive fibers to gastric and duodenal nutrients Relaxes the proximal stomach to increase its reservoir capacity, inhibits GE and acid secretion, gallbladder contraction, and exocrine pancreatic secretion Limits amount of food consumed during an individual meal
CCK1R	Vagal afferents	Induces fullness and nausea in response to duodenal lipid, gastric distention CCK acts on CCK1R to delay GE (antral inhibition, pyloric stimulation) and induce satiation despite increasing gastric accommodation
CCK2R	Hypothalamic nuclei	Controls satiety and appetite
Ghrelin	Acylated 28-AA peptide hormone expressed mostly in stomach (21% sequence identity to motilin)	Growth hormone secretagogue that stimulates pituitary release of GH Stimulates food intake; stimulates appetite via secretion of NPY and orexin and by inhibiting anorexic effects of POMC/α-MSH system Induces metabolic changes, increases weight, fat mass through NPY/AgRP Circulating levels surge shortly before meals and are suppressed by ingested nutrients (carbohydrates > protein > fat) Effects mediated through vagus nerve Stimulates GE and intestinal MMC-like activity, contracts gastric fundus Other actions: stimulates gastric acid, vasodilatation, inhibition of insulin secretion, and antiproliferative effects

(continued)

Table 6.2   Continued

Peptide/Hormone/Receptor[a]	Predominant Site of Synthesis/ Release	Main Functions
GHS-R	G protein–coupled receptor	Distributed in hypothalamus and pituitary, adrenal, thyroid, pancreas, myocardium, spleen, ovary, enteric neurons, and stomach
Leptin	Circulating 16-kDa protein (167 AA) hormone secreted by adipose tissue, placenta, skeletal muscle	Central regulation (arcuate nucleus and other) of food intake and energy balance, storage of fat and insulin signaling Secretion is proportionate to fat stores of the body Decreased leptin induces hunger; starvation reduces leptin levels and increases appetite Regulates feeding behavior and short- and long-term satiation by providing information to brain on availability of external (food) and internal (fat) energy resources
Gastric leptin	Fundic glands and chief cells	Reduced during fasting, rapidly released after food intake by vagal cholinergic stimulation, CCK and secretin, or in response to satiety factors (eg, CCK and insulin)
GLP-1	Hormone co-secreted with PYY from intestinal L cells: GLP-1$_{7-36\,amide}$ is located in the PVN, DMV, NTS, pituitary, and thalamus	Two equipotent biologically active forms: GLP-1$_{7-37}$ and GLP-1$_{7-36\,amide}$ (the major circulating form) cleaved from proglucagon (expressed in gut, pancreas, brain) and rapidly inactivated in the circulation by DPP-4 Incretin hormone that enhances insulin secretion stimulated by oral nutrients; reduces postprandial glucose by ↓ glucagon and ↑ insulin secretion Control of appetite and energy intake in humans Enhanced satiety and fullness after an energy-fixed breakfast, reduced energy intake at an ad libitum lunch, retarded GE, inhibited antral motility, reduced postprandial glycemia, and increased gastric volume (reservoir capacity) ↓ GE and secretion by inhibiting vagal activity
NPY	36-AA peptide hormone in hypothalamus and intestinal neurons	Appetite induction through NPY network in the PVN-ARC of hypothalamus; opposing hormonal signals, such as leptin and ghrelin, regulate secretion of NPY in PVN-ARC Antisecretory effects in small intestine and especially colon; motor inhibitory effects
NPY (Y) receptors	Multiple receptor subtypes Y$_1$ to Y$_5$	Y$_1$, Y$_2$, and Y$_5$ receptor subtypes mediate NPY-induced feeding; central NPY delays GE in rats (through Y$_2$ receptors); intravenous NPY had no effect on human GE
PP	36-AA peptide hormone from D cells in pancreas	Experimentally, anorectic effects with peripheral PP, central PP stimulates food intake; circulating PP levels inversely proportional to adiposity; higher levels with anorexia nervosa, reductions in circulating PP in some studies in obese patients; PP may delay GE
Amylin	37-AA peptide hormone co-secreted with insulin	Inhibits GE and acid and glucagon secretion; decreases meal size and food intake. Functions through vagal inhibition, primarily on area postrema
PYY	Hormone co-secreted with GLP-1 from ileocolonic L cells; active form, PYY$_{3-36}$, results from DPP-4 proteolysis of PYY$_{1-36}$	Secreted postprandially in proportion to calorie load, fat > carbohydrate > protein Stimulates Y$_2$ receptors in hypothalamic ARC nucleus circuitry to regulate food intake; lessened hunger, decreased buffet-meal intake by 36% Activates ileal brake and other feedback control of regional motor function Inhibits gastric acid, pancreatic exocrine, and bile acid secretion Delays GE
OXM	37-AA peptide hormone from intestinal L cells	Acts via GLP-1 receptors to decrease food intake and inhibit gastric acid secretion and GE
Apo A-IV	46-kDa protein hormone from small bowel enterocytes	Synthesized and secreted in response to lipid absorption; exogenous Apo A-IV decreased food intake (mediated centrally) and inhibited gastric acid secretion and motility in rodents

Abbreviations: AA, amino acid; AGRP, agouti-related protein; Apo A-IV, apolipoprotein A-IV; ARC, arcuate nucleus; CCK, cholecystokinin; DMV, dorsal motor nucleus of the vagus nerve; DPP-4, dipeptidyl peptidase 4; EC, enterochromaffin cells; GE, gastric emptying; GH, growth hormone; GHS-R, growth hormone secretagogue receptor; GLP-1, glucagon-like peptide-1; MMC, migrating motor complex; NPY, neuropeptide Y; NTS, nucleus of the tractus solitarius; OXM, oxyntomodulin; POMC/αMSH, pro-opiomelanocortin/α-melanocyte-stimulating hormone; PP, pancreatic polypeptide; PVN, paraventricular nucleus of the hypothalamus; PVN-ARC, paraventricular and arcuate nuclei of the hypothalamus; PYY, peptide tyrosine-tyrosine; ↓, decreased; ↑, increased.

[a] Entries in *italics* are receptors of peptides or hormones.

Modified from Camilleri M. Peripheral mechanisms in appetite regulation. Gastroenterology. 2015 May;148(6):1219-33; used with permission.

Figure 6.17   Motilin Reduces Proximal Stomach Accommodation and Increases Satiation

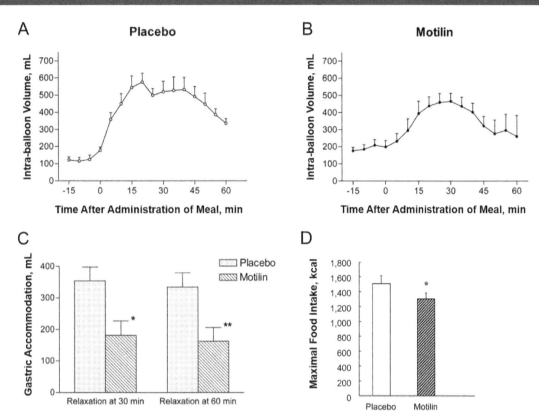

Gastric fundus accommodation to a liquid meal during administration of placebo (A) or motilin (B) in a double-blind, randomized, crossover design. C, Mean gastric relaxation at 30 and 60 minutes after the liquid meal. * $P<.05$ and ** $P<.01$ vs placebo group. D, Influence of motilin on meal-induced satiety in healthy controls. Maximum ingested calories were significantly lower with motilin than with placebo (* $P<.05$ vs placebo).

(From Cuomo R, Vandaele P, Coulie B, Peeters T, Depoortere I, Janssens J, et al. Influence of motilin on gastric fundus tone and on meal-induced satiety in man: role of cholinergic pathways. Am J Gastroenterol. 2006 Apr;101(4):804-11; used with permission.)

hormones released in response to feeding and satiety in humans. Specific effects of several cyclic variations in blood levels of the hormones motilin and ghrelin are shown in Figures 6.17 through 6.19.

Ghrelin is a unique orexigenic hormone that is an acylated 28-amino acid peptide produced (80%-90%) by the stomach and proximal small bowel; it is the endogenous ligand for the growth hormone secretagogue receptor. The effects of ghrelin are summarized in Figure 6.20, and its effects on stimulating interdigestive motility, increasing gastric tone, and accelerating GE are shown in Figures 6.21 and 6.22. At infused doses that mimic physiologic circulating blood levels, ghrelin does not significantly impede gastric accommodation (Figure 6.23).

CCK is a major mediator of satiation, retarding GE, at least in part by fundic relaxation and antral inhibition (Figures 6.24 through 6.27). A CCK-antagonist, dexloxiglumide, reduces postprandial fullness induced by a lipid load into the duodenum (Figure 6.28).

GLP-1 is an incretin that modulates glucose control and retards GE. It is derived from the enzymatic processing of a precursor molecule that also results in production of glucagon and GLP-2 (Figure 6.29). Thus, it inhibits GE (Figures 6.30 and 6.31), and a GLP-1 antagonist increases antral motility and inhibits pyloric tone (Figure 6.32). In the proximal stomach, GLP-1 inhibits gastric tone, and thus gastric accommodation is increased after meals (Figure 6.33).

Figure 6.18   Relationship Among Migrating Motor Complex (MMC) Phases, Plasma Motilin, and Hunger Scores

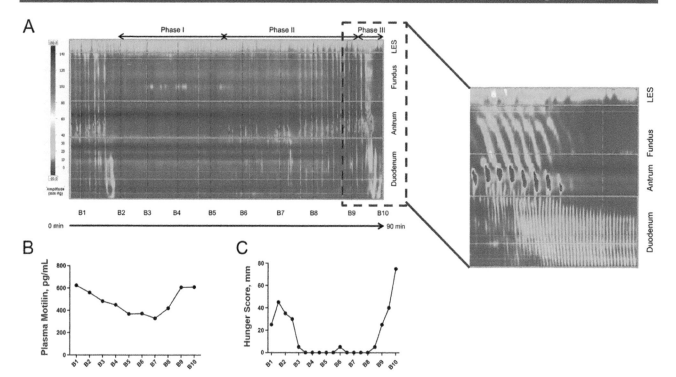

A, Contractions in the MMCs are identified by the dense, light-blue propagated contractions. Phase I refers to motor quiescence; phase II, intermittent contractile activity; and phase III, the propagated contractile activity with contractions occurring at the maximum frequency at each location (3 per minute in the stomach and up to 11 per minute in the small bowel). In the phase III activity front (inset), antral contractions have higher amplitude (red) than fundal and duodenal contractions. Plasma motilin concentration (B) and hunger scores (C) illustrate peaking that coincides with phase III of the MMC. B1-B10 indicate timing of blood samples; LES, lower esophageal sphincter.

(Modified from Deloose E, Tack J. Redefining the functional roles of the gastrointestinal migrating motor complex and motilin in small bacterial overgrowth and hunger signaling. Am J Physiol Gastrointest Liver Physiol. 2016 Feb 15;310(4):G228-33; used with permission.)

The sum total of these effects of GLP-1 on gastric function is illustrated by the effects of liraglutide (GLP-1 analog), which retards GE over 16 weeks of treatment and results in weight loss (Figures 6.34 and 6.35).

PYY is involved in appetite control, the ileal brake, and negative feedback to the stomach and thus delays GE (Figures 6.36 and 6.37). Another ileal hormone, oxyntomodulin, induces weight loss in obesity (Figure 6.38).

Adiposity and Glycemia-Related Hormones

The pancreatic satiation peptide amylin and its analog, pramlintide, which also control glycemia, are associated with retardation of GE (Figure 6.39).

Insulin from the pancreatic ß cells and leptin from white adipocytes (and also the stomach and other tissues) are secreted in direct proportion to body fat. Both hormones cross the blood-brain barrier and access hypothalamic and other brain neurons to influence energy homeostasis. In contrast to satiation signals, which primarily influence calories eaten during individual meals, adiposity signals show how much fat the body carries and maintains. Insulin systemically elicits hypoglycemia, which increases food intake. All these hormones are released postprandially (Figure 6.40), in contrast to ghrelin, which is reduced after meal ingestion.

In obesity, there is insulin and leptin resistance (manifested by higher circulating levels of insulin and leptin), unlike in overweight and normal-weight controls.

Figure 6.19   Preprandial Plasma Ghrelin Level Compared With Insulin and Leptin Levels

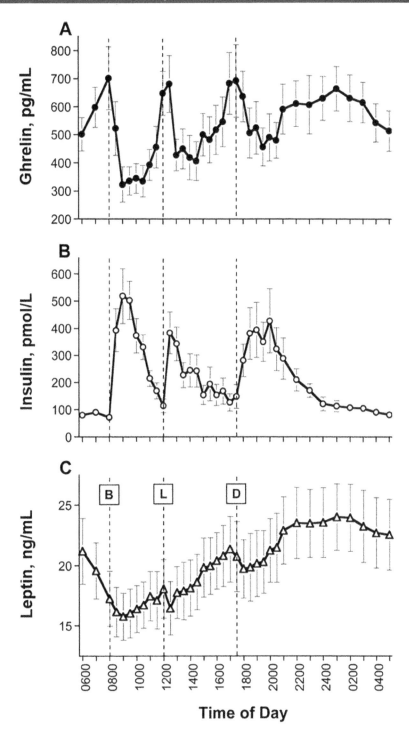

Increase in ghrelin suggest a role in meal initiation and suppression after meals in humans. Average plasma ghrelin (A), insulin (B), and leptin (C) concentrations during a 24-hour period in 10 patients consuming breakfast (B), lunch (L), and dinner (D) at the times indicated (0800, 1200, and 1730, respectively).

Figure 6.20   Summary of Actions of Ghrelin in Gastrointestinal Functions

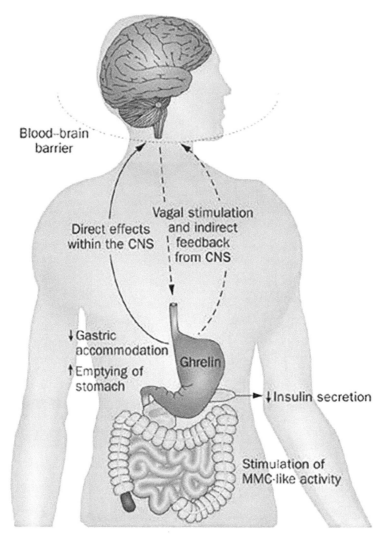

CNS indicates central nervous system; MMC, migrating motor complex.

(From Camilleri M, Papathanasopoulos A, Odunsi ST. Actions and therapeutic pathways of ghrelin for gastrointestinal disorders. Nat Rev Gastroenterol Hepatol. 2009 Jun;6(6):343-52.)

Lessons From Effects of Bariatric Surgery on Gut Hormones, Appetite, and Weight Loss

The most commonly performed bariatric procedures are shown in Figure 6.41, and the main hormonal changes in response to these surgical procedures are shown in Figure 6.42. The main changes in gut hormones after bariatric surgery affect ghrelin, leptin, GLP-1, and PYY.

The effect of restricting gastric volume on weight loss is illustrated by the success of sleeve gastrectomy in reducing dietary intake and inducing weight loss with almost comparable efficacy relative to Roux-en-Y gastric bypass (RYGB): percentage excess weight loss, reduced daily energy and macronutrient intake, and restoration of glycemic control (Ikramuddin 2013; see suggested reading). Both procedures also enhance activation of

Figure 6.21   Intravenous Ghrelin Induces Premature Phase III Interdigestive Motility and Increased Gastric Tone in Healthy Volunteers

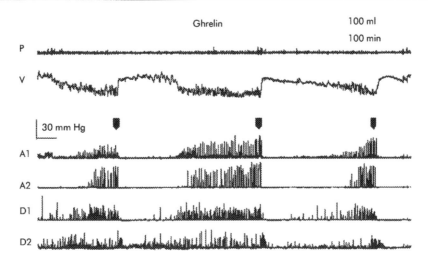

Two antral and 2 duodenal recording sites are shown. All traces begin at the start of the recording. A1 indicates first antral manometry channel; A2, second antral manometry channel; D1, first duodenal manometry channel; D2, second duodenal manometry channel; P, intraballoon pressure; V, intraballoon volume.

(From Tack J, Depoortere I, Bisschops R, Delporte C, Coulie B, Meulemans A, et al. Influence of ghrelin on interdigestive gastrointestinal motility in humans. Gut. 2006 Mar;55(3):327-33; used with permission.)

Figure 6.22   Effect of Ghrelin (10 pmol/kg per minute) on Scintigraphic Gastric Emptying in Healthy (n=8) and Growth Hormone–Deficient (n=6) Patients

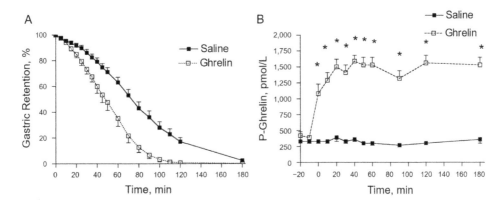

A, Emptying is accelerated with ghrelin compared with saline. B, Increase in plasma (P) concentrations of total ghrelin during infusion of ghrelin (10 pmol/kg per minute) compared with saline after intake of a solid meal (310 kcal) in 8 healthy human volunteers. * indicates significant increases in plasma ghrelin compared with comparable samples during saline infusion.

(From Levin F, Edholm T, Schmidt PT, Gryback P, Jacobsson H, Degerblad M, et al. Ghrelin stimulates gastric emptying and hunger in normal-weight humans. J Clin Endocrinol Metab. 2006 Sep;91(9):3296-302; used with permission.)

Figure 6.23   Effect of Physiologic Levels of Ghrelin (0.33 µg/kg bolus) on Gastric Volume

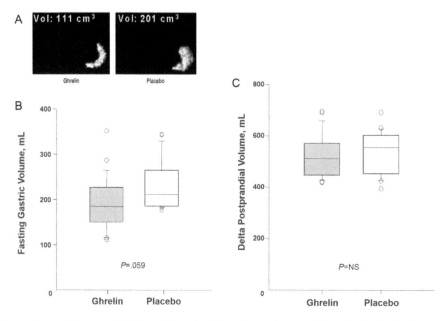

A, Fasting gastric volume images from a patient receiving placebo and another receiving ghrelin. B, Fasting gastric volume. C, Post-prandial change in gastric volume. NS indicates not significant.

(A, From Cremonini F, Camilleri M, Vazquez Roque M, McKinzie S, Burton D, Baxter K, et al. Obesity does not increase effects of synthetic ghrelin on human gastric motor functions. Gastroenterology. 2006 Nov;131(5):1431-9; used with permission. B and C, Data from Cremonini F, Camilleri M, Vazquez Roque M, McKinzie S, Burton D, Baxter K, et al. Obesity does not increase effects of synthetic ghrelin on human gastric motor functions. Gastroenterology. 2006 Nov;131(5):1431-9.)

Figure 6.24   Intraduodenal Lipid Infusion Dose-Dependently Increases Gastric Volume and Plasma Cholecystokinin

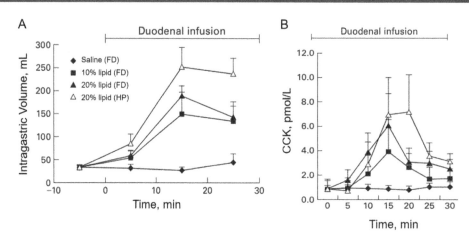

A, Gastric volume responses in patients with functional dyspepsia (FD) and in healthy patients (HP) (n=6). B, Plasma cholecystokinin (CCK) levels (baseline levels normalized) in patients with FD and in HP.

(From Feinle C, Meier O, Otto B, D'Amato M, Fried M. Role of duodenal lipid and cholecystokinin A receptors in the pathophysiology of functional dyspepsia. Gut. 2001 Mar;48(3):347-55; used with permission.)

Figure 6.25   Dose-Related Effects of Infusion of Cholecystokinin-8 (CCK, at doses of ng/kg⁻¹/min⁻¹) on Antropyloric Pressure Activity

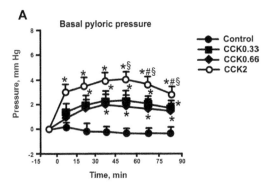

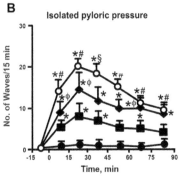

CCK dose-dependently stimulates tonic pressure activity in the pylorus (A) and phasic pressure (contractions) in the pylorus (B). Dose-related statistical comparisons: *CCK0.33, CCK0.66, or CCK2.0 vs control, $P<.01$; φCCK0.66 vs CCK0.33, $P<.05$; #CCK2.0 vs CCK0.33, $P<.05$; §CCK2.0 vs CCK0.66, $P<.001$.

(From Brennan IM, Little TJ, Feltrin KL, Smout AJ, Wishart JM, Horowitz M, et al. Dose-dependent effects of cholecystokinin-8 on antropyloroduodenal motility, gastrointestinal hormones, appetite, and energy intake in healthy men. Am J Physiol Endocrinol Metab. 2008 Dec;295(6):E1487-94; used with permission.)

the farnesoid X receptor pathway in the small bowel; this stimulates FGF-19 production by ileal enterocytes and has been associated with improvements in nonalcoholic steatohepatitis.

With RYGB, the part of the stomach that secretes ghrelin is removed, and weight loss and appetite loss are partly attributed to the reduced plasma levels of ghrelin. Ghrelin induction of hunger may be attenuated in patients who have had vagotomy.

Leptin is produced in the stomach and in adipose tissue. Leptin levels typically decrease after RYGB and sleeve gastrectomy; this effect may reflect reduced gastric production or reduced body fat mass. Whether reduced leptin levels affect energy intake after bariatric surgery is unclear.

Increased GLP-1 (associated in some studies with a blunted GIP or ghrelin response) is one mechanism whereby RYGB induces weight loss and enhances glucose control, and these effects are also enhanced by the diet and weight loss per se, but the latter do not cause the higher GLP-1 levels. GLP-1 levels and insulin sensitivity are higher after RYGB or sleeve gastrectomy than after gastric banding. The increased GLP-1 levels may be insufficient to maintain longer-term glycemic control in obese type 2 diabetes mellitus, in part related to the pancreatic islet cell fatigue before the bariatric surgery is performed.

PYY levels, which are lower in the postprandial period in obese than in normal-weight controls, increase after both RYGB and sleeve gastrectomy. However, because of the concomitant changes in GLP-1, GIP, and other hormones, whether the increased PYY contributes to weight loss, dietary intake, or glycemic control is unclear. Changes in appetite are generally attributed to increased postprandial PYY levels.

Network Meta-analysis of Current Therapies for Obesity

Five medications are approved for the management of obesity: orlistat, lorcaserin, naltrexone-bupropion, phentermine-topiramate, and liraglutide. To compare weight loss and adverse events among drug treatments for obesity, a systematic review and network meta-analysis (Khera 2016; see suggested reading) compared their treatment effects of at least 1 year with those of another active agent or placebo. In 28 randomized clinical trials with 29,018 patients with median baseline BMI of 36.1 kg/m², the percentages of participants who had at least 5% weight loss were 23% with placebo, 75% with phentermine-topiramate, 63% with liraglutide, 55% with naltrexone-bupropion, 49% with lorcaserin, and 44% with orlistat. All active agents were associated with substantial excess weight loss at 1 year compared with placebo (Figures 6.43 through 6.45). The conclusion from the network meta-analysis was that, among overweight or obese adults, phentermine-topiramate and liraglutide were associated with the highest odds of achieving at least 5% weight loss, and liraglutide and naltrexone-bupropion were associated with the highest odds of adverse event–related treatment discontinuation.

Figure 6.26   Cholecystokinin Induces Antral Inhibition and Pyloric Stimulation (B) Compared With Saline (A)

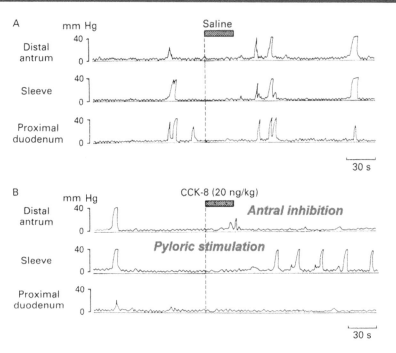

CCK-8 indicates cholecystokinin octapeptide.

(Modified from Fraser R, Fone D, Horowitz M, Dent J. Cholecystokinin octapeptide stimulates phasic and tonic pyloric motility in healthy humans. Gut. 1993 Jan;34(1):33-7; used with permission.)

Figure 6.27   Effect of Cholecystokinin (CCK)-1 Agonist on Gastric Volumes

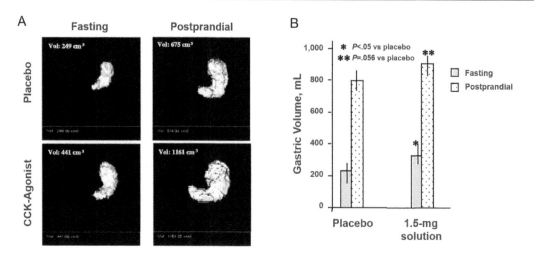

A, Whole stomach volumes measured with single-photon emission computed tomography after treatment with placebo or 1 of 4 doses of GI181771X. A 1.5-mg oral solution had meaningful overall drug effect with increase in fasting and postprandial volumes compared with placebo. B, Reconstructed gastric volumes with placebo and 1.5-mg solution of GI181771X.

(Modified from Castillo EJ, Delgado-Aros S, Camilleri M, Burton D, Stephens D, O'Connor-Semmes R, et al. Effect of oral CCK-1 agonist GI181771X on fasting and postprandial gastric functions in healthy volunteers. Am J Physiol Gastrointest Liver Physiol. 2004 Aug;287(2):G363-9.)

Figure 6.28   Reduction of Duodenal Lipid-Induced Fullness With Cholecystokinin Antagonist Dexloxiglumide

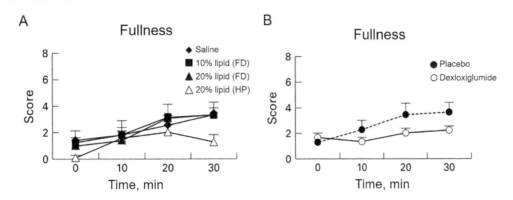

A, Scores for dyspeptic symptom of fullness during duodenal infusion of isotonic saline or 10% or 20% lipid in patients with functional dyspepsia (FD) and 20% lipid in healthy patients (HP). B, Scores for dyspeptic symptom of fullness during duodenal infusion of 20% lipid given with intravenous placebo or dexloxiglumide in patients with functional dyspepsia.

(From Feinle C, Meier O, Otto B, D'Amato M, Fried M. Role of duodenal lipid and cholecystokinin A receptors in the pathophysiology of functional dyspepsia. Gut. 2001 Mar;48(3):347-55; used with permission.)

Figure 6.29   Structure of Glucagon and Glucagon-Like Peptides After Enzymatic Processing

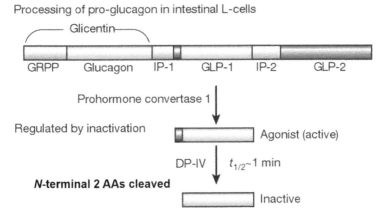

AA indicates amino acids; DP-IV, dipeptidyl peptidase IV; GLP-1, glucagon-like peptide-1; GLP-2, glucagon-like peptide-2; GRPP, glicentin-related polypeptide; IP-1, intervening polypeptide-1; IP-2, intervening polypeptide-2; $t_{1/2}$, gastric emptying of half of radio-activity in a test meal.

(Modified from Moller DE. New drug targets for type 2 diabetes and the metabolic syndrome. Nature. 2001 Dec 13;414(6865):821-7; used with permission.)

Figure 6.30   Glucagon-Like Peptide-1 (GLP-1) Inhibition of Gastric Emptying

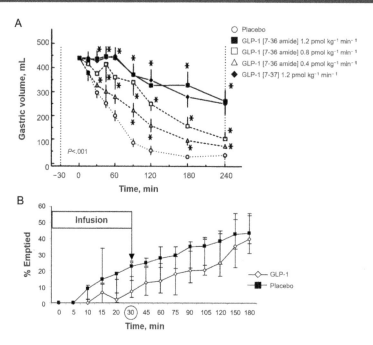

A, Residual gastric volume after mixed liquid meal (8% amino acids [AAs] plus 50 g sucrose in 400 mL) during intravenous infusion of GLP-1-(7-36) amide or -(7-37). B, Gastric emptying of a radiolabeled nutrient liquid meal (30 kcal/min to maximum tolerated volume). The primary end point was the proportion emptied at the time the infusion ended, at 30 minutes. Median proportion emptied was 7% in the GLP-1 group and 23% in the placebo group. *P<.05.

(A, From Nauck MA, Niedereichholz U, Ettler R, Holst JJ, Orskov C, Ritzel R, et al. Glucagon-like peptide 1 inhibition of gastric emptying outweighs its insulinotropic effects in healthy humans. Am J Physiol. 1997 Nov;273(5):E981-8; used with permission. B, From Delgado-Aros S, Kim DY, Burton DD, Thomforde GM, Stephens D, Brinkmann BH, et al. Effect of GLP-1 on gastric volume, emptying, maximum volume ingested, and postprandial symptoms in humans. Am J Physiol Gastrointest Liver Physiol. 2002 Mar;282(3):G424-31.)

Figure 6.31   Effect of Different Glucagon-Like Peptide-1 (GLP-1) Regimens on Gastric Emptying

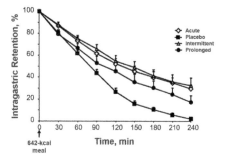

Test meal was 642-kcal homogenized solid meal (72.3 g carbohydrate, 35.5 g fat, 8.1 g protein). Acute GLP-1 increased intragastric retention compared with placebo (P=.001), as did intermittent regimen compared with prolonged infusion (P=.04). Data suggest that prolonged GLP-1 infusion is associated with reduced, although still significant (P=.003 compared with placebo) effect, a finding suggesting tachyphylaxis, subsequently demonstrated with GLP-1 analog liraglutide (see Figure 6.34).

(From Umapathysivam MM, Lee MY, Jones KL, Annink CE, Cousins CE, Trahair LG, et al. Comparative effects of prolonged and intermittent stimulation of the glucagon-like peptide 1 receptor on gastric emptying and glycemia. Diabetes. 2014 Feb;63(2):785-90; used with permission.)

Future Combination Therapies of Hormones, Incretins, and GI Interventions

Experimental pharmacotherapies (Figure 6.46) include combinations of pramlintide (amylin analog) and phentermine as well as amylin and bupropion-naltrexone. Incretin and pancreatic hormones generally inhibit upper GI motor functions, and combinations showing efficacy in obesity are coadministration of GLP-1 with glucagon, a unimolecular dual incretin of pegylated GLP-1/GIP co-agonist, the combination of GLP-1 and PYY3-36, and, in proof-of-concept studies, combined infusions of GLP-1, PYY, and oxyntomodulin. Among bariatric procedures, repeat intragastric balloon treatments are more efficacious than intragastric balloon plus diet, and endoscopic intervention can enhance the effects of RYGB when weight regain occurs. A first trial has provided promising results with the combination of intragastric balloon and the GLP-1 analog liraglutide compared with the balloon alone.

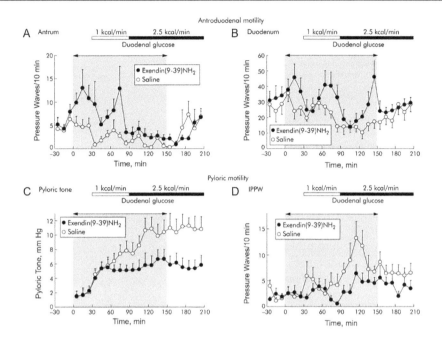

(From Schirra J, Nicolaus M, Roggel R, Katschinski M, Storr M, Woerle HJ, et al. Endogenous glucagon-like peptide 1 controls endocrine pancreatic secretion and antro-pyloro-duodenal motility in humans. Gut. 2006 Feb;55(2):243-51; used with permission.)

Figure 6.33   Effects of Glucagon-Like Peptide-1 (GLP-1) on Gastric Accommodation

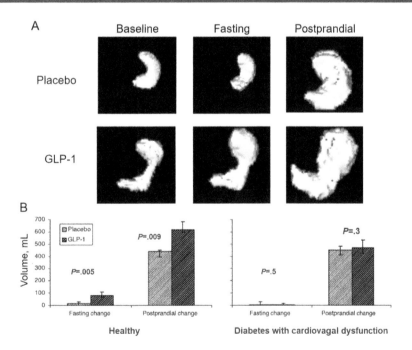

A, Gastric volumes at baseline, during fasting, and during postprandial periods from 2 participants treated with placebo or GLP-1. Volume of the stomach with GLP-1 infusion is visibly larger. B, Gastric volume change in response to placebo or GLP-1 during fasting and postprandially in healthy patients (left) and patients with diabetes and cardiovagal dysfunction. GLP-1 increased gastric volumes in only healthy individuals. Data shown are median (interquartile range).

(A, From Delgado-Aros S, Kim DY, Burton DD, Thomforde GM, Stephens D, Brinkmann BH, et al. Effect of GLP-1 on gastric volume, emptying, maximum volume ingested, and postprandial symptoms in humans. Am J Physiol Gastrointest Liver Physiol. 2002 Mar;282(3):G424-31. B, From Delgado-Aros S, Vella A, Camilleri M, Low PA, Burton DD, Thomforde GM, et al. Effects of glucagon-like peptide-1 and feeding on gastric volumes in diabetes mellitus with cardio-vagal dysfunction. Neurogastroenterol Motil. 2003 Aug;15(4):435-43.)

Figure 6.34   Effects of Treatment With Glucagon-Like Peptide-1 Analog Liraglutide and Placebo on Gastric Emptying (GE) and Weight at 5 and 16 Weeks With Comparison to Baseline Gastric Emptying

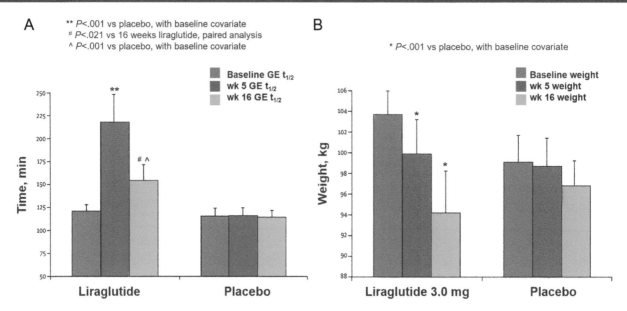

A, GE comparisons between treatment groups were adjusted for baseline GE. Tachyphylaxis is shown by markedly delayed GE at 16 weeks. B, Body weight loss with liraglutide is progressive at 5 and 16 weeks. GE $t_{1/2}$ indicates gastric emptying time for half of radiolabeled meal.

(Modified from Halawi H, Khemani D, Eckert D, O'Neill J, Kadouh H, Grothe K, et al. Effects of liraglutide on weight, satiation, and gastric functions in obesity: a randomised, placebo-controlled pilot trial. Lancet Gastroenterol Hepatol. 2017 Dec;2(12):890-9; used with permission.)

Figure 6.35   Relationship of Gastric Emptying (GE) Delay and Change in Body Weight in Response to Liraglutide at 5 (A) and 16 (B) Weeks

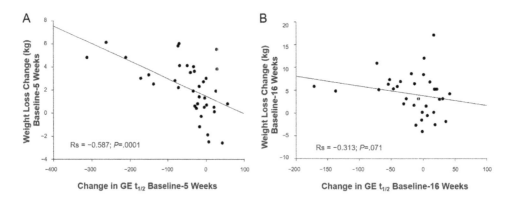

Association between slowing of GE and degree of weight loss was considerable, especially in the 5-week data. GE $t_{1/2}$ indicates gastric emptying time for half of radioactive meal; Rs, Spearman rank correlation coefficient.

(From Halawi H, Khemani D, Eckert D, O'Neill J, Kadouh H, Grothe K, et al. Effects of liraglutide on weight, satiation, and gastric functions in obesity: a randomised, placebo-controlled pilot trial. Lancet Gastroenterol Hepatol. 2017 Dec;2(12):890-9; used with permission.)

Figure 6.36   Effect of Infusion of Peptide Tyrosine Tyrosine (PYY) on Gastrointestinal Transit of Liquid Isotonic Meal

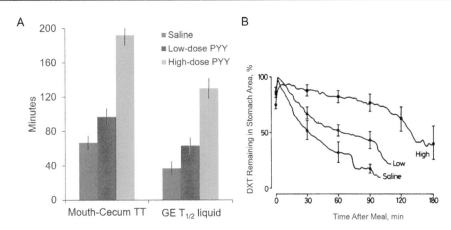

Orocecal transit (A) and gastric emptying (GE) (B) during saline, low-dose PYY, and high-dose PYY infusion. The inhibition of transit and gastric emptying is dose-related. DXT indicates technetium Tc 99m isotopically labeled isotonic liquid meal retained in the stomach; GE $t_{1/2}$, gastric emptying time for half of radioactive meal; TT, transit time.

(From Savage AP, Adrian TE, Carolan G, Chatterjee VK, Bloom SR. Effects of peptide YY (PYY) on mouth to caecum intestinal transit time and on the rate of gastric emptying in healthy volunteers. Gut. 1987 Feb;28(2):166-70; used with permission.)

Figure 6.37   Effect of Intramuscular Peptide Tyrosine Tyrosine (PYY)$_{3-36}$ on 6-Hour Food Intake and Gastric Emptying in Rhesus Monkeys Consuming 1-g Pellets

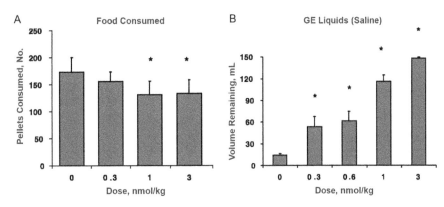

A, Intramuscular PYY$_{3-36}$ (1 and 3 nmol/kg) decreased food intake. B, PYY$_{3-36}$ increased volume of the original test meal remaining in the stomach at the end of the emptying period. Values are mean ± SEM. $P<.05$.

(From Moran TH, Smedh U, Kinzig KP, Scott KA, Knipp S, Ladenheim EE. Peptide YY(3-36) inhibits gastric emptying and produces acute reductions in food intake in rhesus monkeys. Am J Physiol Regul Integr Comp Physiol. 2005 Feb;288(2):R384-8; used with permission.)

Figure 6.38   Effect of Oxyntomodulin (OXM) on Weight Loss in Obesity

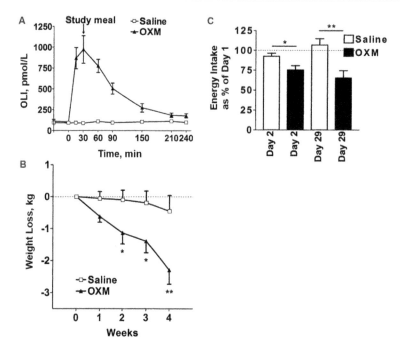

Control (saline, n=12) and treatment (OXM, n=14) groups comparable for body mass index and age at baseline. A, OXM-like immuno-reactivity (OLI) levels for the patients within the treatment group (n=14) after self-administration of subcutaneous saline or OXM. The time of injection was t=0 minute, and study meal was consumed at 30 minutes. B, Change in body weight after self-administration of subcutaneous saline or OXM. Total weight loss was 2.3±0.4 kg by the end of the 4-week study period (* $P<.05$; ** $P=.01$). C, Energy in-take at the study meal, 30 minutes after self-administration of subcutaneous saline or OXM. Intake was reduced at 2 and 29 days with OXM (* $P=.019$; ** $P=.003$).

(From Wynne K, Park AJ, Small CJ, Patterson M, Ellis SM, Murphy KG, et al. Subcutaneous oxyntomodulin reduces body weight in overweight and obese subjects: a double-blind, randomized, controlled trial. Diabetes. 2005 Aug;54(8):2390-5; used with permission.)

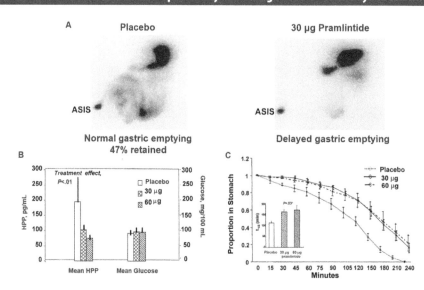

Pramlintide is used for diabetes and causes mild weight loss. A, Abdominal scintiscans 120 minutes after ingestion of radiolabeled meal. Less isotope is emptied from the stomach with 30-µg pramlintide treatment. ASIS indicates radiopaque marker on anterior superior iliac spine. B, Effects of pramlintide on plasma human pancreatic polypeptide (HPP), a surrogate of vagal function, and blood glucose (no drug effect) during first hour postprandially in healthy patients. These data suggest inhibition of vagal function. C, Pramlintide considerably retards gastric emptying.

(Modified from Samsom M, Szarka LA, Camilleri M, Vella A, Zinsmeister AR, Rizza RA. Pramlintide, an amylin analog, selectively delays gastric emptying: potential role of vagal inhibition. Am J Physiol Gastrointest Liver Physiol. 2000 Jun;278(6):G946-51.)

Figure 6.40   Changes in Postprandial Gut Peptides and Leptin in Obesity

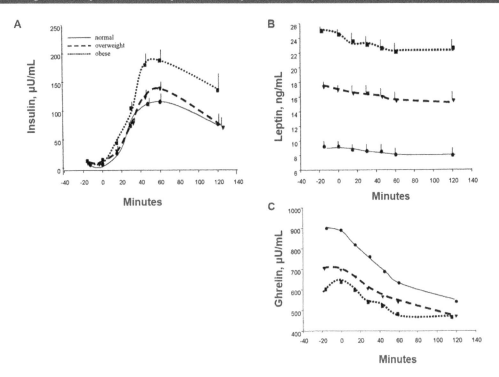

Insulin and leptin values (A and B) are higher and ghrelin value (C) is lower in obesity.

(Modified from Vazquez Roque MI, Camilleri M, Stephens DA, Jensen MD, Burton DD, Baxter KL, et al. Gastric sensorimotor functions and hormone profile in normal weight, overweight, and obese people. Gastroenterology. 2006 Dec;131(6):1717-24; used with permission.)

Figure 6.41   Restrictive and Malabsorptive Surgeries

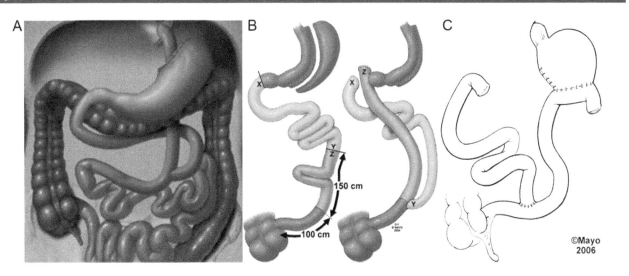

A, Roux-en-Y gastric bypass. B, Duodenal switch: the duodenal bulb is separated from the descending duodenum (X), the switched duodenum is anastomosed to the distal small bowel (Y) 100 cm from the ileocecal valve, and the continuity between the duodenal bulb and the small bowel is restored, 150 cm long (Z). C, Biliopancreatic diversion.

(From Decker GA, Swain JM, Crowell MD, Scolapio JS. Gastrointestinal and nutritional complications after bariatric surgery. Am J Gastroenterol. 2007 Nov;102(11):2571-80; used with permission of Mayo Foundation for Medical Education and Research.)

Figure 6.42   Summary of Effects of Bariatric Surgery on Appetite-Related Gut Hormones

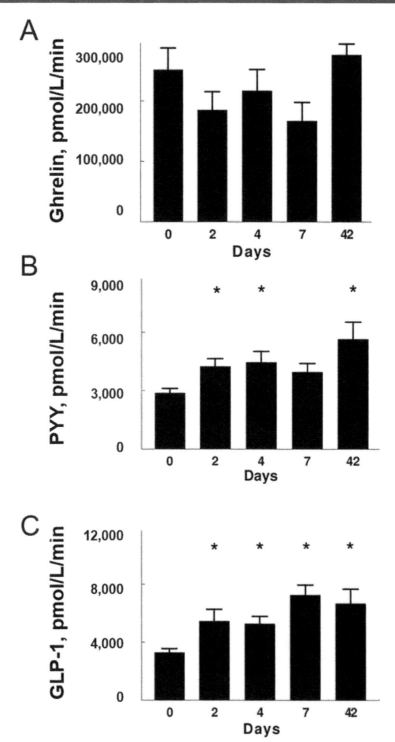

Measurements were taken at different times after the bariatric surgery (days) by the area under the curve (AUC) over a 3-hour period after a 400-kcal meal. A, Ghrelin levels are reduced if part of the stomach is resected. B and C, Peptide tyrosine-tyrosine (PYY) and glucagon-like peptide-1 (GLP-1) are increased compared with preoperative AUC (*$P<.05$).

(From le Roux CW, Welbourn R, Werling M, Osborne A, Kokkinos A, Laurenius A, et al. Gut hormones as mediators of appetite and weight loss after Roux-en-Y gastric bypass. Ann Surg. 2007 Nov;246(5):780-5; used with permission.)

Figure 6.43   **Network Analysis of Drug Therapy for Obesity**

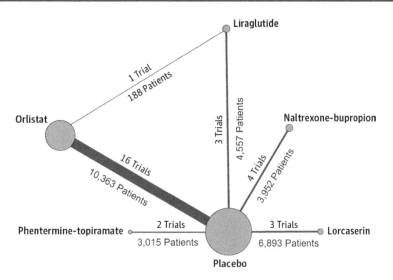

Included studies show available direct comparisons for primary efficacy outcome (≥5% weight loss). The size of the nodes and the thickness of the edges are weighted according to the number of studies evaluating each treatment and direct comparison, respectively.

(From Khera R, Murad MH, Chandar AK, Dulai PS, Wang Z, Prokop LJ, et al. Association of pharmacological treatments for obesity with weight loss and adverse events: a systematic review and meta-analysis. JAMA. 2016 Jun 14;315(22):2424-34; used with permission.)

Figure 6.44   **Comparison of Weight Loss and Adverse Events With Pharmacologic Weight Loss Agents in Network Meta-analysis**

	Odds ratio (95% CrI) for achieving at least 5% weight loss					
	Phentermine-topiramate	1.67 (1.03-2.56)	2.33 (1.54-3.59)	2.98 (1.95-4.54)	3.42 (2.40-4.91)	9.22 (6.63-12.85)
Odds ratio (95% CrI) for discontinuation due to adverse events	0.78 (0.48-1.20)	Liraglutide	1.4 (0.96-2.18)	1.78 (1.22-2.78)	2.06 (1.51-2.96)	5.54 (4.16-7.78)
	0.87 (0.59-1.25)	1.11 (0.74-1.72)	Naltrexone-bupropion	1.28 (0.87-1.84)	1.47 (1.09-1.96)	3.96 (3.03-5.11)
	1.71 (1.14-2.49)	2.2 (1.43-3.39)	1.97 (1.38-2.76)	Lorcaserin	1.15 (0.86-1.55)	3.1 (2.38-4.05)
	1.25 (0.88-1.76)	1.6 (1.10-2.40)	1.44 (1.07-1.95)	0.73 (0.54-1.02)	Orlistat	2.7 (2.34-3.09)
	2.29 (1.71-3.06)	2.95 (2.11-4.23)	2.64 (**2.10-3.35**)	1.34 (1.05-1.76)	1.84 (1.53-2.21)	Placebo

Summary estimate represents odds ratio of achieving at least 5% weight loss (light gray background) and discontinuation due to adverse events (darker gray background). Agents are ordered by rankings for the 5% weight loss outcome. Odds ratio for comparisons are in the cell in common between the column-defining and row-defining treatment. For weight loss outcome, row treatment is compared with column treatment (ie, column treatment is reference). For adverse event outcome, column treatment is compared with row treatment (ie, row treatment is reference). Numbers in parentheses indicate 95% credible intervals (95% CrIs). Numbers in bold are statistically significant results.

(From Khera R, Murad MH, Chandar AK, Dulai PS, Wang Z, Prokop LJ, et al. Association of pharmacological treatments for obesity with weight loss and adverse events: a systematic review and meta-analysis. JAMA. 2016 Jun 14;315(22):2424-34; used with permission.)

Figure 6.45   SUCRAs for Weight Loss and Adverse Event Outcomes: SUCRAs between 0 and 1 represent the probability of being ranked highest

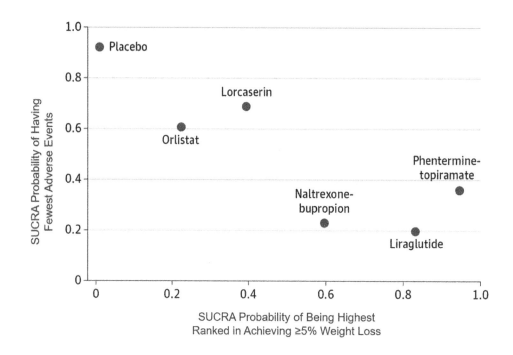

	Placebo	Orlistat	Lorcaserin	Naltrexone-bupropion	Liraglutide	Phentermine-topiramate
Weight loss rank (95% CrI)	6 (6-6)	5 (4-5)	4 (3-5)	3 (2-4)	2 (2-3)	1 (1-1)
Adverse event rank (95% CrI)	1 (1-1)	3 (2-4)	2 (2-3)	5 (5-6)	6 (4-6)	4 (3-6)

For the weight loss outcomes, higher score corresponds to higher proportion achieving at least 5% weight loss with a particular therapy. For the adverse event outcome, higher scores reflect lower probability of discontinuation due to adverse events. The median ranks on both weight loss and adverse event rates (rank 1 through 6 on each scale) are tabulated along with their corresponding 95% credible intervals (95% CrIs). SUCRAs indicates surface under the cumulative rankings.

(From Khera R, Murad MH, Chandar AK, Dulai PS, Wang Z, Prokop LJ, et al. Association of pharmacological treatments for obesity with weight loss and adverse events: a systematic review and meta-analysis. JAMA. 2016 Jun 14;315(22):2424-34; used with permission.)

Figure 6.46   Combination Therapies for Obesity

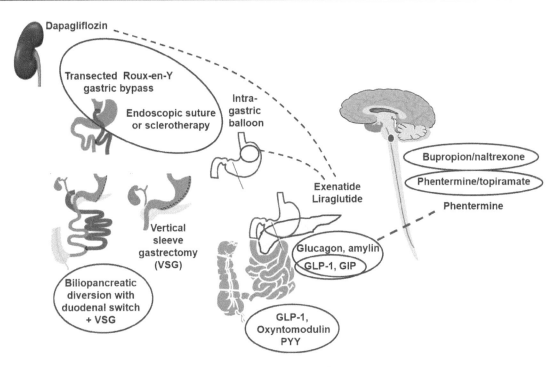

Combination therapies are illustrated by continuous lines when the treatments have a common approach (eg, surgical or pharmacologic, or hormonal) or interrupted lines (that link different therapeutic approaches) combining diverse forms of obesity treatment. GIP indicates glucose-dependent insulinotropic peptide; GLP-1, glucagon-like peptide-1; PYY, peptide tyrosine tyrosine.

(From Camilleri M, Acosta A. Combination therapies for obesity. Metab Syndr Relat Disord. 2018 Oct;16(8):390-4.)

Table 6.3   Phenotypes Associated With Obesity and Potential Therapies

Phenotype	Attributable Contribution, %	Potential Medication	Potential Device	Potential Surgery
Satiety/satiation	21	Phentermine-topiramate ER	VBLOC AspireAssist	–
Psychologic	19	Bupropion-naltrexone	–	–
Gastric sensorimotor	17	GLP-1 agonists	VBLOC	Retrograde pacing
Gastric capacity	14	Motilin or ghrelin agonists	Balloon; POSE or sleeve gastroplasty	Sleeve gastrectomy; RYGB
Postprandial GLP-1, PYY	9	–	Duodeno-jejunal bypass liner	Deep RYGB, duodenal switch

Abbreviations: ER, extended release; GLP-1, glucagon-like peptide-1; POSE, primary obesity surgery endoluminal; PYY, peptide tyrosine-tyrosine; RYGB, Roux-en-Y gastric bypass; VBLOC, vagal nerve blocking.

Data from Camilleri M, Acosta A. Gastrointestinal traits: individualizing therapy for obesity with drugs and devices. Gastrointest Endosc. 2016 Jan;83[1]:48-56.

Thus, combination therapies for the treatment of obesity hold promise for introduction into clinical practice.

Conclusion

Rich and diverse mechanisms are involved in communicating between the gut and the centers in the hypothalamus and brainstem that mediate food intake and digestion. Importantly, the hedonic (pleasures and desires related to food) and higher center responses to food are superimposed on these peripheral mechanisms. Consideration of the different phenotypes in obesity suggests that treatment may be individualized according to the abnormal phenotype detected in individual patients (Table 6.3).

Suggested Reading

Acosta A, Abu Dayyeh BK, Port JD, Camilleri M. Recent advances in clinical practice challenges and opportunities in the management of obesity. Gut. 2014 Apr;63(4):687–95. Epub 2014 Jan 10.

Acosta A, Camilleri M, Shin A, Vazquez-Roque MI, Iturrino J, Burton D, et al. Quantitative gastrointestinal and psychological traits associated with obesity and response to weight-loss therapy. Gastroenterology. 2015;148(3):537–46.

Camilleri M. Integrated upper gastrointestinal response to food intake. Gastroenterology. 2006 Aug;131(2):640–58. Epub 2006 Aug 08.

Camilleri M. Peripheral mechanisms in appetite regulation. Gastroenterology. 2015 May;148(6):1219–33. Epub 2014 Sep 23.

Camilleri M, Acosta A. Gastrointestinal traits: individualizing therapy for obesity with drugs and devices. Gastrointest Endosc. 2016 Jan;83(1):48–56. Epub 2015 Aug 15.

Camilleri M, Malhi H, Acosta A. Gastrointestinal complications of obesity. Gastroenterology. 2017 May;152(7):1656–70. Epub 2017 Feb 14.

Cummings DE, Overduin J. Gastrointestinal regulation of food intake. J Clin Invest. 2007 Jan;117(1):13–23. Epub 2007 Jan 04.

Ikramuddin S, Korner J, Lee WJ, Connett JE, Inabnet WB, Billington CJ, et al. Roux-en-Y gastric bypass vs intensive medical management for the control of type 2 diabetes, hypertension, and hyperlipidemia: the Diabetes Surgery Study randomized clinical trial. JAMA. 2013;309(21):2240–9.

Khera R, Murad MH, Chandar AK, Dulai PS, Wang Z, Prokop LJ, et al. Association of pharmacological treatments for obesity with weight loss and adverse events: a systematic review and meta-analysis. JAMA. 2016;315(22):2424–34.

Vella A, Camilleri M. The Gastrointestinal tract as an integrator of mechanical and hormonal response to nutrient ingestion. diabetes. 2017 Nov;66(11):2729–37. Epub 2017 Oct 25.

Neuromuscular Disorders Causing Gut Dysmotility

Introduction

Gut dysmotility results from disorders of gut muscle (myopathic disorders), disorders of the myenteric plexus and electrical syncytial cells that function as pacemakers (enteric disorders), and diseases of the extrinsic pathways (neuropathic disorders). Some diseases affect both intrinsic and extrinsic neural control. This chapter addresses how to identify extrinsic neurologic disorders, briefly discusses the gut motility presentations in neurologic diseases, and provides examples of classic or syndromic neurologic diseases that include gut dysmotility. The first step in the identification of possible association with neurologic disease is documentation of the presence of a gastrointestinal (GI) dysmotility affecting the upper or lower GI tract. An example of an algorithm for investigation of upper GI dysmotility is shown in Figure 7.1. The diagnosis is typically based on results of GI motility tests, imaging, and autonomic reflex tests.

Figure 7.1   Algorithm for Diagnosis of Neurologic Diseases Presenting With Upper Gastrointestinal Symptoms

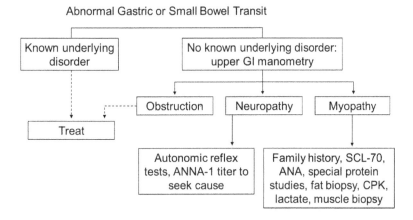

Once an autonomic dysfunction is identified, there needs to be further investigation to identify the cause, such as paraneoplastic neuropathy identified by serologic measurement of ANNA-1. If there is obstruction, or a known underlying disorder, and an abnormality of transit is detected, management should follow standard of care without further investigations. ANA indicates antinuclear antibodies; ANNA-1, antineuronal nuclear antibody type 1; CPK, creatine kinase; SCL-70, anti-topoisomerase 1.

(Modified from Camilleri M, Hasler WL, Parkman HP, Quigley EM, Soffer E. Measurement of gastrointestinal motility in the GI laboratory. Gastroenterology. 1998 Sep;115(3):747-62; used with permission.)

Identification of Extrinsic Neurologic Disease in Patients With GI Symptoms of a Motility Disorder

Diseases at any level of the nervous system may result in GI motor dysfunction. To identify possible causes, further testing is required, particularly if there are features suggestive of autonomic or peripheral nerve dysfunction or a known underlying neuromuscular disease. Medications that influence gut motility must first be excluded as the cause; these include analgesics, central neuromodulators, antihypertensive agents, and amylin and glucagon-like peptide-1 analogs or agonists.

After GI motility and transit measurements are determined to objectively confirm the gut motility disorder, manometry may help distinguish between neuropathic and myopathic disorders if there is no underlying disease that predicts the most likely nature of the disorder. For example, myopathy is likely in patients with scleroderma, and neuropathy is likely in patients with long-standing type 1 diabetes mellitus. Manometry is useful as long as the diameter of the small bowel is not more than 5 cm, because the accuracy of manometry to measure amplitude and patterns of motility decreases with increased luminal diameter (see Chapter 3, "Gastrointestinal Motility: Control Mechanisms and Pathogenesis of Disordered Function"). After these preliminary evaluations, tests of autonomic function are useful to appraise whether the disturbance in extrinsic neural control is central or peripheral and whether it is generalized or selective to sympathetic or parasympathetic systems or both.

There is generally concordance between abnormalities of abdominal vagal function, including the plasma pancreatic polypeptide response to modified sham feeding, and thoracic (cardiovagal) dysfunction in patients with diabetes mellitus. However, if a patient has surgical vagotomy or injury at the level of or below the diaphragm (eg, fundoplication), the cardiovagal test result may be completely normal. Two tests are performed to distinguish preganglionic from postganglionic sympathetic function. The first test is the quantitative sudomotor axon reflex test, in which acetylcholine is applied into skin through iontopheresis and sweat output close by is quantified to determine whether the postganglionic sudomotor cholinergic nerves are intact. The second test distinguishes preganglionic from postganglionic sympathetic function on the basis of plasma norepinephrine levels in response to intravenous edrophonium, which is an acetylcholinesterase inhibitor that stimulates the postganglionic sympathetic nerves to produce norepinephrine, which then appears in the bloodstream. Therefore, the test provides assessment of the integrity of postganglionic sympathetic nerves, many of which supply the digestive tract.

Once visceral autonomic neuropathy is demonstrated, the causes of the neuropathy need to be diagnosed. Specific examples include lung tumors (computed tomography of the chest), amyloidosis (special protein studies in blood and urine, fat, or a rectal biopsy specimen), or a central nervous system lesion (imaging of the brain and spinal cord). A central lesion should be suspected when the result of a thermoregulatory sweat test is abnormal (indicating a lesion somewhere between the hypothalamus and the sweat gland in the skin) and results of tests of postganglionic nerves are normal (eg, the quantitative sudomotor axon reflex test or plasma norepinephrine response to edrophonium).

Neurologic Diseases With Gut Dysmotility

Table 7.1 summarizes neurologic diseases that present with GI dysmotility.

Brain Diseases

Stroke

Dysphagia is a common consequence of stroke and results from cranial nerve involvement; it may cause malnutrition or aspiration pneumonia. A videoflouroscopic barium swallow study is usually performed by speech therapists and may show transfer dysphagia or tracheal aspiration. Percutaneous endoscopic gastrostomy is effective for providing nutrition (by bolus or nocturnal infusion) without interfering with rehabilitation. Swallowing improves, usually within 3 months, in a majority of stroke survivors. Recovery is predicted from the

Table 7.1	Summary of Neurologic Diseases Presenting With GI Dysmotility		
Disease	**GI Dysmotility**	**GI Pathophysiology**	**Comments**
Brain			
Stroke	Dysphagia Malnutrition	Videofluoroscopy: transfer dysphagia, aspiration	PEG until dysphagia resolves
Alzheimer	GI illnesses more prevalent + nausea, vomiting, diarrhea with acetylcholinesterase inhibitors	NA	Consider alternative therapy
Parkinsonism	Dysphagia, impaired GE, constipation, defecatory disorder	Oropharyngeal dysfunction, Lewy bodies (misfolded α-synuclein), delayed transit and abnormal ARM	GE of liquids normal; on-off phenomenon in part due to GE delay
Head injury	Acute nausea or vomiting	Acute delayed GE	Severity of head injury correlates with GE delay
Autonomic epilepsy, migraine	Nausea, vomiting	NA	Treat underlying CNS disease
Amyotrophic lateral sclerosis	Bulbar palsy with dysphagia, aspiration	Videofluoroscopy: transfer dysphagia, aspiration	PEG, radiologically if FVC<50%
Brainstem tumors	Vomiting may be sole presentation	MRI/CT shows mass and distortion of 4th ventricle	
Autonomic System Degeneration			
Dysautonomia	Dysphagia, vomiting, ileus, constipation, CIP	Autonomic reflex screen; esophageal, GI, and colonic transit or manometry	Pan- or selective cholinergic; may follow EBV or influenza A
IOH	Dysphagia, vomiting, ileus, constipation, incontinence	Autonomic reflex screen	CV and sweat abnormalities usually precede GI
POTS	1/3 have GI symptoms, commonest IBS	Dehydration, deconditioning may give false POTS readings	Treat the POTS and GI separately
Shy-Drager syndrome	Parkinsonism and autonomic GI problems	Autonomic reflex screen; esophageal, GI, and colonic transit or manometry	Treat as for GI parkinsonism or dysautonomia
Spinal Cord Lesions			
Cord injury	Cervical: dysphagia Thoracic: GE delay, CIP Lumbar: constipation, impaction, distention Sacral: constipation, incontinence	Esophageal, GI, and colonic transit or manometry	Supportive treatment for region affected; enemas, laxatives, prokinetics; sacral nerve stimulation
Multiple sclerosis	Usually constipation; rarely upper gut	Colonic transit + ARM	Usually with bladder dysfunction
Neuromyelitis optica	Nausea and vomiting	GI may precede eye or cord involvement	Antibody to AQP-4
Acute Peripheral Neuropathy			
Virus infection	Nausea, vomiting, pain, distention, CIP	Abdominal radiography to exclude obstruction	Herpes zoster, EBV, botulism B

(continued)

Table 7.1   Continued

Disease	GI Dysmotility	GI Pathophysiology	Comments
Chronic Peripheral Neuropathy			
Diabetes	Gastroparesis, constipation, diarrhea, incontinence	GI and colonic transit or manometry; ARM; check for SIBO and BAD	Treat underlying cause
Amyloid	Constipation, diarrhea	GI and colonic transit or manometry	Initial neuropathy; later myopathy
Paraneoplastic	Gastroparesis, CIP	GI and colonic transit or manometry, ANNA-1	Treat associated lung cancer
Porphyria	Pain, nausea, vomiting, constipation	NA	
Neurofibromatosis	Constipation and megarectum in childhood	Colon transit, rectal imaging	Surgery when indicated
Autoimmunity	Dysphagia, gastroparesis, CIP, constipation	Anti-ACh ganglionic receptor or voltage-gated potassium channels Ab	Therapeutic trials of corticosteroids or immunoglobulin infusions

Abbreviations: ACh, acetylcholine; ANNA-1, antineuronal nuclear antibody; ARM, anorectal manometry; AQP4, aquaporin-4; BAD, bile acid diarrhea; CIP, chronic intestinal pseudo-obstruction; CNS, central nervous system; CT, computed tomography; CV, cardiovascular; EBV, Epstein-Barr virus; FVC, forced vital capacity; GE, gastric emptying; GI, gastrointestinal; IBS, irritable bowel syndrome; IOH, idiopathic orthostatic hypotension; MRI, magnetic resonance imaging; NA, not applicable; PEG, percutaneous endoscopic gastrostomy; POTS, postural orthostatic tachycardia syndrome; SIBO, small intestine bacterial overgrowth.

severity of the initial neurologic deficit. Colonic pseudo-obstruction occurs rarely in patients with stroke.

Alzheimer Disease

People with Alzheimer disease have a higher incidence of nonmotility and upper and lower GI events, including ulceration, perforation, and bleeding, than matched controls. Treatment of Alzheimer disease with acetylcholinesterase inhibitor medications, such as donepezil or rivastigmine, may be associated with GI symptoms such as nausea, vomiting, and diarrhea, presumably reflecting incoordinated excitation of gut contractility by the increased synaptic acetylcholine.

Parkinson Disease

GI dysfunction is a prominent manifestation of Parkinson disease. The most prevalent symptoms include reduced salivation, dysphagia, impaired gastric emptying, constipation, and defecatory dysfunction. Indeed, constipation may precede the development of somatic motor symptoms of Parkinson disease by several years.

The mechanisms of gut dysfunction in Parkinson disease suggest that the gastrointestinal tract may be critically involved in development of the disease and also is a significant nonmotor manifestation of

the disease. Neuronal death in Parkinson disease is associated with intracellular aggregates of the neuronal protein α-synuclein, known as Lewy bodies. Misfolded α-synuclein is found in enteric nerves and enteroendocrine cells in the gut before it appears in the brain. The digestive tract provides a process by which misfolded α-synuclein could propagate from the gut epithelium to the brain, possibly along vagal afferents. The novel medication squalamine (found in the stomach and liver of the spiny dogfish shark) has been shown to inhibit the initiation of α-synuclein aggregation and suppress its toxicity in neuronal cells and in an animal model of Parkinson disease, and it seemed to reverse constipation and central features of Parkinson disease in a phase 1 clinical trial.

Oropharyngeal dysfunction with impaired swallowing may develop in patients with Parkinson disease or progressive supranuclear palsy. Shy-Drager syndrome, or multiple system atrophy, has a combination of the effects of Parkinson disease and autonomic dysfunction.

In some patients with malnutrition, dysphagia, or aspiration, a percutaneous gastrostomy (placed endoscopically or radiologically) is indicated. Dopamine and its agonists retard gastric emptying of solids. Gastric emptying of liquids is not inhibited by levodopa, a decarboxylase inhibitor, and, therefore, nutrition with liquid supplements is usually feasible.

Constipation is common in patients with Parkinson disease and may be the result of slow colonic transit (aggravated by dopaminergic agents) or, perhaps more frequently, a consequence of pelvic floor or anal sphincter dysfunction.

In summary, several features of Parkinson disease synergize to cause GI hypomotility, including constipation, generalized hypokinesia, associated autonomic dysfunction, and the effects of various anticholinergic and dopamine agonist medications. The bioavailability of other medications can be altered considerably by the effects of Parkinson disease and affect delivery of medications to the small bowel for absorption. Therefore, the gut may contribute to the on-off phenomenon observed in patients with Parkinson disease.

Head Injury

Immediately after moderate to severe head injury, most patients have a transient delay in gastric emptying proportional to the severity of injury or increase in intracranial pressure. These patients may require nutritional support (parenteral initially, enteral later). Typically, gastric stasis resolves completely in 2 to 3 weeks.

Autonomic Epilepsy and Migraine

These disorders are infrequent causes of upper abdominal symptoms such as nausea and vomiting, and, typically, they respond to treatment of the underlying disorder.

Amyotrophic Lateral Sclerosis

The main digestive tract effects of amyotrophic lateral sclerosis and progressive bulbar palsy are dysphagia and respiratory difficulty while eating. These are a result of aspiration or respiratory muscle fatigue due to glossopharyngeal and vagus nerve involvement. Nutrition management usually involves gastrostomy by endoscopy or, when forced vital capacity is less than 50% expected, by radiologic insertion. Decisions on nutrition are guided by overall management of the amyotrophic lateral sclerosis in each patient.

Brainstem Tumors

Brainstem lesions can present with isolated GI motor dysfunction. Whereas nausea and vomiting may result from increased intracranial pressure, they may also occur in its absence as a result of a direct mass effect in the brainstem with distortion of the area postrema (vomiting center) on the floor of the fourth ventricle. Vomiting is the most common symptom; colonic and anorectal dysfunction have also been described with brainstem tumors.

Autonomic System Degenerations

Pandysautonomias or Selective Dysautonomias

Pandysautonomias imply involvement of both the sympathetic and the parasympathetic nervous systems, often affecting both preganglionic and postganglionic pathways. Vomiting, paralytic ileus, constipation, and a chronic pseudo-obstruction syndrome due to involvement of the esophagus, stomach, and small bowel have been reported in acute, subacute, and congenital or familial pandysautonomia. Selective cholinergic dysautonomia, usually after Ebstein-Barr virus or influenza A infection, may also impair upper and lower GI motor activity.

Idiopathic Orthostatic Hypotension

Idiopathic orthostatic hypotension is often associated with more general autonomic involvement, and cardiovascular and sudomotor abnormalities usually precede gut involvement. Motor dysfunction of the gut is manifested as esophageal dysmotility, gastric stasis, alteration in bowel movements, or fecal incontinence. The precise site of the neurologic lesion causing the gut dysmotility is unknown.

Postural Orthostatic Tachycardia Syndrome

About one-third of patients with postural orthostatic tachycardia syndrome have GI manifestations, with typical symptoms consistent with irritable bowel syndrome and, only rarely, chronic intestinal pseudo-obstruction syndrome. It is important to exclude dehydration and deconditioning as a result of the GI manifestations because they could affect assessment of the syndrome.

Shy-Drager Syndrome

The combination of Parkinson disease and autonomic dysfunction may manifest with constipation, fecal incontinence, dysphagia, and feeding intolerance that may result from antral and small bowel dysmotility.

Spinal Cord Lesions

Spinal Cord Injury

The level of injury determines the GI manifestations. Dysphagia with acute cervical spinal cord injury generally improves during the initial hospitalization. Spinal cord injuries result in constipation and associated symptoms such as distention, abdominal pain, or ileus. These manifestations are present soon after injury and typically persist in the chronic phase after injury, especially colonic and anorectal dysfunction (in contrast to upper GI dysfunction). The cause of the motor dysfunction probably results from interruption of supraspinal control of the sacral parasympathetic supply to the colon, pelvic floor, and anal sphincters. The interruption of extrinsic neural control to the colon in patients with thoracic spinal cord injury results in the absence of postprandial colonic motor response.

Patients may rely on reflex rectal stimulation for stool evacuation to avoid fecal impaction, which may also cause anorexia and nausea. Loss of voluntary control of the external anal sphincter commonly results in fecal incontinence in patients with spinal cord injury.

The typical management for irregular bowel function is a combination of laxatives, bulking agents, anal massage, manual evacuation, and scheduled enemas. Electrical stimulation of the sacral anterior roots may restore normal function to the pelvic colon and anorectal sphincters; this anterior sacral root stimulation may need to be used in combination with S2-S4 posterior rhizotomy to avoid autonomic dysreflexia. Transcutaneous electrical stimulation is also being tested. If sacral or transcutaneous electrical stimulation is unavailable or ineffective and severe constipation persists, a colostomy reduces time for bowel care.

Multiple Sclerosis

Multiple sclerosis results in motility disturbances in the lower gut more frequently than in the upper gut. Severe constipation frequently accompanies urinary bladder dysfunction in patients with advanced multiple sclerosis. The cause of constipation is considered to be pelvic colon dysfunction due to impaired function of supraspinal or descending pathways that control the sacral parasympathetic outflow.

Neuromyelitis Optica

The area postrema (vomiting center) may be a selective target of neuromyelitis optica, and involvement of the vomiting center in the same disease process may cause nausea and vomiting often preceding episodes of optic neuritis and transverse myelitis.

Acute Peripheral Neuropathy

Acute viral infections may result in autonomic dysfunction presenting as nausea, vomiting, abdominal cramps, constipation, or a clinical picture of pseudo-obstruction. In the Guillain-Barré syndrome, visceral involvement may include gastric distention or adynamic ileus.

Persistent GI motor disturbances due to acquired dysautonomias may occur in association with herpes zoster, Epstein-Barr virus infection, or botulism B. Diarrhea induced by HIV may also result from autonomic dysfunction.

Chronic Peripheral Neuropathy

Chronic peripheral neuropathy is the most common extrinsic neurologic disorder causing GI motor dysfunction.

Diabetes

Diabetic autonomic neuropathy of the gut, typically in patients with type 1 diabetes mellitus, may present with gastroparesis, constipation, diarrhea, or anorectal dysfunction. The cellular pathogenesis of the injury due to the diabetes is the subject of ongoing research. The pathophysiologic mechanisms of constipation in patients with diabetes may be diverse and include the 3 main categories observed in nondiabetic patients: slow transit, normal transit, or pelvic floor dysfunction. Diarrhea or fecal incontinence (or both) may result from several mechanisms: osmotic diarrhea from bacterial overgrowth due to small bowel stasis, rapid transit from uncoordinated small bowel motor activity, associated gluten-sensitive enteropathy or pancreatic exocrine insufficiency or bile acid diarrhea (aggravated by metformin treatment), or, perhaps most frequently, dysfunction of the anorectal sphincters or abnormal rectal sensation. Optimal treatment requires identification of the cause.

Paraneoplastic neuropathy in association with small cell carcinoma of the lung or pulmonary carcinoid may present with constipation, gastroparesis, or esophageal dysmotility (spasm or achalasia). It is associated with a circulating immunoglobulin G antibody (called type 1 antineuronal antibody [anti-Hu]) directed against enteric neuronal nuclei.

Amyloid Neuropathy

This condition may lead to constipation, diarrhea, and steatorrhea with initial neuropathic features and ultimately smooth muscle failure and features of myopathy.

Porphyria

Acute intermittent porphyria and hereditary coproporphyria may present with abdominal pain, nausea, vomiting, and constipation. Porphyric polyneuropathy may lead to dilatation and impaired motor function in any part of the intestinal tract.

Neurofibromatosis Type I

This condition (von Recklinghausen disease) typically presents in childhood with constipation, megarectum, and prolonged colonic transit time.

Autoimmunity

Antibodies to ganglionic acetylcholine receptors are associated with autoimmune GI dysmotility. The antibody effect is considered to be potentially reversible. This possibility led to the suggestion that immunomodulatory therapy directed at lowering immunoglobulin G levels and reducing immunoglobulin G production may be therapeutically effective.

Similarly, antibodies against specific ion channels (voltage-gated potassium channels and α3-acetylcholine receptor) may be associated with esophageal dysmotility, slow transit constipation, and chronic intestinal pseudo-obstruction. Treatment may include corticosteroids or immunoglobulin infusions.

General Muscle Diseases Causing Gut Dysmotility

Disorders affecting the smooth muscle component of the gut may involve the distal two-thirds of the esophagus to the anorectum and present with dysphagia, gastric stasis, chronic intestinal pseudo-obstruction, multiple small bowel diverticula, steatorrhea due to bacterial overgrowth, constipation, incontinence (particularly at night, from involvement of the internal anal sphincter), and rectal mucosal prolapse. Dysphagia may also result from reflux esophagitis and stricture, in addition to dysfunction of the smooth muscle section of the esophagus. Other manifestations reflect the muscle disease itself or, in the case of amyloidosis or mitochondrial cytopathy, the coexistence of peripheral neuropathy.

At an advanced stage, progressive systemic sclerosis and amyloidosis result in an infiltrative replacement of smooth muscle cells in the digestive tract. Rarely, Duchenne or Becker muscular dystrophies and polymyositis or dermatomyositis have been associated with gastroparesis.

Familial disorders represent genetic diseases such as mitochondrial cytopathy, sometimes in association with an external ophthalmoplegia, ptosis, deafness, and white matter lesions in the brain. Small bowel involvement is dominant and results in malnutrition and malabsorption.

Patients with myotonic dystrophy may have megacolon or anal sphincter dysfunction, consistent with effects such as myopathy, muscular atrophy, and neural abnormalities.

Myopathic disorders are associated with low-amplitude contractions at affected levels of the gut, typically less than 40 mm Hg in the stomach and less than 10 mm Hg in the upper small bowel, as in systemic sclerosis. Myopathic disorders may be complicated by bowel diverticula leading to bacterial overgrowth. Pneumatosis cystoides intestinalis and spontaneous pneumoperitoneum sometimes occur in progressive systemic sclerosis. Skeletal muscle electromyography or biopsy may be needed to establish the nature of the generalized neuromuscular disorder, as in mitochondrial cytopathy or polymyositis.

The fundamentals of treatment are restoration of nutrition (which may necessitate total parenteral nutrition), suppression of bacterial overgrowth, and treatment of complications. The treatment of complications includes use of proton pump inhibitors for gastroesophageal reflux and endoscopic dilatation for esophageal strictures. Prokinetics are rarely effective, but they should be tried. Colonic dilatation and intractable constipation may necessitate subtotal colectomy with ileorectostomy. Allogeneic stem cell or liver transplants have been used as treatments of mitochondrial cytopathy for patients who are relatively healthy.

Suggested Reading

Camilleri M. Disorders of gastrointestinal motility in neurologic diseases. Mayo Clin Proc. 1990 Jun;65(6):825–46. Epub 1990 Jun 01.

Camilleri M, Bharucha AE. Disturbances of gastrointestinal motility and the nervous system. In: Aminoff MJ, Josephson SA, editors. Aminoff's neurology and general medicine. 5th ed. London: Elsevier Academic Press; 2014. p. 255–71.

Vassallo M, Camilleri M, Caron BL, Low PA. Gastrointestinal motor dysfunction in acquired selective cholinergic dysautonomia associated with infectious mononucleosis. Gastroenterology. 1991 Jan;100(1):252–8. Epub 1991 Jan 01.

Case Discussions: Neurologic Disorders Presenting With Gastrointestinal Dysmotility

Introduction

The gastrointestinal tract receives extensive autonomic neural input from the nervous system; therefore, neurologic diseases are associated with gut motility disorders. In addition, neurologic diseases may involve the enteric or intrinsic nervous system and result in gut dysmotility. These conditions are reviewed in Chapter 7 ("Neuromuscular Disorders Causing Gut Dysmotility"). This chapter reviews illustrative cases of such neurologic diseases encountered in clinical practice at Mayo Clinic.

Case Examples

Case 1: Multiple Endocrine Neoplasia 2B

Patients with multiple endocrine neoplasia 2B typically present with constipation, obstruction, or megacolon, often in infancy. Patients have a characteristic facies with thickening of the lips, marfanoid habitus, and medullated corneal nerve fibers. Medullary thyroid carcinoma (MTC) (arising in the parafollicular C cells) develop in all patients, and pheochromocytomas develop in some. The defective *RET* gene is expressed in all tissues affected, such as the enteric nervous system, thyroid, and parathyoid. The disease results from gain-of-function mutations in *RET*: 95% of cases from M918T mutation in exon 16 and 5% from a mutation in A833F.

A 60-year-old man with known MEN 2B had previously received treatment for MTC about 20 years previously (thyroidectomy). His father had had MTC. Among 7 siblings, 1 brother had died of MTC, and 1 sister and 1 brother, aged 55 and 40 years, respectively, had had thyroidectomy for MTC. The patient had 6 children, 2 of whom had had thyroidectomy for MTC: a daughter, aged 33 years, and a son, aged 31 years. The son also had gastrointestinal (GI) symptoms. Details of the family pedigree are provided in Figure 8.1. The clinical features of the patient are shown in Figure 1.14,

Figure 8.1 (Case 1) Megacolon and Family Pedigree of Patient With Multiple Endocrine Neoplasia 2B

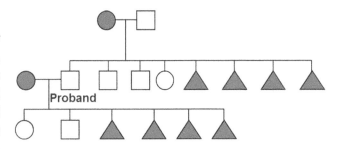

Blue circles indicate unaffected females; blue triangles, unaffected males; yellow circles, affected females; yellow squares, affected males.

and those of the patient and his siblings are listed in Table 8.1. The radiologic and histopathologic features of multiple endocrine neoplasia 2B with megacolon are shown in Figure 1.15.

Table 8.1   Mayo Clinic Series of MEN 2B and Megacolon

	Cases[a]						
	A	B	C	D	E	F	G
Age at diagnosis, y							
MEN 2B	8	20	Not known	3	31	18	51
Megacolon	Infancy	25	60	3	24	18	70 (autopsy)
Sex	M	M	M	F	M	F	M
RET mutation	ND	M918T	M918T	M918T	ND	ND	ND
Family history of MEN	−	−	+	−	+	+	+
Eye signs							
Ganglioneuromas	✓	✓	✓	x	✓	✓	✓
Corneal fibrous nerve	x	x	✓	x	✓	✓	✓
Eyelid eversion	x	x	x	✓	x	x	x
Lips/tongue							
Prominent lips	✓	✓	✓	✓	✓	✓	✓
Ganglioneuromas	✓	✓	✓	✓	✓	✓	✓
Thyroid problems							
MTC	✓	✓	✓	✓	✓	✓	✓
Total thyroidectomy	✓	✓	✓	✓	✓	x	✓
Partial thyroidectomy	x	x	x	x	x	✓	x
Neck dissection	✓	✓	✓	x	x	✓	x
Esophageal problems	x	x	Achalasia	Zenker diverticulum	x	x	Achalasia
Adrenal involvement	x	Cushing syndrome	x	Pheochromocytomas (2)	x	x	x
Colon							
Megacolon	✓	✓	✓	✓	✓	✓	✓
Colectomy	✓	x	✓	✓	x	x	x
Ileosigmoidostomy	✓	x	x	✓	✓	x	x
Anorectal symptoms	✓	x	✓	x	x	x	x
Skeletal							
Marfanoid habitus	✓	✓	✓	✓	✓	✓	✓
Joint laxity	x	x	x	x	✓	✓	x
Scoliosis	x	x	✓	x	x	✓	x
Pes cavus	x	x	x	x	x	x	✓

Abbreviations: F, female; M, male; MEN, multiple endocrine neoplasia; MTC, medullary thyroid cancer; ND, not done.

[a] ✓, clinical feature present; −, absent family history; +, positive family history; x, clinical feature absent.

Modified from Gibbons D, Camilleri M, Nelson AD, Eckert D. Characteristics of chronic megacolon among patients diagnosed with multiple endocrine neoplasia type 2B. United European Gastroenterol J. 2016 Jun;4(3):449-54; used with permission.

Case 2: Multiple Endocrine Neoplasia Type 2B

A 24-year-old man had undergone thyroidectomy for MTC at 10 years of age and underwent a subtotal colectomy with ileosigmoidostomy for megacolon in early adulthood. He presented with persistent abdominal distention and nutritional failure that had been treated with total parenteral nutrition, which was complicated by line sepsis and clots. One month after colectomy and for the next 2 years, he had persistent small bowel dilatation (Figure 8.2).

Physical examination findings suggested a rectal evacuation disorder (0.5-cm perineal descent on straining). This disorder was confirmed by the rectoanal pressure differential of −125 mm Hg and balloon expulsion from the rectum requiring more than 470 g added weight. There was some evidence of reduced rectal sensation (first sensation at 60 mL, desire to defecate at 119 mL, and urgency at 161 mL), but normal rectal compliance excluded megarectum. Because of the rectal evacuation disorder, the patient underwent ileostomy for symptom relief. During

| **Figure 8.2 (Case 2)   Small Intestinal Dilatation 1 Month After Colectomy for Megacolon Due to Rectal Evacuation Disorder** |

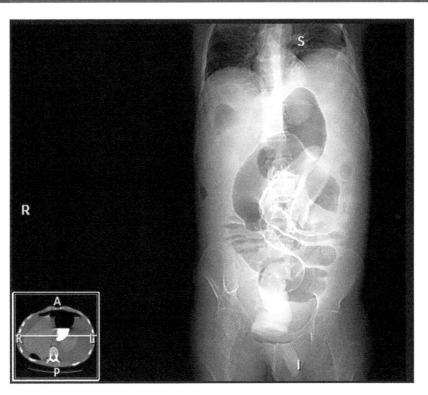

A indicates anterior; I, inferior; L, left; P, posterior; R, right; S, superior.

Figure 8.3 (Case 2) Abdominal Distention in Patient With Multiple Endocrine Neoplasia 2B

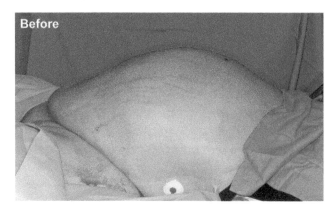

Before

This was the appearance of the abdomen while the patient was receiving general anesthesia, before limited laparotomy for placement of ileostomy.

Figure 8.5 (Case 2) Abdominal Distention Resolved With Ileostomy

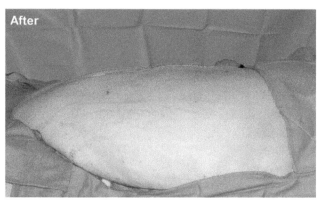

After

Appearance of abdomen while patient was in the operating room after completion of general anesthesia.

the operation, with the patient receiving general anesthesia, his abdominal distention (Figure 8.3) was clearly evident, and, at mini-laparotomy, there were distended intestinal loops (Figure 8.4). After fashioning of the ileostomy, the abdominal distention was no longer evident (Figure 8.5).

At follow-up 1 year after ileostomy, the patient had gained 16 pounds, was not taking any supplementation, was tolerating a full diet, and was emptying his ileostomy bag about 6 times a day.

This case exemplifies the importance of excluding a rectal evacuation disorder before assuming that the intestinal dilatation is exclusively due to the megacolon.

Figure 8.4 (Case 2) Distended Intestinal Loops

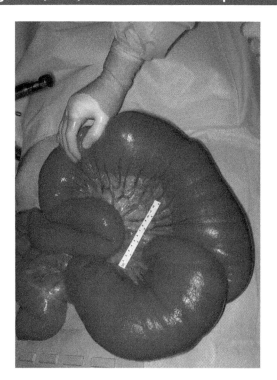

Diameter of the small bowel is compared with the hand of the surgeon.

Case 3: Localized Megacolon

A 19-year-old woman presented with abdominal pain and constipation that had been present since childhood.

Abdominal radiographs showed distention of the splenic flexure (Figure 8.6), and barium enema showed an ahaustral, dilated left colon (Figure 8.7). An

Figure 8.6 (Case 3)   Splenic Flexure Distention on Abdominal Radiographs

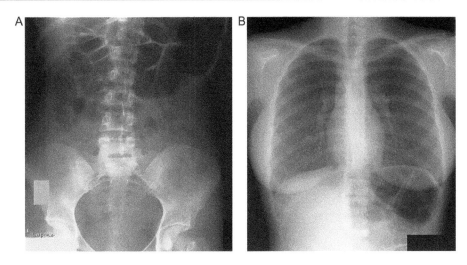

A, Gas-filled distended loops of colon in left upper quadrant of the abdomen. The slight scoliosis that is seen often occurs in patients with congenital segmental or total colonic aganglionosis. B, Gas-filled distention of the splenic flexure.

Figure 8.7 (Case 3)   Ahaustral, Dilated Left Colon on Barium Enema in a Patient With Megacolon of the Hindgut

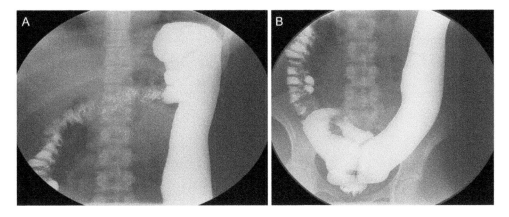

A, Ahaustral and distended splenic flexure and upper descending colon, in contrast to the normal-diameter, contracting ascending and transverse colon. B, Ahaustral and distended descending and sigmoid colon with normal haustrations evident in the ascending colon.

(From Sweetser S, Camilleri M. Clinical challenges and images in GI: hindgut dysgenesis with megacolon. Gastroenterology. 2008 May;134(5):1293, 1635; used with permission.)

Figure 8.8 (Case 3)   Dilated Colon on Excretory Urogram Obtained During Childhood

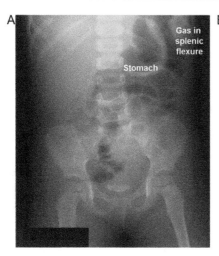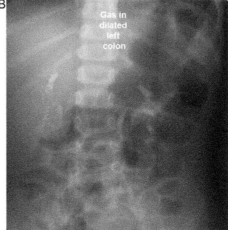

The finding suggested that the disease was congenital. A, Gas distention of the splenic flexure appears separate from the air in the stomach. B, The excretory urogram shows no obstruction or dilatation of the ureters, pelves, or calyces in the kidneys; however, gas distention in the left side of the colon is noted.

excretory urogram obtained when the patient was a child showed colonic dilatation (Figure 8.8).

A motility study of the colon showed no contractions (Figure 8.9), and morphologic studies showed reduced numbers of interstitial cells of Cajal compared with those in control tissue (Figure 8.10).

Figure 8.9 (Case 3)   Reduced Phasic Pressure Activity and Tone on Colonic Manometry

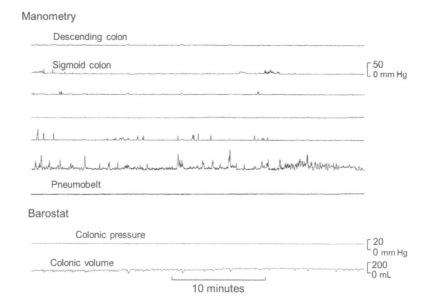

(From Sweetser S, Camilleri M. Clinical challenges and images in GI: hindgut dysgenesis with megacolon. Gastroenterology. 2008 May;134(5):1293, 1635; used with permission.)

Figure 8.10 (Case 3)   Reduction in Interstitial Cells of Cajal (ICC) Relative to Control

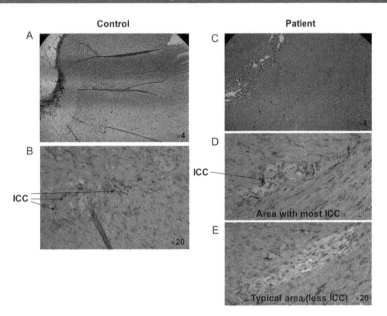

ICCs were reduced 40% to 50% (c-kit stain).

Case 4: Chronic Intestinal Pseudo-obstruction in an Elderly Patient

A 73-year-old man with no significant GI history presented with a 25-pound weight loss, anorexia, and paresthesia in both hands. Barium studies showed dilatation of the stomach and of loops of the small intestine. There was no demonstrable obstruction, and the mucosal appearance on esophagogastroduodenoscopy was normal. These features were suggestive of a disorder of GI motor function, which was confirmed by motor incoordination, but amplitude contractions in the antrum and small bowel were normal. During the next 5 months, severe constipation and sensorimotor peripheral neuropathy involving all extremities developed.

The diagnosis was paraneoplastic chronic intestinal pseudo-obstruction (CIPO) due to a small cell carcinoma of the lung associated with a circulating antineuronal nuclear (anti-Hu) antibody and inflammatory plexopathy of the myenteric plexus in the stomach (Figure 8.11).

Paraneoplastic GI dysmotility syndrome is usually associated with small cell lung cancer and type 1 antineuronal antibody. It may result in diverse GI dysmotilities, from achalasia to constipation and usually CIPO. This syndrome typically affects middle-aged smokers, who have rapid development of intolerance of food and weight loss. The result of chest radiography is usually negative, and mediastinal computed tomography (CT) is essential if the diagnosis is suspected. A circulating antibody to an epitope is shared by the tumor and myenteric neurons; histologic ganglionitis confirms the immune destruction of the myenteric plexus.

Figure 8.11 (Case 4)   Paraneoplastic Chronic Intestinal Pseudo-obstruction Due to a Small Cell Carcinoma of the Lung

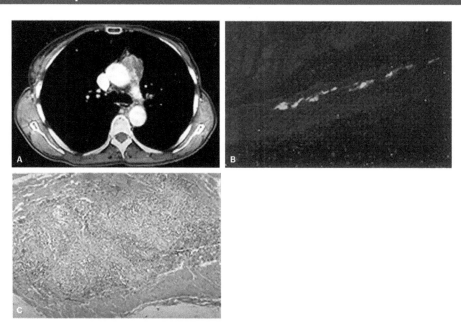

The carcinoma was a mediastinal mass to the left of the blood vessels (A), and it was associated with a circulating antineuronal nuclear (anti-Hu) antibody (showing positive immunofluorescent staining of rat myenteric plexus [B]) and inflammatory plexopathy of the myenteric plexus in the stomach (C). Marked inflammatory cell infiltrate expanding the myenteric plexus is seen between muscle cell layers.

Case 5: GI Dysmotility After Infectious Mononucleosis in a College Student

A 23-year-old woman presented with a 3-year history of nausea, distention, and constipation that had been present since a diagnosis of acute mononucleosis. Symptoms started acutely, 1 week after diagnosis. She had been a track athlete in college and had been hospitalized for heat stroke after an 800-m run. She also had blurred vision; dry mouth,

eyes, and vagina; and bladder emptying problems. On physical examination, she had a distended tympanic abdomen but no succussion splash. She had dilated pupils with no accommodation response and minimal reaction to light. Plain abdominal radiograph (Figure 8.12) showed air-fluid levels suggestive of obstruction or pseudo-obstruction, and gastroduodenal manometry suggested neuropathy with normal-amplitude incoordinated contractions and postprandial antral hypomotility (Figure 8.13).

Figure 8.12 (Case 5) **Megacolon (A) and Air-Fluid Levels (B) During Acute Episode in a 23-Year-Old Woman With Postinfectious Mononucleosis**

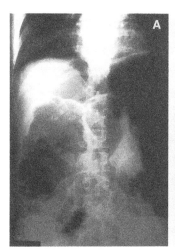 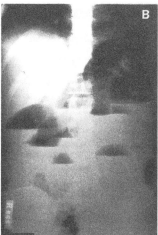

(From Vassallo M, Camilleri M, Caron BL, Low PA. Gastrointestinal motor dysfunction in acquired selective cholinergic dysautonomia associated with infectious mononucleosis. Gastroenterology. 1991 Jan;100(1):252-8; used with permission.)

Figure 8.13 (Case 5) **Gastroduodenal Manometry: Neuropathy**

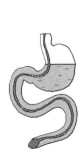 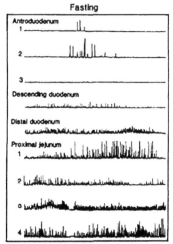 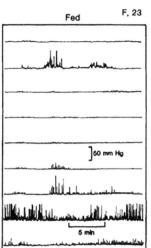

(Modified from Vassallo M, Camilleri M, Caron BL, Low PA. Gastrointestinal motor dysfunction in acquired selective cholinergic dysautonomia associated with infectious mononucleosis. Gastroenterology. 1991 Jan;100(1):252-8; used with permission.)

Table 8.2   Results of Autonomic Tests for the Patient With Acute Infectious Mononucleosis

Test	Results	Normal Values Corrected for Age (23) and Sex (F)
Valsalva ratio	1.97	>1.5
Orthostatic Δ BP, mm Hg	Systolic: 0 Diastolic: 6	<25 <15
Plasma norepinephrine, pg/mL (lying; standing levels)	309; 1,093	70-750; 200-1,700
Heart rate beats/min Δ to deep breathing	15	>18
ΔPanc polypeptide to sham feed, pg/mL	8	22-65
Thermoregulatory sweat test	>95% anhidrosis	<3
Q-SART sweat output, μL/cm³	L forearm: 0.05 L foot: 0	0.34-1.33 0.25-1.95
Pupils		
Initial size, mm	R: 6.29; L: 6.68	<3
Response to light		
Latency, s	2; 0.43	0.2-0.3
Contraction Δ, mm	0.42; 1.52	2-4
Psychosensory response	Normal both eyes	Prompt dilatation after constriction
Contraction to 0.125% pilocarpine (muscarinic cholinergic agonist), mm	3.42; 3.43 (denervation supersensitivity)	<0.05

Abbreviations: BP, blood pressure; L, left; panc, pancreatic; Q-SART, quantitative sudomotor axon reflex test; R, right.

Modified from Vassallo M, Camilleri M, Caron BL, Low PA. Gastrointestinal motor dysfunction in acquired selective cholinergic dysautonomia associated with infectious mononucleosis. Gastroenterology. 1991 Jan;100(1):252-8; used with permission.

On special autonomic tests, normal adrenergic but abnormal vagal function and abnormal sympathetic cholinergic function were suggestive of postganglionic denervation and abnormal pupillary parasympathetic cholinergic function (Table 8.2).

In addition, results of bladder function tests were consistent with denervation hypersensitivity (Figure 8.14). The patient underwent colectomy. Pathologic examination of the enteric neurons found no inflammation, no intranuclear inclusions, and normal transmitter content (Figure 8.15), findings confirming that the motility disorder reflected extrinsic cholinergic denervation.

The diagnosis was Ebstein-Barr virus–induced selective cholinergic dysautonomia, a form of demyelinating neuropathy associated with herpes family virus infection.

Figure 8.14 (Case 5)   Results of Autonomic Pharmacologic Stimulation of the Urinary Bladder

System/test	Patient's result		Normal value
	Right	**Left**	<0.05
Pupil contraction (mm) to 0.125% pilocarpine*	3.42	3.43	

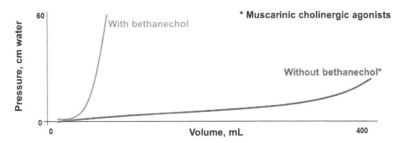

Increased pressure with cholinergic stimulus (bethanechol) indicates cholinergic denervation supersensitivity.

(Data from Vassallo M, Camilleri M, Caron BL, Low PA. Gastrointestinal motor dysfunction in acquired selective cholinergic dysautonomia associated with infectious mononucleosis. Gastroenterology. 1991 Jan;100(1):252-8.)

Figure 8.15 (Case 5)   Pathologic Results for Enteric Neurons

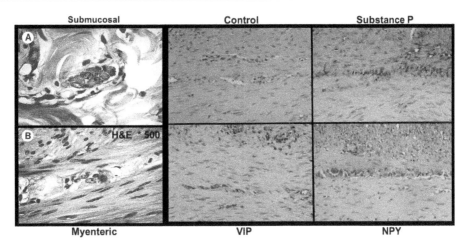

Lack of inflammation and intranuclear inclusions and normal transmitter content confirm that the motility disorder reflected extrinsic cholinergic denervation. Preserved ganglion cells are in the submucosal (A) and myenteric (B) plexus. On the right: normal staining (neurotransmitter content) in the ganglion cells within the plexus. H&E indicates hematoxylin-eosin stain; NPY, neuropeptide Y; VIP, vasoactive intestinal peptide.

(From Vassallo M, Camilleri M, Caron BL, Low PA. Gastrointestinal motor dysfunction in acquired selective cholinergic dysautonomia associated with infectious mononucleosis. Gastroenterology. 1991 Jan;100(1):252-8; used with permission.)

Case 6: Weight Loss and Food Intolerance

A 72-year-old man presented with weight loss and food intolerance. See Case 1 of Chapter 5, "Case Discussions: Nausea and Vomiting."

Case 7: Known Macrodystrophia Lipomatosa Involving the Right Lower Extremity and Diffuse Fibrolipomatous Hypertrophy of the Right Hemipelvis

A 33-year-old woman presented with bowel and bladder symptoms. At the age of 3 years, the patient had undergone appendectomy and was found to have multiple lipomas within the pelvis. During late adolescence and young adulthood, she experienced diarrhea and abdominal pain. At age 23 years, she had obstruction of the lower left colon caused by extrinsic masses that were compressing the bladder and the colon; she also had descending colon diverticula, for which she had a 6-cm resection of the colon.

The patient's symptoms included severe constipation associated with lack of urge, need to strain excessively to pass bowel movements, and spontaneous bowel movements approximately once per month that require weekly large doses of senna or magnesium salts. She denied perineal support of anal or vaginal digitation or use of enemas to facilitate evacuation of the rectum. She had a sense of incomplete evacuation of the rectum and the bladder, urinary frequency was about once per hour and 3 or 4 times an hour when she had caffeinated beverages.

The patient also experienced neuropathic pain in the right foot that was slowly extending up the right lower limb and degenerative joint disease in the right foot and ankle. She required daily treatment with amitriptyline (150 mg), gabapentin (100 mg), and nonsteroidal anti-inflammatory drugs.

The patient's father also had had abdominal lipomas, and they were surgically removed when he was a child. A cousin of the father had a skeletal abnormality possibly related to the familial macrodystrophia lipomatosa.

On examination, anal sphincter pressure at rest was normal, squeeze pressure was normal, and there was normal descent of the perineum but tender puborectalis muscle. No palpable pelvic masses were appreciated from the rectal examination. There was enlargement of the calf and thigh with fatty infiltration and some wasting of the gluteus maximus (Figure 8.16).

Gastric emptying and small bowel transit were normal. Colonic transit was delayed (Figure 8.17), and colonic manometry showed features of colonic inertia (Figure 8.18).

Figure 8.16 (Case 7)   Involvement of Right Sciatic Nerve With Macrodystrophia Lipomatosis in a 33-Year-Old Woman

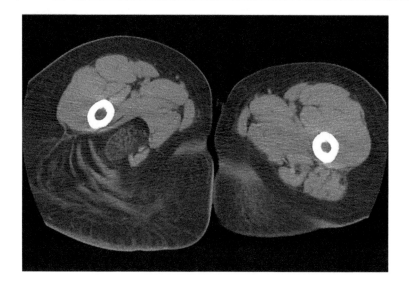

Figure 8.17 (Case 7)   Colonic Transit Study Shows Virtually No Movement of Isotope Over 20 Hours

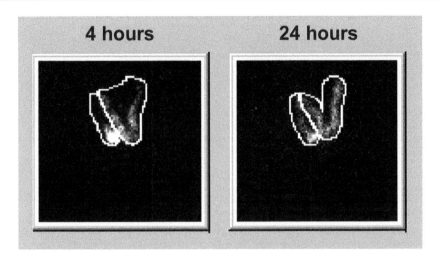

Figure 8.18 (Case 7)   Modest Phasic and Tonic Motor Responses to a Meal and a Fair Response to Intravenous Neostigmine, 1 mg, on Colonic Manometry

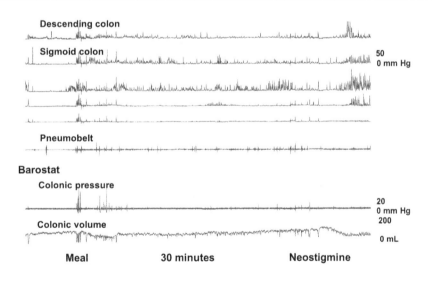

Figure 8.19 (Case 7)   Comparison of Intrinsic Colonic Nerves of Control (A) and Patient With Macrodystrophia Lipomatosis (B)

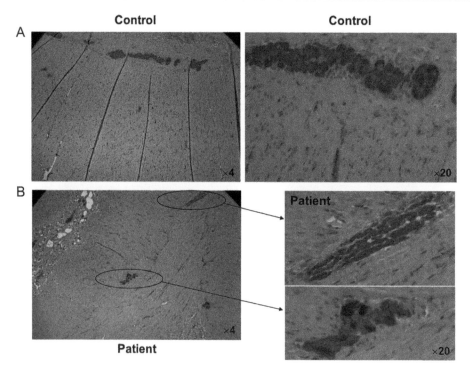

Results on staining with protein G product 9.5 were normal.

The patient underwent colectomy, which showed normal intrinsic nerves (Figures 8.19 and 8.20). There were no intraluminal lipomas or masses compressing or obstructing the colon. Colonic intrinsic innervation was normal.

In summary, the patient had macrodystrophia lipomatosa with involvement of the right lower limb and buttock and lipomas in the retrorectal area and around the sacral nerves. The colonic inertia was associated with prolonged hyperpolarization (inhibition) of nerve attributed to extrinsic denervation of sacral parasympathetic supply to the colon.

Figure 8.20 (Case 7)   Intrinsic Colonic Nerves in Sigmoid (A) and Ascending Colon (B) in a Patient With Macrodystrophia Lipomatosis

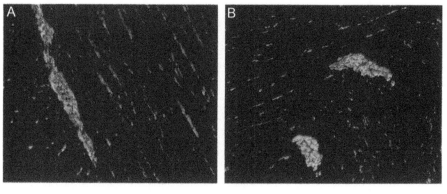

Specimens were stained with protein G product 9.5.

Cases 8 and 9: Mitochondrial Cytopathy and Gut Dysmotility

Mitochondrial cytopathy is an autosomal recessive disorder in which GI and hepatic manifestations may present at any age: hepatomegaly and hepatic failure in neonates; seizures or diarrhea in infancy; and hepatic failure, CIPO, or oculo-GI dystrophy in childhood or adulthood. The finding of small bowel diverticulosis at a young age (<40 years), as seen on gamma camera scanning in case 8 (Figure 8.21), should raise suspicion for mitochondrial cytopathy.

The condition can be suspected from screen tests showing acidosis with lactate, increased pyruvate level, or increased creatine kinase level consistent with skeletal muscle damage. Biopsies of skeletal muscle and rectal submucosa show mega-mitochondria, and genetic studies prove the diagnosis. Because mitochondria are involved in oxidative phosphorylation in every organ, mitochondrial cytopathy can involve almost every organ in the body (see Figure 1.16).

In case 9, a 43-year-old man presented with pigmentary retinopathy causing blindness, sensorineural hearing loss, myoclonus epilepsy, mild ptosis and ophthalmoparesis, migraine headaches, and mild sensorimotor peripheral neuropathy. He had previously undergone drainage of intra-abdominal abscesses related to multiple small bowel diverticuli. He also had hypothyroidism, testosterone insufficiency, sleep apnea, lack of energy, and, in his GI system, transfer dysphagia, diarrhea, and incontinence with weakness of both internal and external anal sphincters. Skeletal muscle biopsy showed ragged red fibers from subsarcolemmal mitochondria. The fibers were positive for succinate

Figure 8.21 (Case 8)   Multiple Small Bowel Diverticula and Abscesses on Gamma Camera Scan

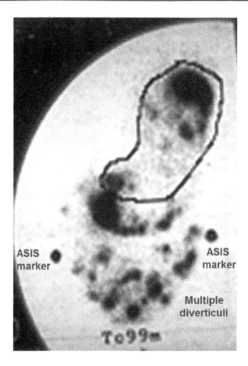

Scan was obtained after ingestion of a radiolabeled egg meal in a 23-year-old man with mitochondrial neurogastrointestinal encephalomyopathy. ASIS indicates anterior superior iliac spine; Tc99m, technetium Tc 99m.

dehydrogenase, and the defect in mitochondrial function in cytochrome c oxidase based on immunocytochemistry (see Figure 1.17).

Mega-mitochondria have also been identified in submucosal neurons on rectal biopsy (see Figure 1.18, left panels). In this patient with mitochondrial cytopathy (case 9), other manifestations included delayed

Figure 8.22 (Case 9)   Delayed Gastric Emptying in a Patient With Mitochondrial Encephalopathy With Ragged Red Fibers

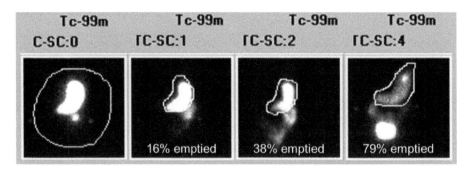

Tc-99m indicates technetium Tc 99m.

gastric emptying (Figure 8.22), diffuse brain atrophy and calcification of basal ganglia, skeletal muscle disorders of mitochondrial enzyme chain (Figure 8.23), small bowel diverticulosis on coronal CT abdominal (Figure 8.24), and colonic wide-mouthed diverticula on barium enema (Figure 8.25).

The small bowel bacterial overgrowth due to diverticulosis was treated with rotating antibiotics (initially 1 week per month): ciprofloxacin, doxycycline, and metronidazole at half the recommended adult dose daily. This regimen relieved the diarrhea and restored the continence of stool.

Figure 8.23 (Case 9)   Brain and Skeletal Muscle Images

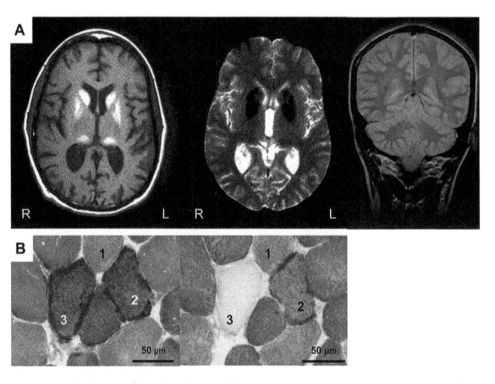

A, Diffuse brain atrophy and calcification of basal ganglia. B, Defect in mitochondrial enzyme chain with lack of cytochrome c oxidase on skeletal muscle biopsy. 1 indicates cytochrome c oxidase, nonragged red fiber (normal); 2, cytochrome oxidase–positive, ragged red fiber; 3, cytochrome oxidase–negative, ragged red fiber.

(Modified from Nishigaki Y, Tadesse S, Bonilla E, Shungu D, Hersh S, Keats BJ, et al. A novel mitochondrial tRNA(Leu(UUR)) mutation in a patient with features of MERRF and Kearns-Sayre syndrome. Neuromuscul Disord. 2003 May;13(4):334-40; used with permission.)

Figure 8.24 (Case 9)   Dilated Stomach and Small Bowel Diverticulosis (arrows) on Coronal Computed Tomography in a Patient With Mitochondrial Encephalopathy With Ragged Red Fibers

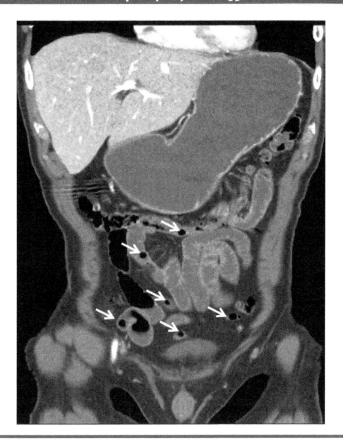

Figure 8.25 (Case 9)   Wide-Mouthed Diverticula and Extensive Involvement of Right Colon on Barium Enema

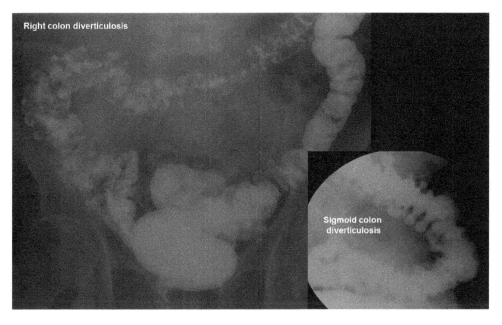

Diarrhea was controlled with rotating antibiotics resulting in no further incontinence.

Case 10: Suspected CIPO

A 26-year-old woman presented with a distended abdomen. Eighteen years previously, a full-thickness biopsy at laparotomy suggested a diagnosis of hollow visceral myopathy with lymphocytic infiltrate of the circular muscle and fibrous connective tissue in the outer layer of the stomach, duodenum, and jejunum but normal myenteric plexus. She reported having had 3 prior surgeries for CIPO, she was taking antibiotics for small bowel bacterial overgrowth, and she has a venting gastrostomy. Physical examination showed marked abdominal distention, tympanic percussion note, no succession splash, and very infrequent bowel sounds. Her pupils were markedly dilated with no reaction to light. External ocular movements and eyelids functioned normally. Results of rectal examination were normal. Abdominal CT showed dilated bowel (Figure 8.26) and dilated ureter and kidney collecting system (Figure 8.27). Antroduodenal manometry showed marked hypomotility (Figure 8.28), and small bowel aspirate was positive for bacterial overgrowth (Figure 8.29).

Figure 8.26 (Case 10)   Abdominal Findings in Patient With Hollow Visceral Myopathy

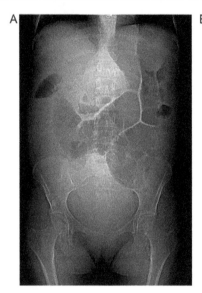 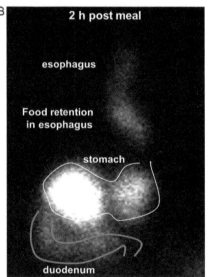

A, Dilated bowel on abdominal computed tomogram. B, Isotopically labeled egg meal retained in the dilated esophagus, stomach, and duodenal loop 2 hours after meal ingestion.

Figure 8.27 (Case 10)   Ureteropelvicaliectasis associated with hollow visceral myopathy showing the dilated left renal pelvis (A, arrow) and the dilated ureter (B, arrow)

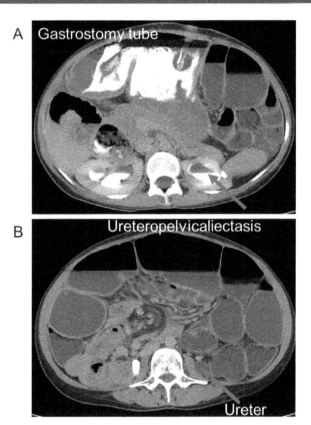

Decompressing gastrostomy tube is seen in A.

Figure 8.28 (Case 10)   Postprandial Gastroduodenal Motility Findings

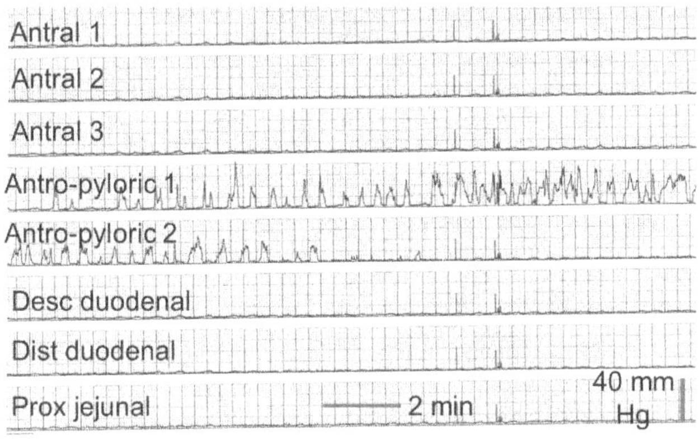

The pylorus is the only segment contracting in the upper gastro-intestinal tract. The pylorus is identified by the intermittent tonic elevation of baseline pressure and the combination in the same recording level of wider antral contractions and slender duode-nal contractions. Desc indicates descending; Dist, distal; Prox, proximal.

Figure 8.29 (Case 10)   Small Bowel Aspirates and Biopsy Stained With Hematoxylin-Eosin

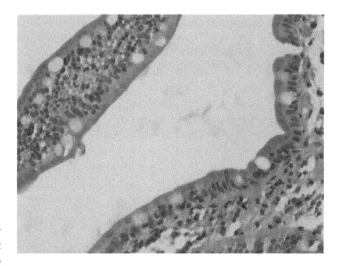

Total intestinal flora, >100,000 cfu/mL; aerobic gram-negative bacilli, >100,000 cfu/mL; yeast, 100,000 cfu/mL; no parasites seen; intraepithelial lymphocytes and cuboidal enterocytes are seen. The shortening of columnar enterocytes is associated with small intestinal bacterial overgrowth.

Case 11: 12-Year History of Progressive Constipation

A 22-year-old woman presented with a 12-year history of progressive constipation. The patient had increased joint flexibility, hyperextensible skin, and excessive perineal descent on physical examination. Features were consistent with Beighton criteria for hypermobility syndrome (palms flat on the ground when patient touches toes with knees fully extended), mild scoliosis, and slow colonic transit. Retained

rectal gas was consistent with rectal evacuation disorder (Figure 8.30).

Radiologic studies confirmed evidence of rectal evacuation disorder due to descending perineum syndrome, enterocele, and rectocele (Figure 8.31).

In a wide genetic screen (611,000 single nucleotide polymorphisms), 4 variations were identified in *COL1A1* gene (Figure 8.32). These mutations result in an increase in the number of base pairs in the C′ end and replacement of the glycine amino acid in the N′ end, changes leading to incomplete cleavage of procollagen by proteases and resulting in collagen weakness.

Figure 8.30 (Case 11)   Features Consistent With Beighton Criteria for Hypermobility Syndrome

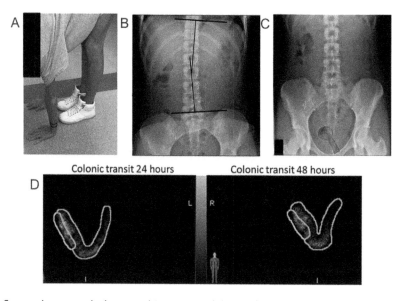

Patient can place palms flat on the ground when touching toes with knees fully extended (A) and has mild scoliosis (B). Retained rectal gas (outlined with red shape) is consistent with rectal evacuation disorder (C), and slow colonic transit, shown by the isotope retained in the ascending and transverse colon at 48 hours, is virtually unchanged from the appearance at 24 hours (D). I indicates inferior; L, left; R, right.

(From Vijayvargiya P, Camilleri M, Cima RR. COL1A1 mutations presenting as descending perineum syndrome in a young patient with hypermobility syndrome. Mayo Clin Proc. 2018 Mar;93(3):386-91; used with permission.)

Figure 8.31 (Case 11)   Radiologic Results for Patient With 12-Year History of Progressive Constipation

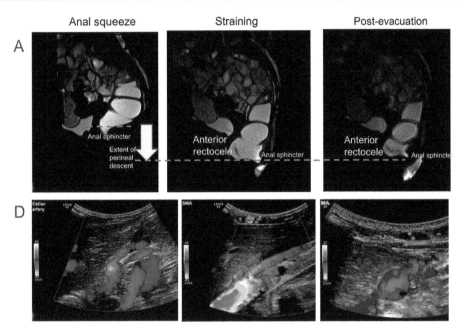

A, Excessive perineal descent on magnetic resonance defecography. B, Normal blood vessels and exclusion of vascular variant of Ehlers-Danlos Syndrome on Doppler ultrasonography. IMA indicates inferior mesenteric artery; SMA, superior mesenteric artery.

(From Vijayvargiya P, Camilleri M, Cima RR. COL1A1 mutations presenting as descending perineum syndrome in a young patient with hypermobility syndrome. Mayo Clin Proc. 2018 Mar;93(3):386-91; used with permission.)

Figure 8.32 (Case 11)   *COL1A1* Gene Variants Resulting in Ehlers-Danlos Syndrome–Hypermobility Variant

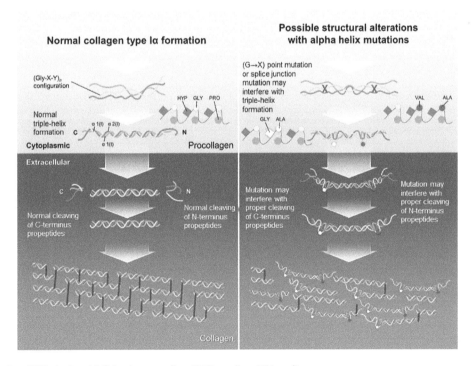

ALA indicates alanine; GLY, glycine; HYP, hydroxyproline; PRO, proline; VAL, valine.

(From Vijayvargiya P, Camilleri M, Cima RR. COL1A1 mutations presenting as descending perineum syndrome in a young patient with hypermobility syndrome. Mayo Clin Proc. 2018 Mar;93(3):386-91; used with permission.)

Ehlers-Danlos Syndrome and GI Manifestations: A 20-Year Experience at Mayo Clinic

Among 687 patients with Ehlers-Danlos syndrome (EDS), 56% had GI manifestations, 86.8% were female, and the mean age at diagnosis was 29.6 years. The frequencies of GI manifestations, by EDS categories, were 58.9% in EDS classic, 57.5% in EDS hypermobility, and 47.3% in EDS vascular subtypes.

The most common GI symptoms were abdominal pain (56.1%), nausea (42.3%), constipation (38.6%), heartburn (37.6%), and irritable bowel syndrome–like findings (27.5%). GI symptoms were more prevalent in EDS hypermobility than in the other subtypes. The most common abnormalities on esophagogastroduodenoscopy, performed on 37.8% of patients, were gastritis, hiatal hernia, and reflux esophagitis.

Gastric emptying was abnormal in 22.3% of 76 patients tested: slow in 11.8% and fast in 10.5% (see Figure 1.20). Colonic transit was abnormal in 28.3% of 46 tested: delayed in 19.6% and accelerated in 8.7% (see Figure 1.21). Rectal evacuation disorder was found in 60% of patients who underwent anorectal manometry. Patients with the vascular subtype of EDS have intraabdominal aneurysms. Proton pump inhibitors (38%) and drugs for constipation (23%) were the most commonly used medications. A minority of patients underwent colectomy (2.9%) or small bowel surgery (4%) (Nelson 2015; see suggested reading).

Case 12: Anorexia, Weight Loss, and 3 Years of Recurrent Hiccups

A 28-year-old woman presented with anorexia, weight loss, and a 3-year history of recurrent hiccups. She acknowledged a diagnosis of bulimia in an effort to control her weight when she was in college. She has a 3-year-old son, is unable to work, is depressed, and has experienced recurrent hiccups and vomiting on and off for 3 years associated with weight loss of 25 pounds (current weight 98 pounds). She had undergone several tests, including abdominal CT, ultrasonography, and upper GI endoscopy 3 times, including tests for *Helicobacter pylori* infection (serologic and gastric biopsies). Results of all the tests were negative. She has achieved no response with antidepressants and psychologic counseling and was referred to the eating disorders clinic. Her husband volunteered the information that her "hiccups continue while she is asleep." The abdominal CT showed no signs of disease around the diaphragm. Brain and brainstem magnetic resonance imaging showed a large brainstem tumor (Figure 8.33).

The patient underwent surgical removal of the brainstem tumor (Figure 8.34).

When seen 3 months postoperatively, the patient had no hiccups, no belching, an excellent appetite, a weight gain of 40 pounds, some tongue weakness and wasting, and speech and swallow weakness at the end of the day.

Figure 8.33 (Case 12)   Large Brainstem Tumor on Preoperative Magnetic Resonance Imaging in a Patient With 3-Year History of Recurrent Hiccups

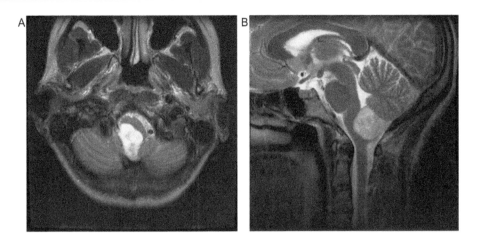

Figure 8.34 (Case 12)   Three-Month Postoperative Results on Magnetic Resonance Imaging

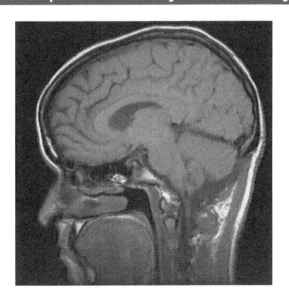

Case 13: Nausea and Vomiting for 7 Months

A previously healthy 49-year-old man presented to our clinic with a 7-month history of chronic anorexia, nausea, and occasional vomiting. Nausea was present throughout the day, and bile-stained vomiting usually occurred within minutes of eating. Evaluation elsewhere included upper GI endoscopy, barium upper GI series, stool examination for ova and parasites, and CT of the head, all of which had negative results. Separate therapeutic trials with doxepin and metoclopramide failed to relieve his symptoms. Five months after the onset of symptoms, CT of the abdomen suggested an enlarged pancreatic head; however, exploratory laparotomy and pancreatic biopsy were negative.

On initial evaluation, the patient had experienced a profound weight loss (21 kg in 7 months), and he described low-grade occipital-frontal headaches, frequent episodes of hiccups, and yawning spells. On physical examination, he was cachectic and had depressed affect, orthostatic hypotension, and normal results of neurologic examination. Autonomic testing showed a Valsalva ratio of 1.12 (normal >1.5), heart period response during deep breathing of 12 beats per minute (normal >15), and abnormal sweating on the abdomen and lower limbs, findings suggesting central autonomic denervation.

Manometry was consistent with a neuropathic process (Figure 8.35), autonomic reflexes suggested a central dysautonomic process, and brain magnetic resonance imaging showed a brainstem tumor (Figure 8.36).

Figure 8.35 (Case 13)   Delayed Gastric Emptying of Solids and Liquids in a Patient With 7-Month History of Nausea and Vomiting

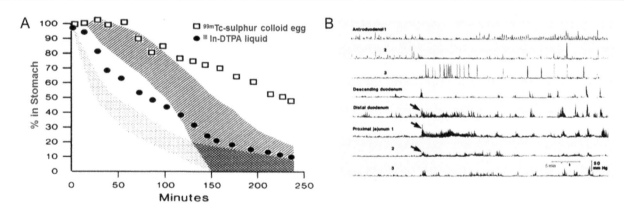

A, Gastric emptying test. Shaded areas show normal values for emptying of solids (darker shading) and liquids (lighter shading). B, Gastroduodenojejunal manometry. Postprandial motility shows incoordinated, simultaneous onset of phase III–like activity front in the small bowel. DTPA indicates diethylenetriamine pentaacetic acid, to which the isotope ^{111}In is bound; ^{111}In, indium In 111; ^{99m}Tc, technetium Tc 99m.

Figure 8.36 (Case 13)   Tumor in the Medulla Oblongata (arrow) on Computed Tomography of the Brain

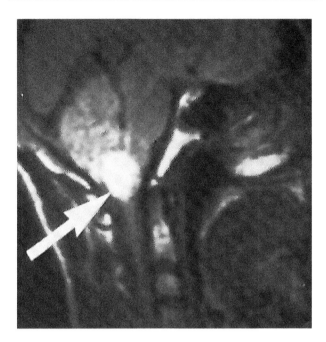

(From Wood JR, Camilleri M, Low PA, Malagelada JR. Brainstem tumor presenting as an upper gut motility disorder. Gastroenterology. 1985 Dec;89(6):1411-4; used with permission.)

Suggested Reading

Chedid V, Camilleri M. Autonomic nervous system dysfunction and the gastrointestinal tract. In: Kuipers EJ, ed. Encyclopedia of Gastroenterology. 2nd ed. Oxford: Academic Press; 2020:197–212.

Gibbons D, Camilleri M, Nelson AD, Eckert D. Characteristics of chronic megacolon among patients diagnosed with multiple endocrine neoplasia type 2B. United European Gastroenterol J. 2016;4(3):449–54.

Nelson AD, Mouchli MA, Valentin N, Deyle D, Pichurin P, Acosta A, et al. Ehlers Danlos syndrome and gastrointestinal manifestations: a 20-year experience at Mayo Clinic. Neurogastroenterol Motil. 2015;27(11):1657–66.

Vassallo M, Camilleri M, Caron BL, Low PA. Gastrointestinal motor dysfunction in acquired selective cholinergic dysautonomia associated with infectious mononucleosis. Gastroenterology. 1991;100(1):252–8.

Vijayvargiya P, Camilleri M, Cima RR. COL1A1 mutations presenting as descending perineum syndrome in a young patient with hypermobility syndrome. Mayo Clin Proc. 2018;93(3):386–91.

Chronic Diarrhea[a]   9

Introduction

Acute diarrhea is most often caused by infection. In contrast, chronic watery, nonbloody diarrhea, which is defined by a duration of more than 4 weeks, can result from decreased absorption, increased secretion, reduced barrier function, and various extra-epithelial mechanisms. This chapter addresses clinical evaluation and investigation that guide therapy of patients presenting with chronic diarrhea.

Chronic diarrhea may have diverse causes. It is important to define the frequency and consistency of bowel movements and, in some patients, to measure stool weight over 24 hours. Chronic diarrhea is unlikely to be infectious, and a first step in assessment is based on the appearance of stool: fatty, bloody, or watery.

Chronic watery diarrhea is the most common form of chronic diarrhea and includes the highly prevalent functional diarrhea (or diarrhea-predominant irritable bowel syndrome [see Chapter 11, "Irritable Bowel Syndrome: Peripheral Mechanisms, Biomarkers, and Management"]) and disaccharidase deficiencies. In general, chronic watery diarrhea may result from effects of autocrine, luminal, paracrine, immune, neural, and endocrine factors. These different mechanisms induce diarrhea through their effects on intestinal permeability, ion transport, and motility, mediated through altered functions of the paracellular pathway, epithelium, muscle, and vasculature. The archetype of chronic watery diarrhea, typically characterized by large volume and persistence with fasting, is produced by neuroendocrine tumors, which are exceedingly rare. Given the change in stool consistency or the watery nature of stool in chronic diarrhea, it is essential to understand the physiology of fluid and ion transport at the cellular and organ level.

Physiology

Intestinal Cellular Mechanisms of Fluid and Ion Transport

The content of solutes affects the volume of stool. In patients with chronic watery diarrhea, there is insufficient absorption of solutes or, rarely, they may actually be actively secreted into the lumen, or both. A normal epithelial barrier function is required to prevent the back diffusion of electrolytes and other solutes once they have been absorbed across the epithelium. Therefore, normal epithelial transport and barrier functions in the small bowel and colon are essential to avoid diarrhea.

Fluid fluxes in the intestine involve secretion, generally in crypt cells, and absorption occurs in villous cells (Figure 9.1). Enteroendocrine cells in the crypt produce a number of peptide and amine bioactive substances that have paracrine or neurocrine effects. Diarrhea is associated with net fluid secretion, most often active chloride secretion, and inhibition of active absorption of sodium and chloride. These effects involve intracellular second messengers, such as cyclic adenosine monophosphate (cAMP), which are coupled sodium-hydrogen exchange and chloride-bicarbonate exchange. These processes are under enteric neural and hormonal regulation (Figures 9.1 and 9.2).

---

[a] Portions previously published in Camilleri M. Chronic diarrhea: a review on pathophysiology and management for the clinical gastroenterologist. Clin Gastroenterol Hepatol. 2004 Mar;2(3):198-206; used with permission; and Camilleri M, Sellin JH, Barrett KE. Pathophysiology, evaluation, and management of chronic watery diarrhea. Gastroenterology. 2017 Feb;152(3):515-532; used with permission.

Figure 9.1   Regulation of Absorption and Secretion in the Intestine

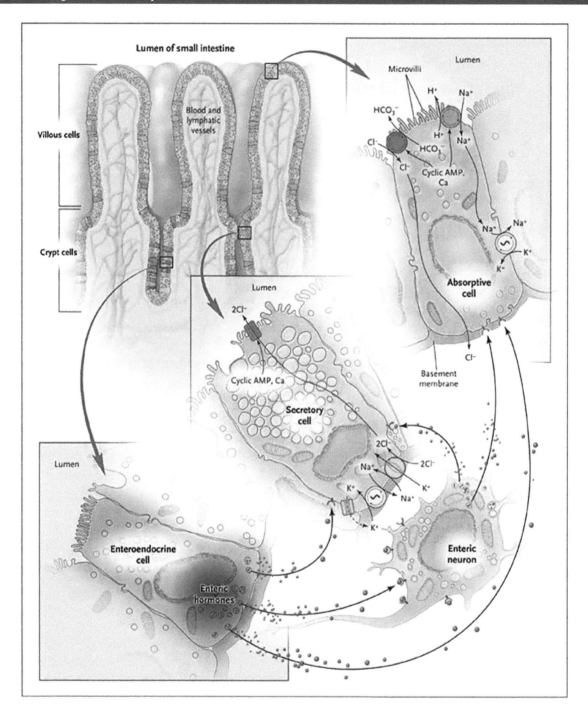

Secretory processes generally occur in crypt cells, whereas absorptive processes are located in villous cells. Enteroendocrine cells are predominantly in the crypts. Almost all diarrheal disorders are associated with net fluid secretion, most often due to the stimulation of active Cl^- secretion and to the inhibition of active absorption of Na^+ and Cl^- (by second messengers such as cyclic AMP) which involves the coupling of Na^+–H^+ exchange and Cl^-–HCO_3^- exchange. Regulation is provided by both the enteric nervous system and the enteric hormones. AMP indicates adenosine monophosphate; Ca, calcium; Cl^-, chloride; K^+, potassium; H^+, hydrogen; HCO_3^-, bicarbonate; Na^+, sodium.

(From Binder HJ. Causes of chronic diarrhea. N Engl J Med. 2006 Jul 20;355(3):236-9; used with permission.)

Figure 9.2 Cellular Mechanisms for Intestinal Absorption and Secretion

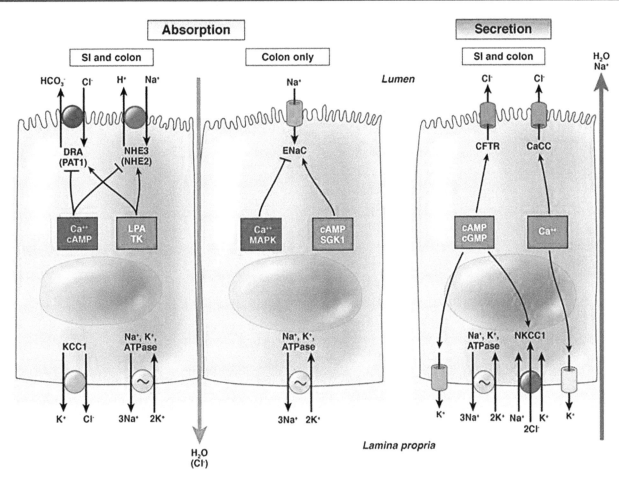

Factors that reduce the amount or function of a specific transporter are shown in red boxes; those that increase levels of activity are shown in green boxes. Long vertical arrows indicate the paracellular absorption or secretion of water, with or without an appropriate counterion. ATPase indicates adenosine triphosphatase; Ca^{++}, calcium; CaCC, calcium-activated chloride channel; cAMP, cyclic adenosine monophosphate; CFTR, cystic fibrosis transmembrane conductance regulator; cGMP, cyclic guanosine monophosphate; Cl^-, chloride; DRA, down-regulated in adenoma; ENaC, epithelial sodium channel; H^+, hydrogen; HCO_3^-, bicarbonate; K^+, potassium; KCC1, potassium-chloride cotransporter-1; LPA, lysophosphatidic acid; MAPK, mitogen-activated protein kinase; Na^+, sodium; NHE, sodium-hydrogen exchanger; NKCC1, sodium-potassium-2 chloride cotransporter-1; PAT1, putative anion transporter-1; SGK1, serum and glucocorticoid-regulated kinase 1; SI, small intestine; TK, tyrosine kinase.

(From Camilleri M, Sellin JH, Barrett KE. Pathophysiology, evaluation, and management of chronic watery diarrhea. Gastroenterology. 2017 Feb;152(3):515-32; used with permission.)

Sodium Chloride Absorption

Coupled sodium and chloride ion absorption is prominent throughout the small and large bowels, particularly in the interdigestive period. Transporters expressed in the apical membrane of enterocytes include the cation sodium-hydrogen exchanger and the anion exchanger (chloride-bicarbonate), and they allow sodium and chloride ions to enter the cell. Subsequently, they exit respectively across the basolateral membrane by way of the sodium-potassium adenosine triphosphatase and

a potassium-chloride cotransporter. The activity of the apical transporters is coordinated and regulated in parallel by neural signals or hormones.

Electrogenic Sodium Absorption

In distal colonocytes, apical membranes express the heterotrimeric epithelial sodium channel (ENaC), which absorbs sodium ions without concomitant uptake of chloride. The sodium ions then exit by way of basolateral sodium-potassium adenosine triphosphatase. ENaCs are stimulated by neurohumoral agents that increase cAMP and are inhibited by cytoplasmic calcium or mitogen-activated protein kinases. ENaC is downregulated in microscopic colitis, a cause of chronic watery diarrhea. In addition, bile acids are natural modulators of ENaC activity.

Chloride Secretion

In the healthy gut, fluidity of luminal content facilitates digestion, absorption, and movement of contents. The healthy small bowel contributes 3 L/day of the 8 to 9 L of fluid that typically enter the gut every day. This fluid flux in the small bowel is in response to osmotic load within the lumen, and it facilitates digestion, absorption, and movement of intestinal contents. However, in addition to paracellular water diffusion along osmotic gradients, active secretion of chloride from crypt epithelial cells is regulated by neurohormonal triggers that increase cAMP, cyclic guanosine monophosphate, or calcium.

For chloride to be secreted, it has to first be taken across the basolateral membrane by way of a sodium-potassium-2 chloride cotransporter. The activity of this transporter is driven by the presence of low intracellular sodium, which occurs as a result of extrusion of sodium by the basolateral sodium-potassium adenosine triphosphatase. Potassium ions also enter across the basolateral membrane by cAMP- or calcium-activated channels. Chloride ions move from the cytosol to the luminal side of the enterocyte and exit through the apical surface by way of cystic fibrosis transmembrane conductance regulator and calcium-activated chloride channels. As chloride ions transfer to the intestinal lumen, sodium and water follow through the paracellular space.

Active chloride secretion is stimulated in some acute, infectious diarrheas (cholera or rotavirus), bile acid diarrhea, some neuroendocrine tumors (vasoactive intestinal polypeptide [VIPoma] and carcinoid), and the rare familial chronic diarrhea due to a gain-of-function mutation in the *GUCY2C* (guanylate cyclase 2C) gene. Many agents that stimulate chloride secretion simultaneously inhibit sodium chloride absorption.

These specific ion transport mechanisms may be responsible for different types of congenital diarrhea (Figure 9.3) due to rare defects in specific carriers. Examples include congenital chloridorrhea, which causes defective chloride-bicarbonate exchange; congenital diarrhea with alkalosis, which results from a mutated *DRA* (down-regulated in adenoma) gene; and

congenital sodium diarrhea, which results from a mutation in the *NHE3* (defective sodium-hydrogen exchanger) gene and results in acidosis.

Intestinal Barrier Function

The gut barrier allows the uptake of beneficial substances, specifically solutes, through tight-junction pores, while excluding pathogens and toxins. This function requires careful control of the paracellular transport of solutes by the barrier, predominantly provided by tight junctions between epithelial cells and intercellular junctions (Figure 9.4).

A family of claudin molecules establishes the permeability properties of the tight junctions and other membrane-bound components, such as occludin and tricellulin, limiting permeability to larger molecules. These membrane-bound components of the tight junctions interact with the actomyosin ring that encircles just below the apical poles of epithelial cells.

Reduced epithelial barrier function has to be coupled with defects in ion transport to cause diarrhea. Reduced tight junction expression of the sealing claudin-1 has been reported in biopsy specimens from the ileum and colon of patients with irritable bowel syndrome with diarrhea (IBS-D).

Physiology at the Organ Level: Intestinal Ion and Water Transport

Ions and water move in both directions across the intestinal mucosa, and net ion flux determines the overall direction of transport. The active transport of sodium, chloride, and bicarbonate across enterocyte epithelium provides the electrical and chemical forces that drive the coupled active (energy-requiring) transport of solutes (eg, glucose through the sodium-glucose coupled active transporter [GLUT-1]) through channels and transporters and also the net transmucosal flow of water. Endocytotic uptake from the lumen is followed by exocytotic delivery to the basolateral compartment. This sets up the concentration and osmotic gradients to absorb water through the intercellular tight junctions (paracellular pathway). Thus, 80% of water transport uses

Figure 9.3   Pathogenesis of Congenital Diarrheal Disorders

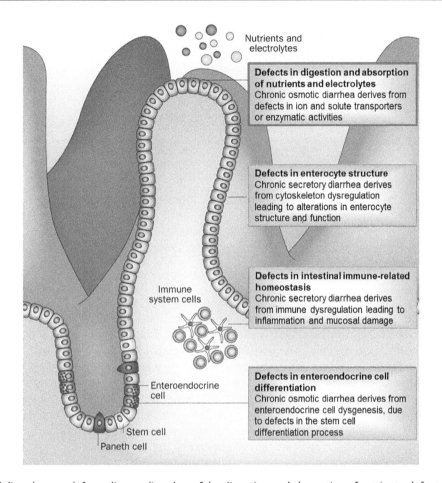

Congenital diarrheal disorders result from diverse disorders of the digestion and absorption of nutrients, defects in enterocyte structure, intestinal immunity, and enteroendocrine cell dysgenesis.

(Modified from Canani RB, Castaldo G, Bacchetta R, Martín MG, Goulet O. Congenital diarrhoeal disorders: advances in this evolving web of inherited enteropathies. Nat Rev Gastroenterol Hepatol. 2015 May;12(5):293-302; used with permission.)

the paracellular pathway through osmotic gradients. There is considerable variation in the net ion and fluid movement across the epithelium at different levels of the small bowel, and this may parallel the differences in intestinal permeability, which are higher in the jejunum than in the ileum.

Daily Fluid Fluxes in the Gastrointestinal Tract

Each day, 7 to 8 L of fluid arrive in the gastrointestinal tract (Table 9.1, Figure 9.5); contributions are approximately equal from oral intake and saliva and gastric, pancreatic, and biliary secretions. Fluid influx during intestinal digestion occurs along osmotic gradients through the highly permeable jejunal mucosa and contributes 3 L of fluid. This results in initial loss of fluids from the intravascular space, to be followed later by reabsorption of 5 L of water (and electrolytes) and only about 1.2 L of fluid entering the colon each day. The colon recovers 1 L of fluid, although it has a reserve absorptive capacity of up to 3 L per day, and stool volume rarely exceeds 200 mL per day in health. The amount of fluid entering the colon and transit rates determine stool form.

The small bowel can absorb fluid at a rate of 5 to 7 mL per minute, and the colon at 2.7 mL per minute, but the colon is 5 to 15 times as efficient in fluid absorption per unit area and thus has a vast reserve capacity to absorb fluid. As a result, moderate secretory states or malabsorption may not result in chronic diarrhea.

Figure 9.4   Intestinal Epithelial Barrier

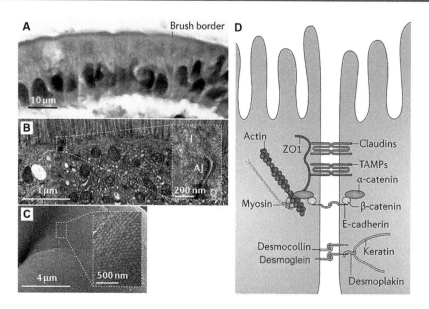

This epithelial barrier constitutes one layer in the barrier that governs intestinal permeability, including (not shown) surface mucus, defensins produced by Paneth cells, and immune mechanisms in the lamina propria. A, A single layer of intestinal epithelial cells separates the luminal contents (apical) from the underlying lamina propria (basal). Bar = 10 µm. B, Intercellular junctions and a dense microvillus brush border on transmission electron microscopy. Membranous organelles are excluded from the dense band of actin just beneath the brush border. Bar = 1µm. Inset: Apical junctional complex, composed of the tight junction (TJ), adherens junction (AJ), and desmosome (D). Bar = 200 nm. C, Continuous brush border surface of the small intestine on scanning electron microscopy. Bar = 4 µm. Inset: Dense, tightly packed microvillus array. Bar = 500 nm. D, Individual epithelial cells are held together and communicate with one another through a series of junctions within the apical junctional complex comprised of the tight junction, adherens junction, and desmosomes. TAMPs indicates tight junction-associated MARVEL proteins.

(Modified from Odenwald MA, Turner JR. The intestinal epithelial barrier: a therapeutic target? Nat Rev Gastroenterol Hepatol. 2017 Jan;14(1):9-21; used with permission.)

Motility of the Small Bowel and Colon, Including Storage and Salvage Functions

Gut motility facilitates the digestion, mixing, and absorption of digesta and the fluids secreted. Normally,

Table 9.1   Daily Fluid Flux Into the Gastrointestinal Tract

Type of Fluid	Amount, L
Oral intake	1.5
Saliva	0.5
Gastric secretions	1.0
Bile	1.0
Pancreatic secretion	1.0
Small bowel secretion	3.0

Modified from Camilleri M. Chronic diarrhea: a review on pathophysiology and management for the clinical gastroenterologist. Clin Gastroenterol Hepatol. 2004 Mar;2(3):198-206; used with permission.

transit of solids or liquids through the small bowel takes 3 hours. The distal ileum acts as a reservoir, emptying intermittently by bolus movements, which allow time for salvage of fluids, electrolytes, and nutrients. Segmentation by haustra compartmentalizes the colon and facilitates mixing, retention of residue, and formation of solid stools.

The ascending and transit regions of the colon function as reservoirs, facilitating the reabsorption of fluid and electrolytes. The descending colon serves as a conduit, and the sigmoid and rectum are volitional reservoirs. The colon produces segmenting or mixing contractions about 6 times per day (early in the morning and after meals). In an average healthy person, high-amplitude propagated contractions occur and result in mass movements in the colon.

Abnormal motility of the bowel results in transit alteration that may influence absorption of fluid by affecting time of contact of luminal content to the absorptive surface. The colon is efficient at conserving

> **Figure 9.5   Daily Fluid Fluxes in the Gut**

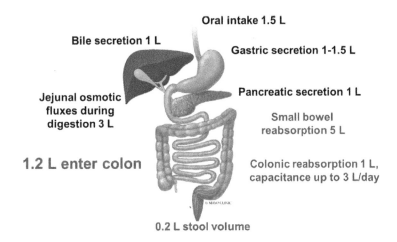

Oral intake 1.5 L

Bile secretion 1 L

Gastric secretion 1-1.5 L

Jejunal osmotic
fluxes during
digestion 3 L

Pancreatic secretion 1 L

Small bowel
reabsorption 5 L

1.2 L enter colon

Colonic reabsorption 1 L,
capacitance up to 3 L/day

0.2 L stool volume

The entire gastrointestinal system absorbs 6 to 7 L of fluid daily and 7 to 8 L leave the body daily.

(Used with permission of Mayo Foundation for Medical Education and Research.)

sodium and water under influence from aldosterone, and this ability is particularly important in sodium-depleted patients, in whom the small bowel alone is unable to maintain sodium balance.

Peptides and Amines Produced by Enteroendocrine Cells, Mast Cells, or Submucosal Neurons

Several peptides and amines are released from enteroendocrine cells by components in the diet, bacterial metabolites of nutrients (eg, short-chain fatty acids [SCFAs]), and endogenous chemicals (bile acids). Enteroendocrine mediators of secretion or absorption and their potential roles in the development of IBS-D and neuroendocrine diarrhea are listed in Table 9.2.

Categories of Chronic Diarrhea Based on Pathophysiology

Chronic diarrhea may result from inflammatory, osmotic, secretory, iatrogenic, motility, and functional diseases, and most often it is pathophysiologically multifactorial (Figure 9.6). For example, secretion,

inflammation, and motility all contribute to diarrhea due to *Clostridioides difficile* toxin.

Watery diarrheas may be osmotic or secretory (discussed below) and frequently have a component of rapid transit, which limits the contact time for fluid and electrolyte absorption through a normal epithelium.

Iatrogenic Causes of Chronic Diarrhea

The commonest iatrogenic causes of chronic watery diarrhea are cholecystectomy, vagal injury, ileal resection, and medications. Diarrhea develops after cholecystectomy in 5% to 10% of patients, in part due to bile acid diarrhea. Diarrhea due to vagal injury is associated with fundoplication, gastric bypass procedures, or esophageal resection. Positive test results for vagal malfunction include lack of sinus arrhythmia on electrocardiography if the vagal injury is above the level of the heart or plasma pancreatic polypeptide in response to modified sham feeding for dysfunction of the abdominal vagus (Figure 9.7). Pancreatic polypeptide (PP) is secreted by pancreatic D cells, which are controlled by vagal and intrapancreatic cholinergic neurons; sham feeding stimulates the brainstem vagal nuclei to induce PP secretion (increase >25 pg/mL over fasting baseline).

Table 9.2   Altered Functions of Peripheral Hormones, Amines, and Peptides in Patients With Chronic Diarrhea

Mechanism	Pathophysiology	Release, Distribution, or Action	Biologic and Clinical Correlates in IBS	Tumors Causing Diarrhea
Granins	Cgs and Sgs in secretory granules mobilize release of peptide hormones from enteroendocrine cells	Release of, for example, 5-HT, PYY, SS from secretory granules	IBS-D or IBS-alternating: higher fecal CgA, SGII and III, and duodenal CgA cell density; changes not specific for IBS; higher CgA and Sg associated with faster colonic transit and weakly with symptoms	
Serotonin	Primarily from EC and neurons: mediates intrinsic reflexes that stimulate motility, secretion, and vasodilatation; activates extrinsic afferents that mediate extrinsic reflexes and sensation	Circulating 5-HT represents 5-HT that does not undergo reuptake by SERT in epithelial cells or platelets	Plasma postprandial 5-HT elevated in IBS-D and IBS-PI; reduced in IBS-C; Platelet SERT uptake disrupted in IBS-D; Mucosal 5-HT elevated in IBS-C and IBS-PI; Mucosal SERT mRNA expression and immune-reactivity varies between studies	Carcinoid diarrhea arises when tumor mass produces sufficient 5-HT or other peptides to induce secretion, accelerated transit, and colonic hypermotility
Substance P	Derived primarily from EC and neurons	Excitatory neurotransmitter stimulating motility		Co-secreted with 5-HT from carcinoid tumors
Prostaglandins	Derived primarily from immune cells and subepithelial myofibroblasts	Stimulate fluid secretion and motility		Co-secreted with 5-HT from carcinoid tumors
PYY	Derived primarily from EC	Intraluminal PYY induces small bowel and colon fluid/electrolyte absorption	Rectal biopsy PYY elevated during acute *Campylobacter* enteritis; normal IBS-PI by 12 weeks; lower PYY in colonic mucosa in IBS	
NPY	Derived from enteric neurons	NPY Y2 receptor agonists reduce intestinal fluid secretion (mice)	NPY levels in both plasma and the sigmoid slower in IBS patients than controls	
SS	Derived primarily from EC and neurons	SS inhibits NHE1 (basolateral in enterocytes), involved in secretion of HCO_3^-	Expression of SS in serum and colonic or rectal mucosa of IBS higher compared with controls; SS in mucosa in IBS-C greater than in IBS-D	
VIP	Derived mainly from gut secretomotor neurons	Increases secretion and vasodilatation	Sigmoid mucosa and plasma levels of VIP higher in IBS than controls; rectosigmoid mucosal expression of VIP mRNA increased	VIP-associated tumors (usually pancreatic) cause watery diarrhea, hypokalemia, achlorhydria
Gastrin	Derived from parietal cells and pancreatic tumors	Intestinal secretion, some malabsorption caused by altered duodenal pH		Gastrinoma diarrhea
Calcitonin	Derived from thyroid parafollicular C cells	Intestinal secretion		Medullary cancer diarrhea

Table 9.2 Continued

Mechanism	Pathophysiology	Release, Distribution, or Action	Biologic and Clinical Correlates in IBS	Tumors Causing Diarrhea
Serine proteases	Derived from mast cells and other immune cells	Visceral hypersensitivity	Increased mast cell numbers and greater visceral afferent sensitivity to proteases from mucosa of IBS patients	Systemic mastocytosis
Purines	P1 and P2 receptors activated by adenosine and extracellular nucleotides, eg, ATP	$P1A_{2B}$ receptor regulates colonic Cl^- and water secretion; P2Y activates K^+, Cl^-, HCO_3^- secretion; inhibits Na^+ absorption	Rectosigmoid mucosal expression of *P2RY4* mRNA	

Abbreviations: ATP, adenosine triphosphatase; Cg, chromogranin; Cl^-, chloride; EC, enteroendocrine cells; 5-HT, 5-hydroxytryptamine (serotonin); HCO_3^-, bicarbonate; IBS, irritable bowel syndrome; IBS-C, IBS with constipation; IBS-D, IBS with diarrhea; IBS-PI, postinfectious IBS; K^+, potassium; Na^+, sodium; NHE1, sodium-hydrogen antiporter 1; NPY, neuropeptide Y; $P1A_{2B}$, purinoceptor 1A2B; PYY, peptide YY; SERT, serotonin receptor; Sg, secretogranin; SS, somatostatin; VIP, vasoactive intestinal peptide.

Modified from Camilleri M, Sellin JH, Barrett KE. Pathophysiology, evaluation, and management of chronic watery diarrhea. Gastroenterology. 2017 Feb;152(3):515-32; used with permission.

Figure 9.6 Multifactorial Pathophysiologic Nature of Diarrhea

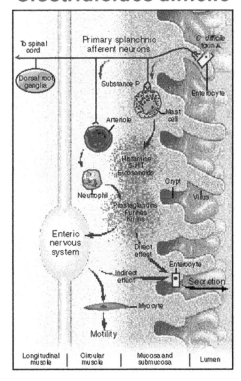

No cause is truly unifactorial: even toxin-related diarrheas are associated with secretion, inflammation, and motility. The two examples show the multifactorial pathophysiologic nature in response to infections with cholera (A) and *Clostridioides difficile* (B). Inset: The original hypothesis that cholera toxin induced intestinal secretion by stimulation of cyclic adenosine monophosphate–dependent mechanisms in the enterocyte. A, Secretomotor actions of cholera toxin are shown, including activation of intrinsic afferents and submucosal reflexes involving cholinergic and VIP-ergic stimulation of enterocyte secretion and mucosal vasodilation. Diarrhea results from actions of the toxin at 3 distinct sites (numbered circles). 5-HT stimulates intrinsic afferent neurons (open circle) that activate 3 groups of interneurons (open squares) that active at 3 groups of interneurons (lettered squares) in myenteric ganglia. B, Secretomotor and inflammatory actions of *C difficile* toxin A lead to secretion through activation of inflammatory mediators such as histamine, 5-HT, eicosanoids prostaglandins, and purines that induce secretion. ACh indicates acetylcholine; ECC, enterochromaffin cell; 5-HT, 5-hydroxytryptamine (serotonin); NE, norepinephrine; SOM, somatostatin; VIP, vasoactive intestinal polypeptide.

(From Goyal RK, Hirano I. The enteric nervous system. N Engl J Med. 1996 Apr 25;334(17):1106-15; used with permission.)

Figure 9.7   Testing Vagal Function

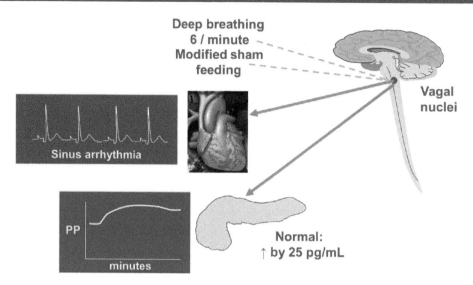

Electrocardiographic R-R interval in response to deep breathing and pancreatic polypeptide (PP) response to modified sham feeding. Potential pitfalls: inadequate sham feeding, high basal PP value with uremia, or swallowed food. The presence of sinus arrhythmia is indicative of normal cardiovagal function.

The PP response may be false-positive if the patient does not adequately sham feed or has a high baseline PP level due to uremia. Alternatively, the response is false-negative with swallowed food, which activates enterally mediated PP secretion.

The extent of ileal resection determines the manifestations of diarrhea: with resections of less than 100 cm, diarrhea results from colonic secretion induced by di-α-hydroxy bile acids; with resections greater than 100 cm, chronic depletion of bile acids results in diarrhea as a result of the malabsorption of fat and induction of colonic secretion.

Medication-associated causes of chronic diarrhea include surreptitious laxative abuse, supplements or salts, artificial sweeteners that induce osmotic diarrhea, and antibiotics through *C difficile* colitis.

Inflammatory Chronic Diarrhea

Inflammatory diseases may cause chronic diarrhea. Exudative, secretory, or malabsorptive components due to changes in both innate and acquired immunity (Figures 9.8 and 9.9) interact with dietary and bacterial antigens on a background of genetic predisposition.

Inflammatory causes of chronic diarrhea may present with either features that suggest malabsorption (which depend on the regions affected) or rectal bleeding due to ulcerations.

The presence of mucus and blood in the stool; problems in skin, eyes, and joints; and abnormal results on bowel imaging and tissue biopsies are indicative of an inflammatory cause of chronic diarrhea.

Osmotic Chronic Diarrhea

In osmotic diarrheas, fluid flows through the highly permeable jejunal epithelium following the osmotic gradient (higher osmolality in the lumen), typically due to malabsorption and maldigestion states and osmotic laxatives. Osmotic diarrheas may result in passage of fat and nitrogenous substances into the stool and typically no rectal bleeding. Normally, the stool water has equal numbers of anions and cations, and an osmotic gap is present when measured osmolality = $2(Na^+ + K^+)$ + >50 mOsm/kg. When stool water pH is less than 5, the osmotic diarrhea factor is likely from disaccharide fermentation by colon bacteria.

Osmotic diarrhea due to carbohydrate; wheat; and fermentable oligosaccharides, disaccharides,

Figure 9.8   The Intestinal Immune System

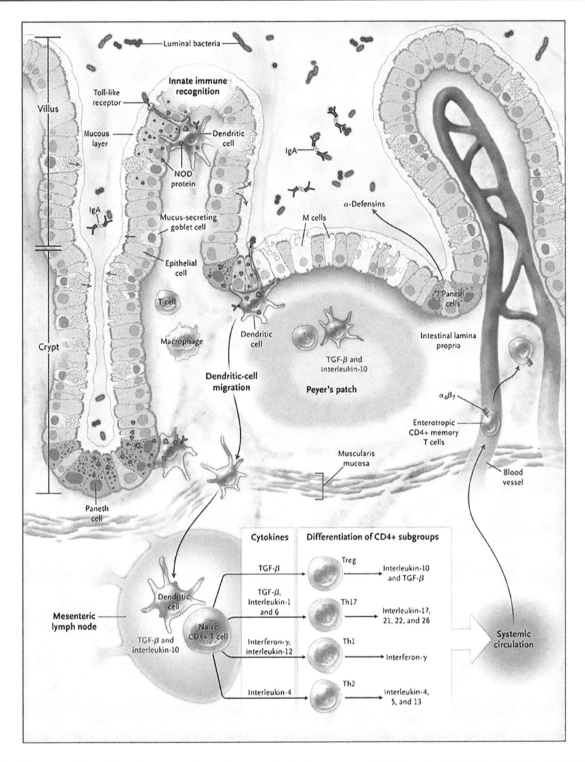

In the healthy state, the goblet cells secrete a layer of mucus that limits exposure of the intestinal epithelial cells to bacteria. Both the secretion of antimicrobial peptides (eg, α-defensins) by Paneth cells and the production of immunoglobulin A (IgA) provide additional protection from luminal microbiota. Innate microbial sensing by epithelial cells, dendritic cells, and macrophages is mediated through pattern-recognition receptors, such as toll-like receptors and nucleotide oligomerization domain (NOD) proteins. Dendritic cells present antigens to naive CD4+ T cells in secondary lymphoid organs (Peyer patches and mesenteric lymph nodes), where factors such as the phenotype of the antigen-presenting cells and the cytokine milieu (transforming growth factor β [TGF-β] and interleukin-10) modulate differentiation of CD4+ T-cell subgroups with characteristic cytokine profiles (regulatory T cells [eg, Treg] and helper T cells [eg, Th1, Th2, and Th17]), and enterotropic molecules (eg, α4β7) are induced that provide for gut homing of lymphocytes from the systemic circulation. These activated CD4+ T cells then circulate to the intestinal lamina propria, where they carry out effector functions.

(From Abraham C, Cho JH. Inflammatory bowel disease. N Engl J Med. 2009 Nov 19;361(21):2066-78; used with permission.)

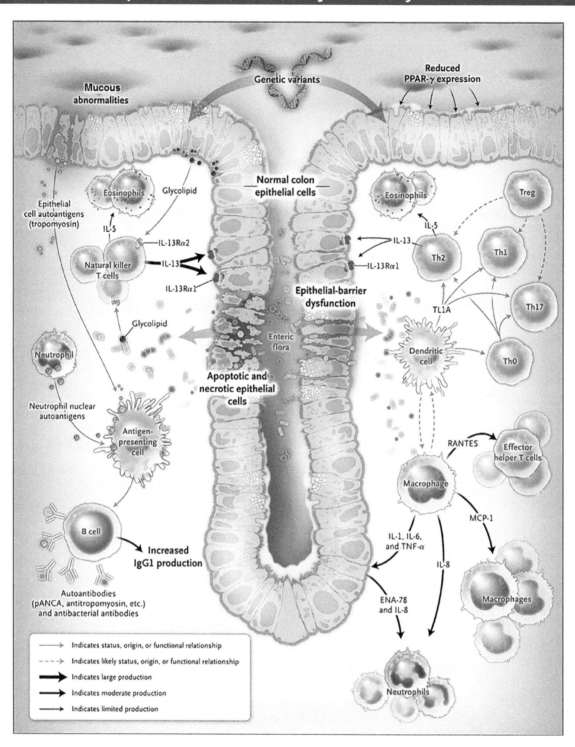

Normal epithelium, with its highly evolved tight junctions and products of goblet-cell populations, most notably trefoil peptides and mucin glycoproteins, provides an effective barrier against luminal agents. The integrity of the barrier may be compromised by genetic variations in key molecular determinants, a diminished reparative response to injury, or exogenous agents, such as nonsteroidal anti-inflammatory drugs. Chronic, recurrent intestinal inflammation seems to result from stimulation of the mucosal immune system by products of commensal bacteria in the lumen. Antigens from dietary sources may also contribute. Stimulation may occur as a result of the penetration of bacterial products through the mucosal barrier, leading to their direct interaction with immune cells, especially dendritic cells and lymphocyte populations, to promote a classic adaptive immune response. Alternatively, bacterial products may stimulate the surface epithelium, possibly through receptors that are components of the innate immune response system; the epithelium can, in turn, produce cytokines and chemokines that recruit and activate mucosal immune cells. ENA-78 indicates epithelial neutrophil-activating peptide 78; IgG, immunoglobulin G; IL, interleukin; MCP-1, monocyte chemoattractant protein 1; pANCA, perinuclear antineutrophilic cytoplasmic antibodies; PPAR-γ, peroxisome proliferator-activated receptor-γ; RANTES, regulated upon activation, normal T cell expressed and secreted; Th, helper T cells; TNF-α, tumor necrosis factor α; Treg, regulatory T cells.

monosaccharides, and polyols intolerance-lactase deficiency affects three-fourths of nonwhites worldwide and 5% to 30% of persons in the United States. The total lactose load at any one time influences the symptoms experienced. Most patients learn to avoid milk products without requiring treatment with enzyme supplements. Some sugars, such as sorbitol, lactulose, or fructose, in medications, gum, or sweetened candies may also cause diarrhea.

Chronic diarrhea, bloating, and abdominal pain are symptoms of nonceliac intolerance of gluten and fermentable oligosaccharides, disaccharides, monosaccharides, and polyols due to interaction with the colonic bacteria.

Secretory Chronic Diarrhea

In secretory diarrheas, iso-osmolar fluid is secreted into the small bowel. Other electrolyte abnormalities may coexist: Hypokalemia and acidosis are associated with Verner-Morrison syndrome (VIPoma); loss of chloride in stool occurs in congenital chloridorrhea, due to a genetic abnormality in chloride-bicarbonate exchange in the ileum. Another example of secretory diarrhea is the loss of α_2-adrenergic function in enterocytes in diabetic autonomic neuropathy. Colonic secretion may occur from bile acid malabsorption or topical effects of fatty acids, and intestinal secretion results from neuroendocrine tumors secreting VIP, gastrin, serotonin, calcitonin, prostaglandins, and others. The secretory potential of the mediators and hormones is typically demonstrated in Ussing chamber studies, which measure short-circuit current reflection chloride ion secretion in response to extracellular mediators, such as prostaglandins or acetylcholine (mimicked pharmacologically by carbachol [also called carbamyl choline]), or to intracellular mediators, such as cyclic adenosine monophosphate (mimicked pharmacologically by 8-bromo-cyclic adenosine monophosphate) (Figure 9.10).

These hormones or transmitters may also alter motor functions (Figure 9.11), including accelerated small bowel and proximal colonic transit times and changes in the colon's capacitance or reservoir function, and the motor response to ingestion of a meal (Figure 9.12) in carcinoid syndrome. Diagnosis of neuroendocrine tumors is based on measurements of the hormone or metabolites in plasma or urine and imaging (magnetic

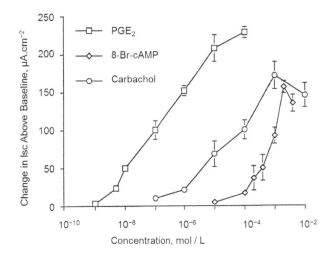

Figure 9.10   **Change in Short-Circuit Current (Isc) of the Human Colonic Epithelium in Response to Secretagogues**

Increasing concentrations of prostaglandin (PGE_2), 8-Br-cAMP, and carbachol in biopsy specimens obtained from 16 patients. Each point represents the mean of 4 or more tissues from separate patients. 8-Br-cAMP indicates 8-bromo-cyclic adenosine monophosphate.

(From Arn M, Butt G, Lubcke R, Ross I, Grigor M, Warhurst G, et al. Somatostatin and octreotide stimulate short-circuit current in human colonic epithelium. Dig Dis Sci. 2000 Nov;45(11):2100-7; used with permission.)

resonance imaging, endoscopic ultrasonography or octreotide scanning or gallium Ga 68-dotatate positron emission tomography).

Secretory diarrhea is characterized by persistence of diarrhea during fasting; the absence of steatorrhea, azotorrhea, or blood rectally; and a stool osmotic gap less than 50 mOsm/kg.

Secretomotor Disorders Causing Chronic Diarrhea

Secretion Due to Intraluminal Factors: Bile Acids and SCFAs

Bile Acids

Abnormal enterohepatic circulation of bile acids is common in patients with ileal disease (eg, Crohn disease and radiation enteritis) or resection, both of which result in delivery of secretory bile acids to the colon

Figure 9.11   *Carcinoid Diarrhea: Motor Dysfunction*

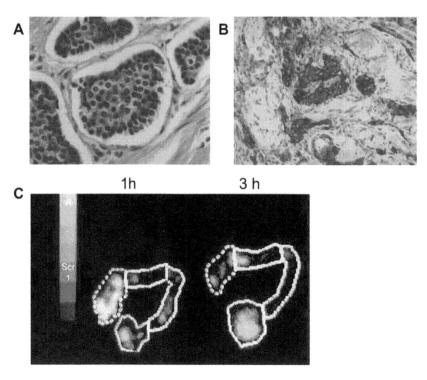

A, Hematoxylin-eosin and B, chromogranin stains of carcinoid tumor. C, Abdominal scintiscans obtained 1 and 3 hours after the beginning of colonic transit test in a patient with carcinoid syndrome and diarrhea show extremely rapid transit (whole colon traversed in 2 hours).

(From von der Ohe MR, Camilleri M, Kvols LK, Thomforde GM. Motor dysfunction of the small bowel and colon in patients with the carcinoid syndrome and diarrhea. N Engl J Med. 1993 Oct 7;329(15):1073-8; used with permission.)

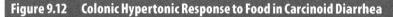

Figure 9.12   Colonic Hypertonic Response to Food in Carcinoid Diarrhea

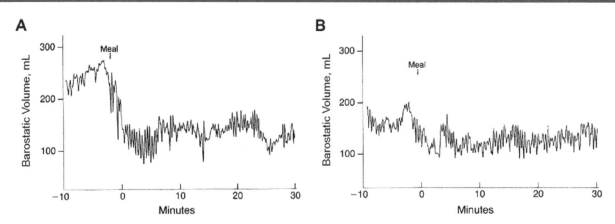

The change in volume of a 10-cm infinitely compliant balloon under clamped pressure after ingestion of a standard 1,000-kcal meal was larger in a patient with carcinoid (A) than in a healthy control (B).

(From von der Ohe MR, Camilleri M, Kvols LK, Thomforde GM. Motor dysfunction of the small bowel and colon in patients with the carcinoid syndrome and diarrhea. N Engl J Med. 1993 Oct 7;329(15):1073-8; used with permission.)

Figure 9.13   Structure of Primary and Secondary Bile Acids (BAs), the Chemistry of Which Determines Effects on Colonic Mucosa

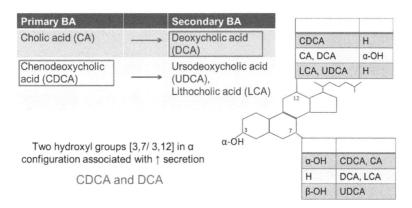

Primary BA		Secondary BA
Cholic acid (CA)	→	Deoxycholic acid (DCA)
Chenodeoxycholic acid (CDCA)	→	Ursodeoxycholic acid (UDCA), Lithocholic acid (LCA)

CDCA	H
CA, DCA	α-OH
LCA, UDCA	H

Two hydroxyl groups [3,7/ 3,12] in α configuration associated with ↑ secretion

CDCA and DCA

α-OH

α-OH	CDCA, CA
H	DCA, LCA
β-OH	UDCA

The primary BAs produced in the liver are cholic acid and chenodeoxycholic acid, which undergo 7 α-D hydroxylation by colonic bacteria to form the secondary bile acids: deoxycholic acid, ursodeoxycholic acid, and lithocholic acid. α-OH indicates hydroxyl group in α configuration; β-OH, hydroxyl group in α configuation (generally, α configuration has the hydroxy pointing down, and β has the hydroxy pointing up; H, hydrogen. The hydrogen or hydroxyl groups are attached to a carbon at the 3, 7, and 12 positions of the bile acid "backbone" structure. The di-α hydroxylated bile acids (DCA and CDCA) induce colonic secretion.

(Modified from Vijayvargiya P, Camilleri M, Shin A, Saenger A. Methods for diagnosis of bile acid malabsorption in clinical practice. Clin Gastroenterol Hepatol. 2013 Oct;11(10):1232-9; used with permission.)

(Figure 9.13). With ileal resection of less than 100 cm, these di-α-hydroxy bile acids (chenodeoxycholic acid and deoxycholic acid) induce colonic secretion, increasing permeability or cAMP. Ileal resection of more than 100 cm causes chronic depletion of bile acids with poor micellar formation and steatorrhea (Figure 9.14).

Malabsorption of bile acids (types 1-3) (Figure 9.14) increases the bile acid concentration in the colon and leads to watery diarrhea. The extent of ileal resection determines whether the result is watery diarrhea (<100 cm resection) or steatorrhea (>100 cm resection). Thus, only bile acid–induced (watery) diarrhea responds to cholestyramine (Figure 9.15).

Primary bile acid diarrhea (type 2 bile acid malabsorption) accounts for approximately 30% of cases of functional diarrhea or IBS-D. It is thought to result from defective fibroblast growth factor 19 signaling in ileal enterocytes (Figure 9.16), which leads to increased hepatocyte synthesis of bile acids resulting in diarrhea. An alternative mechanism results from genetic variation in the genes controlling the receptor proteins (β-klotho and fibroblast growth factor receptor 4) on the hepatocyte to which the portal hormone fibroblast

growth factor 19 attaches to cause downregulation of hepatocyte bile acid synthesis (Figure 9.17).

Bile acids also stimulate colonic motility and transit and increase mucosal permeability, chloride secretion, and apical chloride-bicarbonate exchange. Many of the effects of bile acids are mediated by the receptor G-protein–coupled bile acid receptor 1 (also known as Takeda G-protein–coupled receptor 5) (Figure 9.17). Bile acids and, particularly, primary bile acids in stool are associated with diarrhea (when bile acids are in excess) or constipation (when deficient) (Figures 9.18 and 9.19).

Short-Chain Fatty Acids

Even in healthy adults, up to 20% of dietary starch escapes absorption in the small bowel; fermentation of starch by bacteria generates SCFAs (<6 carbon-chain length) and increases delivery of water to the colon. Mechanisms of secretion include SCFA stimulation of colonic enteroendocrine cells to release serotonin and propionate-induced chloride secretion. Despite these secretory effects, overall, SCFAs are rapidly absorbed in the colon and most stimulate absorption rather than secretion. In fact, fecal SCFA profiles from patients with IBS-D are characterized

Figure 9.14   Bile Acid Malabsorption (Types 1-3)

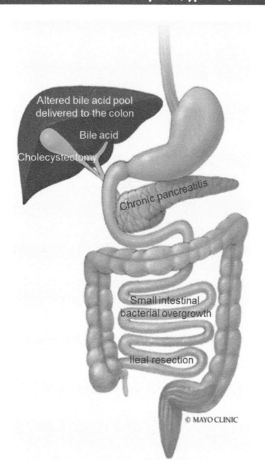

Type 1, ileal dysfunction and impaired reabsorption (eg, Crohn disease). Type 2, primary or idiopathic bile acid diarrhea produces a similar combination of increased fecal bile acids, watery diarrhea, and response to bile acid sequestrants in the absence of ileal or other obvious gastrointestinal disease. Type 3, other gastrointestinal disorders that affect absorption, such as small intestinal bacterial overgrowth, celiac disease, or chronic pancreatitis.

(Used with permission of Mayo Foundation for Medical Education and Research.)

by lower total SCFAs, acetate, and propionate and higher *n*-butyrate.

Motor Disorders Causing Chronic Diarrhea

Rapid transit delivers fluid secreted during digestion to the distal small bowel or colon and may be associated with high-amplitude propagated contractions overwhelming the reabsorption capacity of the colon. Alternatively, slow small bowel transit may result in small intestinal bacterial overgrowth (SIBO) with bile

acid deconjugation, poor micelle formation, and steatorrhea. Fecal fat up to approximately 14 g/day may result from experimental induction of intestinal secretion by an osmotic laxative.

Chronic diarrhea resulting from motility disorders is often associated with increased frequency of colonic high-amplitude contractions (Figure 9.20). Typically, the chronic diarrhea is nonbloody and may be due to underlying neuropathic or myopathic diseases such as diabetes mellitus and scleroderma, which are associated with the classic triopathy of diabetes mellitus (peripheral neuropathy, retinopathy, and nephropathy) or peripheral manifestations affecting skin, eyes, mouth, and joints.

Diabetic diarrhea and steatorrhea (Table 9.3) may also result from associated exocrine pancreatic insufficiency, celiac sprue, SIBO, bile acid malabsorption, loss of α_2-adrenergic tone in enterocytes, small bowel or colonic dysmotility, and incontinence due to anorectal dysfunction from either sensory neuropathy, sympathetic neuropathy causing weak internal anal sphincter, or pudendal neuropathy causing weakness of the external anal sphincter.

In systemic sclerosis, chronic diarrhea typically results from SIBO because of small bowel dilatation, wide-mouthed diverticulosis (Box 9.1 and Figure 9.21), or incontinence (typically starting nocturnally, because of weakness of the internal anal sphincter.

Functional Diarrhea and IBS

Functional diarrhea and diarrhea associated with IBS affect 3% to 5% of people in Western countries (see Chapter 11, "Irritable Bowel Syndrome: Peripheral Mechanisms, Biomarkers, and Management") and result from diverse pathophysiologic mechanisms, including accelerated colonic transit and rectal hypersensitivity. When there is a secretory component, bile acid diarrhea may be responsible. Visual aids such as the Bristol Stool Form Scale (Figure 9.22) are used in clinical practice to assess stool consistency. Characterizing the rapidity of colonic transit (Figure 9.23) can help selection of agents for normalizing transit as part of the strategy to treat the diarrhea (eg, loperamide vs alosetron, vs octreotide).

Figure 9.15   Chronic Diarrhea After Ileal Resection

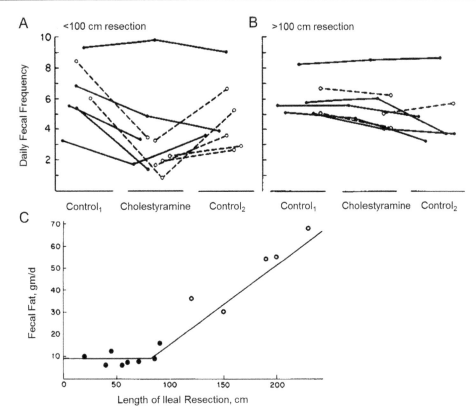

Extent of resection determines mechanism and manifestations. A, With less than 100 cm resection, di-α-hydroxy bile acids induce colonic secretion (by increasing permeability or cyclic adenosine monophosphate); responds well to bile acid sequestrants. B, With more than 100 cm resection, there is chronic depletion of bile acids with poor micellar formation and steatorrhea (C) and poor response to bile acid sequestrant.

(From Hofmann AF, Poley JR. Cholestyramine treatment of diarrhea associated with ileal resection. N Engl J Med. 1969 Aug 21;281(8):397-402; used with permission.)

There is some evidence of increased expression of ion secretory mechanisms in the colorectal mucosa of patients with IBS-D, such as levels of GUC2AB mRNA and PDZD3 protein, which facilitate chloride ion secretion.

Incontinence: The Unspoken Symptom

Several factors may predispose to incontinence, including weak anal sphincters, poor rectal sensation, decreased rectal compliance, and urge resulting from high propulsion or delivery of large-volume liquid stool in the distal colon (see also Chapter 14, "Gastrointestinal Physiology and Motility Problems in Older Persons: Constipation, Irritable Bowel Syndrome, and Diverticulosis").

Many patients with incontinence of stool report it as chronic diarrhea because of embarrassment. The strength of the anal sphincter at rest and during squeeze should be evaluated with a digital rectal examination. A low anal sphincter tone at rest predisposes to nocturnal incontinence or stool seepage; diarrhea with urgency or incontinence from stress or physical activity suggests weakness of the external sphincter.

Clinical Appraisal of the Patient

The common causes of diarrhea are functional gastrointestinal disorders (or IBS), inflammatory bowel disease, and, when associated with steatorrhea, celiac disease,

Figure 9.16   Defective Fibroblast Growth Factor 19 (FGF-19) Signaling in Bile Acid (BA) Diarrhea

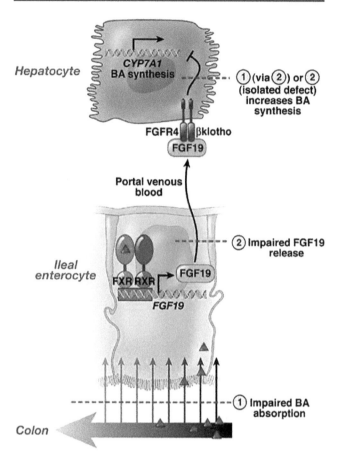

Patients with BA diarrhea have reduced serum FGF-19 associated with increased BA synthesis, manifested as an increase in serum 7αC4. This mechanism is pivotal for the reduced serum FGF-19. Bile acids traversing the ileal enterocyte normally activate FXR, the nuclear receptor for bile acids (shown as a heterodimer with RXR, the retinoid X receptor). FXR activation promotes the synthesis of FGF-19, a protein that exits the ileal enterocyte by an unknown mechanism and travels to the liver in portal venous blood. FGF-19 activates the dimeric receptor fibroblast growth factor receptor 4 (FGFR4)/ß-klotho on the hepatocyte basolateral surface, inducing transcriptional repression of the gene encoding cholesterol 7α-hydroxylase, the rate-limiting enzyme in bile acid biosynthesis. Ileal dysfunction causes defective ileal transport of bile acids and decreased FGF-19 formation and release, changes leading to increased hepatic bile acid biosynthesis that, in turn, causes diarrhea.

(From Hofmann AF, Mangelsdorf DJ, Kliewer SA. Chronic diarrhea due to excessive bile acid synthesis and not defective ileal transport: a new syndrome of defective fibroblast growth factor 19 release. Clin Gastroenterol Hepatol. 2009 Nov;7(11):1151-4; used with permission.)

pancreatic insufficiency and SIBO. Clinical appraisal should search for features suggestive of these diseases.

History

Key questions to ask a patient and other information to obtain are listed in Box 9.2, and a management algorithm is shown in Figure 9.24.

Physical Examination

The main features to be assessed during physical examination are summarized in Table 9.4. Abdominal mass or tenderness suggests inflammatory bowel disease or a neoplasm. Hepatomegaly with nodularity suggests carcinoid diarrhea; flushing is also present in approximately 80% of patients with carcinoid diarrhea.

Rectal examination is mandatory to assess the mucosa, wall defects (eg, rectocele), occult intussusception that may cause overflow diarrhea, anal sphincters, perianal excoriation or moisture, and a patulous anus or puborectalis spasm, which may cause retention with overflow or encopresis in childhood. Excessive perineal descent during straining may reflect a long history of excessive straining for constipation, which may stretch the pudendal nerves and lead to sphincter weakness and incontinence.

Tests and Therapies

The algorithm in Figure 9.24 provides a practical approach to select patients for specific testing, to determine the diagnosis of functional diarrhea with relatively inexpensive screening tests, and to efficiently introduce therapy.

Initial investigations are necessary to exclude organic, structural, metabolic, or infectious diseases. Among the initial investigations are full colonic imaging for patients older than 40 years or with a first-degree relative with colon polyps or cancer, a barium enema, or colonoscopy.

Abnormal hemoglobin, mean corpuscular volume, potassium, calcium, or albumin values should lead to further investigation to exclude malabsorption (stool fat, small bowel aspirate, and biopsy) or a

Figure 9.17   Updates in Bile Acid Malabsorption

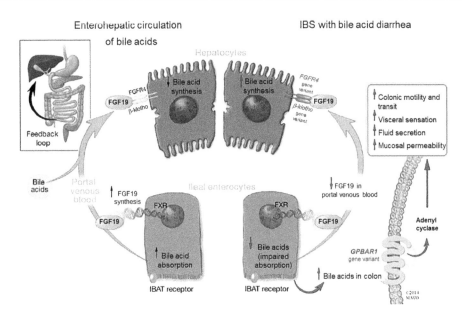

In addition to disorders of fibroblast growth factor 19 (FGF-19) synthesis by ileal enterocytes, genetic variations of *FGFR4* or *β-klotho* result in excess bile acid concentration in the colon. This activates the G-protein–coupled bile acid receptor 1 (GPBAR1, also called TGR5 or Takeda G-protein–coupled receptor 5) with enteroendocrine cell stimulation (eg, release of serotonin) and stimulation of colonic motility with acceleration of colonic transit, activation of visceral sensation, and fluid secretion. Gene variation in *GPBAR1* is associated with increased colonic transit in irritable bowel syndrome (IBS) with diarrhea. FGFR4 indicates fibroblast growth factor receptor 4; FXR, farnesoid X receptor; IBAT, ileal bile acid transporter.

(From Camilleri M. Physiological underpinnings of irritable bowel syndrome: neurohormonal mechanisms. J Physiol. 2014 Jul 15;592(14):2967-80; used with permission of Mayo Foundation for Medical Education and Research.)

Figure 9.18   Increased Bile Acid Synthesis (Serum C4) and Increased Fecal Bile Acid Excretion in IBS-D and Decreased Bile Acid Synthesis/Excretion in IBS-C

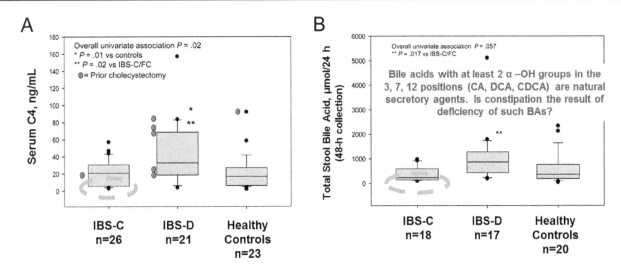

A, Fasting serum C4. B, Total 48-hour stool bile acid. BA indicates bile acids; CA, cholic acid; CDCA, chenodeoxycholic acid; DCA, deoxycholic acid; FC, functional constipation; IBS-C, irritable bowel syndrome with constipation; IBS-D, irritable bowel syndrome with diarrhea.

(Modified from Wong BS, Camilleri M, Carlson P, McKinzie S, Busciglio I, Bondar O, et al. Increased bile acid biosynthesis is associated with irritable bowel syndrome with diarrhea. Clin Gastroenterol Hepatol. 2012 Sep;10(9):1009-15; used with permission.)

Figure 9.19   Primary and Secretory BAs in Stool Are Significantly Associated With Group

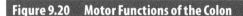

Primary BAs are increased in IBS-D (A), secretory secondary BA deoxycholic acid is reduced in IBS-C (B). BA indicates bile acid; IBS-C, irritable bowel syndrome with constipation; IBS-D, irritable bowel syndrome with diarrhea.

(From Camilleri M. Advances in understanding of bile acid diarrhea. Expert Rev Gastroenterol Hepatol. 2014 Jan;8(1):49-61; used with permission.)

secretory/hormonal diarrhea, which requires further tests to identify the cause with measurements of plasma VIP, gastrin, calcitonin, or 24-hour urine 5-hydroxyindoleacetic acid.

Mucosal lesions in the colon at endoscopy or barium enema require further assessment and specific therapy. Stool fat is not routinely measured in patients with chronic diarrhea unless there are features to suggest malabsorption. A more detailed dietary history may identify intolerance of lactose, fructose, or sorbitol.

Colonoscopy and Endoscopy

The diagnostic yield of colonoscopy for chronic watery diarrhea has been reported to range from 2% to 15%, and the test has limited benefit for detecting microscopic colitis in patients suspected to have functional diarrhea. The microscopic colitis may result from use of high-risk medications such as proton-pump inhibitors, nonsteroidal anti-inflammatory drugs, and serotonin reuptake inhibitors; celiac disease; or bile acid malabsorption.

Figure 9.20   Motor Functions of the Colon

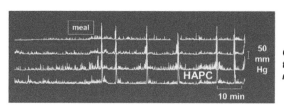

Contractions recorded in the left colon after a meal may result in defecation

In addition to the reservoir functions of the ascending and transverse colon, the descending colon functions as a conduit, rapidly transporting contents from the ascending and transverse colon to the sigmoid and rectum, which function as volitional reservoirs until the urge and the opportunity to defecate coincide. High-amplitude propagating contractions (HAPC) recorded in the left colon after a meal may result in defecation. Such contractions are more prevalent in patients with IBS-diarrhea and colonic autonomic neuropathies, such as those due to diabetes mellitus.

Table 9.3   Gastrointestinal Manifestations of Diabetes Mellitus and Associated Diseases

GI Manifestations	Clinical Presentation
Diabetes mellitus	
Gallbladder motility	Gallstones
Antral hypomotility pylorospasm	Gastric stasis, bezoars
α2-Adrenergic tone in enterocytes	Secretory diarrhea
SB dysmotility	Gastric or SB stasis or rapid SB transit
Colonic dysmotility	Constipation or diarrhea
Anorectal dysfunction	Diarrhea or incontinence
Sensory neuropathy	
IAS-sympathetic	
EAS-pudendal neuropathy	
Associated disease	Diarrhea, steatorrhea
Exocrine pancreatic insufficiency	
Celiac sprue	
SB bacterial overgrowth	
Bile acid malabsorption	

Abbreviations: EAS, external anal sphincter; GI, gastrointestinal; IAS, internal anal sphincter; SB, small bowel.

If results of serologic tests for tissue transglutaminase-immunoglobin A are negative (assuming the patient is not immunoglobulin A–deficient), upper gastrointestinal endoscopy with biopsy provides only limited benefit for diagnosing celiac disease. Patients with villous atrophy limited to the duodenal bulb are significantly less likely to present with diarrhea than patients with traditional celiac disease.

Box 9.1

Gastrointestinal Manifestations of Systemic Sclerosis

GI Manifestations (%)	Endoscopic or Upper GI Radiographic Findings (%)
Dysphagia (61)	Esophageal peristalsis (34)
	Esophageal stricture (29)
Heartburn (77)	GERD/erosions (53)
	Barrett esophagus (16)
Nausea, vomiting (58)	Small bowel dilatation or diverticula (42)
Pseudo-obstruction (34), diarrhea (53)	Pneumatosis intestinalis (8)
Constipation (31)	Colonic dilatation or diverticula (8)
Fecal incontinence and weak IAS (13)	Atrophy and fibrosis in internal anal sphincter

Abbreviations: GERD, gastroesophageal reflux disease; GI, gastrointestinal; IAS, internal anal sphincter.

Figure 9.21   Diarrhea and Steatorrhea Due to Small Bowel Diverticulosis on Barium Follow-Through

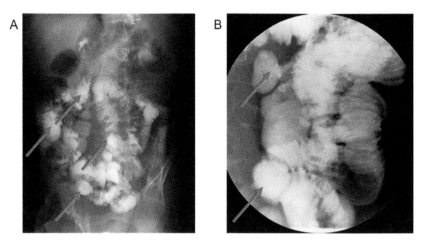

Arrows show diverticula in the small bowel. Small intestinal bacterial overgrowth due to stasis in the diverticula results in fat malabsorption and leads to both steatorrhea and diarrhea.

Figure 9.22   Bristol Stool Form Scale

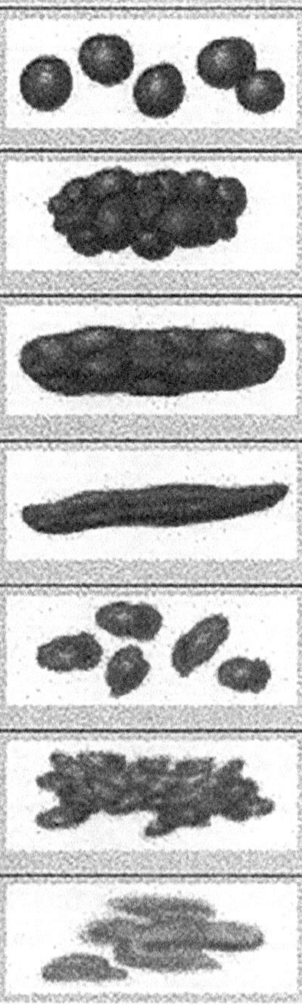

Stool form	Appearance	Type
Separate hard lumps, like nuts (hard to pass). Result of slow transit		1
Sausage-shaped but lumpy		2
Like a sausage but with cracks on its surface		3
Like a sausage or snake – smooth and soft		4
Soft blobs with clear cut edges (easy to pass)		5
Fluffy pieces with ragged edges, a mushy stool		6
Watery, no solid pieces. Result of very fast transit		7

The scale is used to determine whether consistency of stool is abnormal (typically types 1 and 2 in constipation and types 6 and 7 in diarrhea).

(Modified from Lewis SJ, Heaton KW. Stool form scale as a useful guide to intestinal transit time. Scand J Gastroenterol. 1997 Sep;32(9):920-4; used with permission.)

Figure 9.23   Colonic Transit in IBS

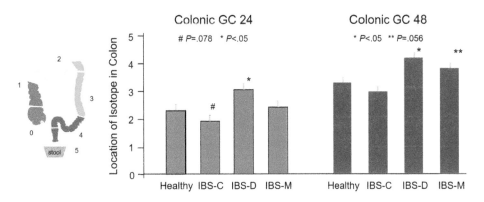

Associations of IBS with colonic transit (IBS-C at 24 hours, IBS-D at 24 and 48 hours, and IBS-M at 48 hours, adjusted for age and BMI). Thirty-two percent IBS had abnormal colonic transit: 12% IBS-C slow and 30% IBS-D fast at 24 hours (GC 24 <1.43 or >3.87). In addition, 4% IBS-C, 16% IBS-D fast, and 14% IBS-M fast at 48 hours (GC 48 <2.0 or >4.91). BMI indicates body mass index; GC, geometric center; IBS, irritable bowel syndrome; IBS-C, IBS with constipation; IBS-D, IBS with diarrhea; IBS-M, mixed IBS.

(Modified from Camilleri M, McKinzie S, Busciglio I, Low PA, Sweetser S, Burton D, et al. Prospective study of motor, sensory, psychologic, and autonomic functions in patients with irritable bowel syndrome. Clin Gastroenterol Hepatol. 2008 Jul;6(7):772-81; used with permission.)

Timed Stool Collection

Neither patients nor laboratory technicians relish the timed stool test (48–72 hours of stool collection; normal stool weight is 200 g/24 h with less than 7 g fat), yet this is the standard for assessing steatorrhea. A fresh stool sample is necessary to differentiate secretory from osmotic diarrhea. Stool weight of more than 1,000 g/24 h leads to a different diagnostic approach (a search for a possible neuroendocrine cause) than a value of 300 g/24 h.

Box 9.2

Basic Information in the Clinical History

1. Is the consistency of the stool altered, or are stools of normal consistency passed more frequently?
2. Does the patient have diarrhea or incontinence? Is incontinence at daytime or nighttime?
3. Does the diarrhea alternate with constipation?
4. What is the diurnal frequency and periodicity of the symptom? Specifically, does the diarrhea occur at night time?
5. Does the patient pass blood per rectum with or without diarrhea?
6. Are there features suggestive of steatorrhea (oily, undigested food, difficult to flush, or weight loss)?
7. Are there other features to positively diagnose irritable bowel syndrome: relationship with abdominal pain, sense of incomplete rectal evacuation?
8. Medications, past medical/surgical history
9. Relationship of diarrhea to meals or dietary factors
10. Symptoms referable to skin, eyes, joints

From Camilleri M. Chronic diarrhea: a review on pathophysiology and management for the clinical gastroenterologist. Clin Gastroenterol Hepatol. 2004 Mar;2(3):198-206; used with permission.

Figure 9.24   Algorithm for Management of Chronic Diarrhea

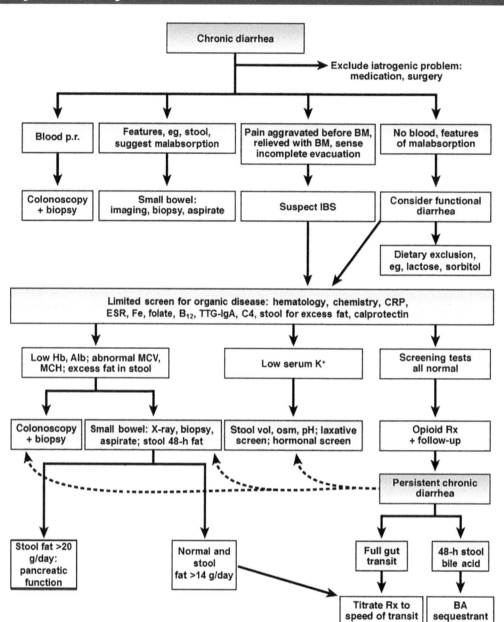

Patients undergo an initial evaluation based on different symptom presentations, leading to selection of patients for imaging, biopsy analysis, and limited screens for organic diseases. Alb indicates albumin; BA, bile acid; BM, bowel movement; CRP, C-reactive protein; ESR, erythrocyte sedimentation rate; Hb, hemoglobin; IBS, irritable bowel syndrome; K+, potassium; MCH, mean corpuscular hemoglobin; MCV, mean corpuscular volume; osm, osmolality; p.r., per rectum; Rx, treatment; TTG-IgA, tissue transglutaminase immunoglobulin A; vol, volume.

(Modified from Camilleri M, Sellin JH, Barrett KE. Pathophysiology, evaluation, and management of chronic watery diarrhea. Gastroenterology. 2017 Feb;152(3):515-32; used with permission.)

The 48-hour stool collection test can also be used to measure fecal fat (normal, 7 g/day) and bile acids (total >2,337 μmol/48 h, or >1,000 μmol/48 h with >4% primary bile acids, or any total bile acids with >10% primary bile acids).

Nonfecal Tests for Bile Acid Diarrhea

Bile acid malabsorption may also be determined by measuring serum levels of 7α-hydroxy-4-cholesten-3-one (C4) or fibroblast growth factor

Table 9.4   Clinical Features in Chronic Watery Diarrhea

Factor	Potential Implications
History	
Family history of celiac disease, IBD, or MEN 2B	Celiac disease, IBD, hormone-induced diarrhea
Drugs (including olmesartan)	Celiac-like disease
Surgery/radiation	
Cholecystectomy	BAD
Intestinal resection	Short bowel syndrome, BAD
Abdominal radiation	Radiation enteritis (BAD)
Vagotomy, bariatric surgery	Rapid transit, motility disorder
Travel	Infections (eg, parasitic)
Immune status	Opportunistic/uncommon infections
Common variable immunodeficiency	Chronic giardiasis/Norwalk virus infection
Diabetes mellitus	Rapid transit, SIBO, celiac disease, pancreatic insufficiency
Associated with diabetes medications and alternative sweeteners	Metformin, acarbose, sorbitol, sugar alcohols
Physical Examination	
Anemia, edema, clubbing	Malabsorption
Raynaud, lung crepitations	Collagen-vascular diseases
Orthostasis, hypotension, pupillary reactions	Autonomic neuropathy (diabetes/amyloid)
Urticaria pigmentosa, dermatographism	Mast cell disease (mastocytosis)
Pinch purpura, macroglossia	Amyloidosis
Migratory necrotizing erythema	Glucagonoma
Leonine facies, flushing, heart murmur, wheezing	Carcinoid syndrome
Dermatitis herpetiformis	Celiac disease
Thyroid nodule, lymphadenopathy	Medullary carcinoma of the thyroid
Tremor, lid lag	Hyperthyroidism
Lymphadenopathy	HIV, lymphoma, cancer
Abdominal mass or tenderness	Inflammation, cancer
Abdominal bruit	Chronic mesenteric ischemia
Hepatomegaly	Neuroendocrine tumor, amyloidosis
Anal sphincter weakness	Fecal incontinence
Abnormalities of rectal mucosa	Cancer, inflammation

Abbreviations: BAD, bile acid diarrhea; IBD, irritable bowel disease; MEN 2B, multiple endocrine neoplasia type 2B; SIBO, small intestinal bacterial overgrowth.

Modified from Schiller LR. Definitions, pathophysiology, and evaluation of chronic diarrhoea. Best Pract Res Clin Gastroenterol. 2012 Oct;26(5):551-62; used with permission, and Camilleri M, Sellin JH, Barrett KE. Pathophysiology, evaluation, and management of chronic watery diarrhea. Gastroenterology. 2017 Feb;152(3):515-32; used with permission.

19 or 7-day retention of ^{75}Se-labeled 23-seleno-25-homotaurocholic acid (available in some countries). The prevalence of bile acid diarrhea is estimated to be similar to that of celiac disease. Thus, it is logical to screen for this condition in patients with chronic watery diarrhea.

Evaluation for SIBO

SIBO presents with diarrhea, bloating, and weight loss and is generally caused by strictures, achlorhydria, or small bowel dysmotility with dilatation or diverticula (eg, scleroderma). Quantitative culture of bowel aspirates is uncommonly performed. The hydrogen breath test with glucose or lactulose has insufficient diagnostic accuracy for clinical decisions.

Appraisal After the Initial Biochemical, Hematologic, and Stool Evaluations

The described appraisal excludes organic disease in the vast majority of patients and leads to symptomatic treatment with antidiarrheal agents such as loperamide, up to 16 mg/day in divided doses, including preprandial dosing.

If patients do not respond to treatment with opioids, further tests of stool osmolality, chemistry tests, and screen for laxatives are indicated to identify disaccharide or other malabsorption or surreptitious laxative abuse, and small bowel and colonic transit studies are done to assess the severity of accelerated transit. Rarely, hormonal diarrhea needs to be excluded. These tests provide the basis for further treatment with drugs for chronic watery diarrhea (Table 9.5).

Table 9.5   Drugs Used for Treatment of Chronic Watery Diarrhea

Drug Class	Agent	Dose
Opioid agonists (μ-receptor selective)	Diphenoxylate	2.5–5 mg, 4 times/day
	Loperamide	2–4 mg, 4 times/day
	Codeine	15–60 mg, 4 times/day
	Opium tincture	2–20 drops, 4 times/day
	Morphine	2–20 mg, 4 times/day
Opioid μ- and κ-agonist and δ-antagonist	Eluxadoline	100 mg twice daily (μ-opioid agonist and δ-opioid antagonist) for IBS-D
α$_2$-Adrenergic receptor agonist	Clonidine	0.1–0.3 mg 3 times/day; weekly patch
Somatostatin analog	Octreotide	50–250 μg 3 times/day (subcutaneously)
Bile acid–binding resin	Cholestyramine	4 g daily or up to 4 times/day
	Colestipol	4 g daily or up to 4 times/day
	Colesevelam	Up to 1,875 mg, up to twice daily
Fiber supplements	Ca polycarbophil	5–10 g daily
	Psyllium	10–20 g daily
Soluble fiber	Pectin	2 capsules before meals
Calcium		1,000 mg twice or 3 times daily
Serotonin 5-HT$_3$ receptor antagonists	Alosetron	0.5–1.0 mg twice daily
	Ondansetron	2–8 mg up to 3 times daily

Abbreviations: Ca, calcium; 5-HT$_3$, 5-hydroxytryptamine (serotonin); IBS-D, irritable bowel syndrome with diarrhea.

Modified from Camilleri M, Sellin JH, Barrett KE. Pathophysiology, evaluation, and management of chronic watery diarrhea. Gastroenterology. 2017 Feb;152(3):515-32; used with permission.

Conclusion

Chronic diarrhea, a frequent diagnosis in gastroenterologic practice, results most commonly from functional or motility disorders rather than from inflammatory, malabsorptive, or secretory diseases. Careful history and rectal examination are essential. The nature of the symptoms should inform the clinician on the choice of initial tests, positive diagnosis, or empiric trials with motility inhibitors.

Suggested Reading

Camilleri M. Chronic diarrhea: a review on pathophysiology and management for the clinical gastroenterologist. Clin Gastroenterol Hepatol. 2004 Mar;2(3):198–206. Epub 2004 Mar 16.

Camilleri M. Physiological underpinnings of irritable bowel syndrome: neurohormonal mechanisms. J Physiol. 2014 Jul 15;592(14):2967–80. Epub 2014 Mar 26.

Camilleri M, Sellin JH, Barrett KE. Pathophysiology, evaluation, and management of chronic watery diarrhea. Gastroenterology. 2017 Feb;152(3):515–32. Epub 2016 Oct 25.

Vijayvargiya P, Camilleri M. Current practice in the diagnosis of bile acid diarrhea. Gastroenterology. 2019 Apr;156(5):1233–8. Epub 2019 Mar 5.

Introduction

Chronic constipation is a common condition affecting quality of life. Three subtypes of primary constipation are generally recognized, although there is overlap among them: normal-transit constipation, rectal evacuation disorders, and slow-transit constipation. The first step in diagnosis is exclusion of alarm symptoms (such as unintentional weight loss or rectal bleeding) that may result from organic diseases (such as polyps or tumors). The second step is a therapeutic trial with dietary changes, lifestyle modifications, and over-the-counter laxatives. If symptoms do not improve, it is important to identify rectal evacuation disorders with digital rectal examination and anorectal testing (including the balloon expulsion test, anorectal manometry, or defecography), followed by colonic motility evaluation, most often with transit tests and less frequently with colonic manometry-barostat study. In addition to diet and lifestyle interventions, the main treatments are pharmacologic and, rarely, surgical.

Definition

The symptoms of constipation reflect difficult, infrequent, or incomplete defecation that is recurrent or chronic. Although most healthy persons have at least 3 bowel movements per week, low stool frequency is only 1 criterion. Other common manifestations are excessive straining, hard stools, lower abdominal fullness, or a sense of incomplete evacuation. A careful and detailed history is essential to understand what the patient means when presenting with constipation or difficulty with defecation.

The Bristol Stool Form Scale (7-point scale) (see Figure 9.22) categorizes stool consistency from separate hard lumps to liquid consistency with no solid pieces. Stool consistency is fairly well correlated with colon transit (anchored by the extremes in stool consistency) and time from the preceding defecation. Excessive straining and need for enemas or digital disimpaction are useful to corroborate a patient's perception of difficult defecation.

Physiology

Motility and Absorption in the Colon

After the distal ileum serves as a reservoir to allow time for fluid, electrolyte, and nutrient salvage and absorption, it empties nondigestible residue and fluids intermittently by bolus movements. Segmentation of the colon by haustra compartmentalizes the colon, facilitating the formation of solid stools. While residue is mixed and fluid is absorbed in the entire colon, the ascending and transverse regions serve as reservoirs (total transit time, about 25 hours), facilitating the reabsorption of most of the fluid and electrolytes that reach the colon (approximately 1.2 L per day). The function of the other regions is summarized as follows: the descending colon serves as a conduit (transit time, 3 hours), and the sigmoid and rectum serve as volitional reservoirs (see Figure 9.20).

Different types of contractions are recorded in the colon: segmenting or mixing contractions, antegrade and retrograde contractions, and occasional high-amplitude propagated contractions (HAPCs), occurring approximately 6 times per day in health, commonly early in the morning on awakening or after the ingestion of a meal. Altered transit may result from abnormal colonic motility and affects absorption of fluid through the contact time of luminal content to the absorptive surface. The colon is efficient at conserving sodium and water and is under control from the mineralocorticoid aldosterone; thereby, some potassium ions are exchanged into the colonic lumen.

Peristalsis

The mechanisms involved in intrinsic and extrinsic neural control of colonic peristalsis generally follow those discussed in Chapter 2 ("Measurement of Gastrointestinal and Colonic Motility in Clinical Practice"); therefore, they are briefly reviewed here.

Regulation by the Enteric Nervous System

Peristalsis, the basic unit of motor function, occurs along the length of the intestine and results in a contractile ring propagating to drive content aborally. Peristalsis is activated by chemical stimuli including nutrients, bile salts, and short-chain fatty acids sensed by enteroendocrine cells and by mechanical stimuli sensed by mechanosensitive neurons in submucosal or myenteric ganglia in response to stretch of the viscera. Peptides and amines released from enteroendocrine cells activate receptors on intrinsic primary afferent neurons, initiating the neural excitatory ascending and inhibitory descending circuitry of the peristaltic reflex. Primary neurotransmitters in the peristaltic reflex are acetylcholine (excitatory), purinergic (adenosine triphosphate), and nitrergic (nitric oxide) factors (inhibitory).

Two types of cells—interstitial cells of Cajal (Figures 10.1 through 10.3) and platelet-derived growth factor receptor α–positive cells—constitute pacemaker networks, altering the state of contraction or relaxation of smooth muscle cells. Enteric glial cells also influence the propulsive motility circuitry, but mechanisms are not fully understood. Deficiencies of these pacemaker cells result in chronic constipation.

Regulation by External Signals

The enteric nervous system is influenced by extrinsic sympathetic and parasympathetic inputs to the gut (see Figure 3.6 and Chapter 3, "Gastrointestinal Motility: Control Mechanisms and Pathogenesis of Disordered Function"). The sympathetic neurotransmitter is norepinephrine released from sympathetic postganglionic projections from prevertebral ganglia and acting on presynaptic α_2-adrenergic receptors on essentially all myenteric nerve terminals, decreases propulsive motility. Sympathetic neural influence on the myenteric plexus can be mediated by prevertebral ganglia or spinal reflexes.

Parasympathetic input (see Figure 3.6) stimulates colonic motility with acetylcholine, the main transmitter.

Figure 10.1   Distribution of Interstitial Cells of Cajal

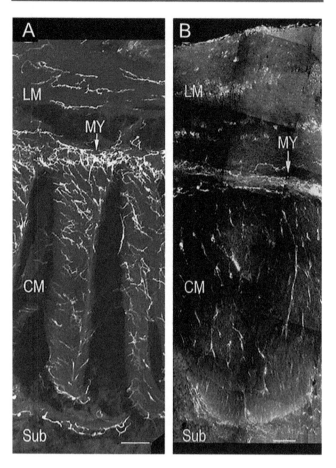

A, Normal human sigmoid colon. B, Sigmoid colon of a patient with slow-transit constipation. CM indicates circular muscle; LM, longitudinal muscle; MY, myenteric plexus; Sub, submucosal plexus.

(From He CL, Burgart L, Wang L, Pemberton J, Young-Fadok T, Szurszewski J, et al. Decreased interstitial cell of cajal volume in patients with slow-transit constipation. Gastroenterology. 2000 Jan;118(1):14-21; used with permission.)

It provides the primary neural drive for defecation, including stimulation from the central nervous system to the defecation center in the spinal cord and in the colonic response to food ingestion.

Colonic Propulsion

Mass Movements

Colonic propulsion largely depends on mass movements, which are associated with the inhibition

Figure 10.2   Interstitial Cells of Cajal (ICCs) in Patients With Slow-Transit Constipation (STC) and Controls

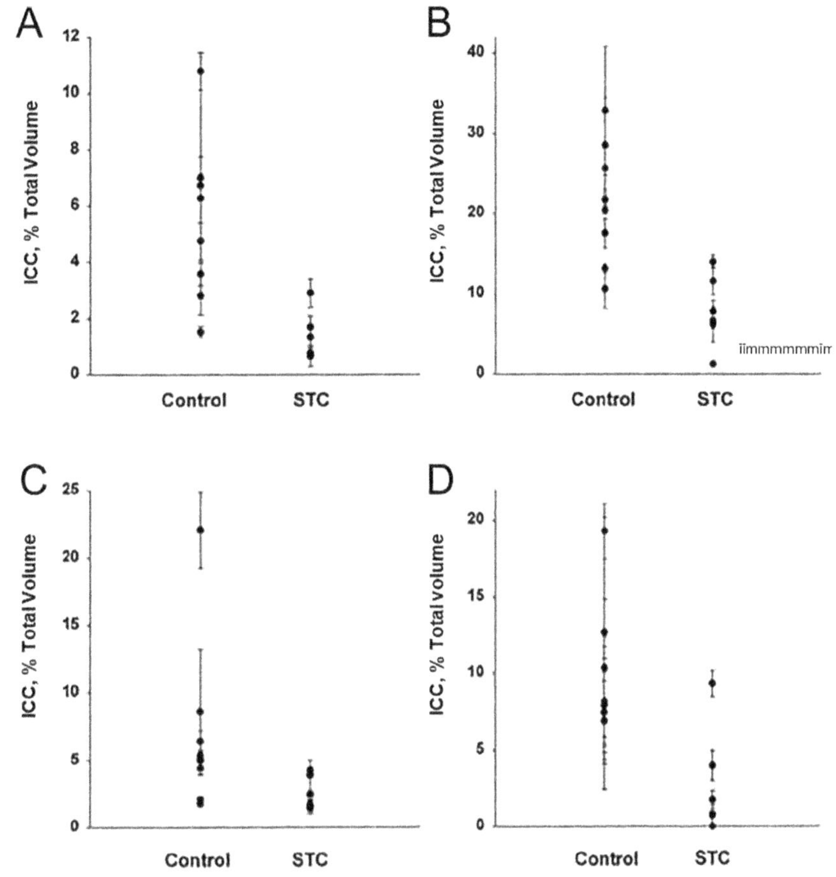

Scatterplots showing the percentage volume occupied by ICCs in the different regions of the sigmoid colon. Each point is the mean ± SEM of 4 areas analyzed for each region. *P*<.05 (controls vs STC) for all 4 regions. A, Longitudinal muscle. B, Myenteric plexus. C, Circular muscle. D, Submucosal plexus. SEM indicates standard error of the mean.

(Modified from He CL, Burgart L, Wang L, Pemberton J, Young-Fadok T, Szurszewski J, et al. Decreased interstitial cell of cajal volume in patients with slow-transit constipation. Gastroenterology. 2000 Jan;118(1):14-21; used with permission.)

of segmentation by haustra, and contraction of the bowel wall, which is characterized by short-lived phasic contractions of sufficient amplitude, tone, and coordination. There are regional differences in the compliance (segmental volume in response to imposed pressure) of the colon; it is higher in the ascending and transverse than in the sigmoid colon (Figure 10.4). HAPCs (Figures 10.5 and 10.6) induce mass movements in response to a high-calorie meal, when waking up from sleep, or in response to chemical stimulation (eg, with bisacodyl or chenodeoxycholic acid). HAPCs cause the mass movement of colonic content, induce urgency and

defecation, and can propagate from the cecum to rectum (see Figure 3.5).

Retrograde Propulsion

Colonic content also moves retrogradely after a meal and when a person withholds defecation (eg, from the descending to the transverse colon, potentially serving as a brake to prevent rectal filling). Retrograde sigmoid phasic contractions reduce the number of defecatory episodes; whereas in functional diarrhea, a reduction in postprandial distal colonic pressure waves is associated

Figure 10.3   High-Magnification View of Interstitial Cells of Cajal (ICCs) in the Circular Muscle Layer of Human Sigmoid Colon

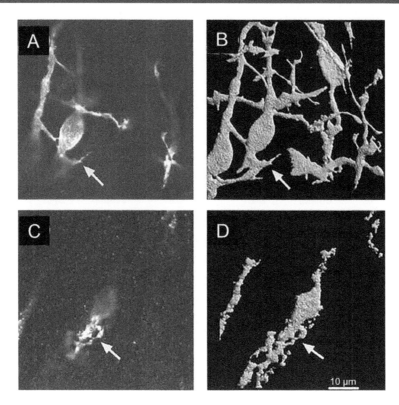

A, Single slice obtained from healthy sigmoid colon. Well-developed fine processes are coming off cell bodies of ICCs (arrow). B, Reconstruction of 20 consecutive slices at 0.5-μm depth increments (z-axis). Fine processes of the individual ICC are seen (arrow). C and D, Similar findings from sigmoid colon of a patient with slow-transit constipation. Surface markings are irregular, and there is loss of fine processes (arrows). Bar = 10 μm.

(From He CL, Burgart L, Wang L, Pemberton J, Young-Fadok T, Szurszewski J, et al. Decreased interstitial cell of cajal volume in patients with slow-transit constipation. Gastroenterology. 2000 Jan;118(1):14-21; used with permission.)

Figure 10.4   Colonic Compliance

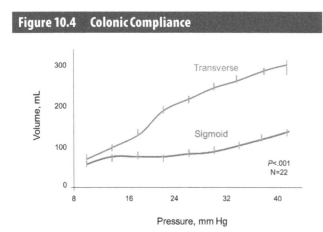

Compliance of the transverse colon is greater than that of the sigmoid colon.

(From Ford MJ, Camilleri M, Wiste JA, Hanson RB. Differences in colonic tone and phasic response to a meal in the transverse and sigmoid human colon. Gut. 1995 Aug;37(2):264-9; used with permission.)

with rapid transport of content into the rectosigmoid region.

Other Mechanisms of Colonic Propulsion

Propulsive events occurring in the absence of propagated contractions are thought to result from longitudinal muscle shortening, nonlumen occluding circular muscle contractions, or alterations in regional wall tone.

Fluid and Ion Transport in the Colon

Excessive colonic fluid absorption is not a primary factor in the cause of constipation; however, fluid and

Figure 10.5   Normal Colonic Motor Function

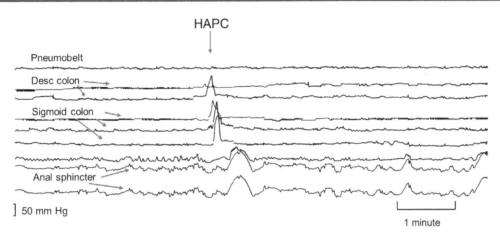

High-amplitude propagating contractions (HAPCs) associated with anal sphincter relaxation and rapid propagation through distal colon. Measurements are based on water-perfused manometry in the distal colon and anal sphincters. Desc indicates descending.

electrolyte secretion or prevention of its absorption in the colon is critical in the treatment of constipation. The main mechanisms associated with fluid and ion fluxes in the small bowel and colon (see Chapter 9, "Chronic Diarrhea") are coupled sodium chloride absorption, electrogenic sodium absorption, and chloride secretion. The ability to dehydrate the stool also depends on normal epithelial barrier function to prevent the back diffusion of electrolytes and water once they have been absorbed across the epithelium.

Figure 10.6   Motor Patterns Recorded With High-resolution Fiberoptic Manometry in a Healthy Adult

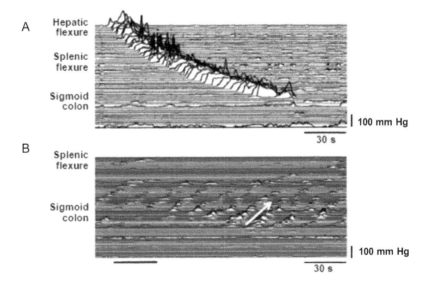

A, High-amplitude propagating sequence. B, Cyclic motor activity showing retrograde propagation in a retrograde (oral) direction (yellow arrow).

(From Dinning PG, Wiklendt L, Maslen L, Gibbins I, Patton V, Arkwright JW, et al. Quantification of in vivo colonic motor patterns in healthy humans before and after a meal revealed by high-resolution fiber-optic manometry. Neurogastroenterol Motil. 2014 Oct;26(10):1443-57; used with permission.)

On an average day, 1.2 liters of fluid reaches the colon, and stool volume is less than 0.2 liters per day. The colon is able to reabsorb up to 4 times the usual fluid volume load, provided the transit is not too fast for colonic absorption to occur.

Epidemiology, Risk Factors, and Associated Features

The pooled global prevalence of self-reported chronic constipation in adults in the community is 14%; with stricter Rome III criteria, it is approximately 7% (Figure 10.7). In community-based US studies (Figure 10.8), the age- and sex-adjusted prevalence (per 100 individuals) of normal-transit constipation was 19.2% (95% CI, 16.1%-22.3%) and that of rectal evacuation disorders was 11.0% (95% CI, 8.7%-13.3%), and rectal evacuation disorders were more frequent in women.

Lifestyle factors, including physical activity, diet, medications, and genetic factors, are considered important but have not been systematically and rigorously examined.

The prevalence of constipation increases modestly with increasing age: between 14% and 16% in persons 65 years or younger and approximately 25% in those older than 65 years. Among African-Americans, the prevalence is approximately 20%. The prevalence in women is almost 2-fold higher than that in men. However, this sex imbalance is not found in children or older persons with chronic constipation.

Low socioeconomic status is a risk factor for chronic constipation compared with higher socioeconomic status (odds ratio, 1.32; 95% CI, 1.11-1.57). Comorbid conditions with chronic constipation are other functional disorders of the gastrointestinal tract, such as dyspepsia, gastroesophageal reflux disease, and irritable bowel syndrome (IBS), and mood disorders, such as anxiety, depression, or somatoform-type behavior. Whether chronic constipation increases the risk of colorectal cancer is still unclear.

Quality of Life

Quality of life (QOL) is impaired in persons with chronic constipation. The condition also poses a considerable economic and health care burden and affects work productivity and school attendance (estimated loss of 0.8 day of work or school per month). In all age

Figure 10.7   Global Prevalence of Constipation

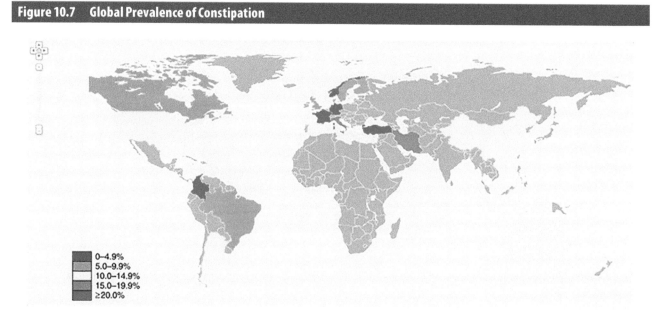

0–4.9%
5.0–9.9%
10.0–14.9%
15.0–19.9%
≥20.0%

(From Suares NC, Ford AC. Prevalence of, and risk factors for, chronic idiopathic constipation in the community: systematic review and meta-analysis. Am J Gastroenterol. 2011 Sep;106(9):1582-91; used with permission.)

Figure 10.8   Epidemiology of Gastrointestinal Symptoms in Olmsted County, Minnesota, United States, in Association With Age in Years

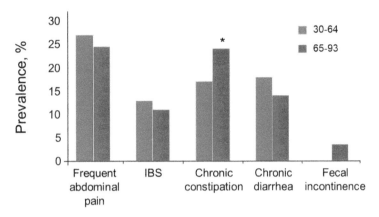

IBS indicates irritable bowel syndrome. Asterisk indicates significantly higher prevalence of chronic constipation in people older than 64 years.

(Data from Talley NJ, O'Keefe EA, Zinsmeister AR, Melton LJ 3rd. Prevalence of gastrointestinal symptoms in the elderly: a population-based study. Gastroenterology. 1992 Mar;102(3):895-901.)

groups, constipation is associated with lower generic QOL scores, and the score is worse for unemployed or retired patients. QOL scores in patients with chronic constipation are comparable to those in patients with functional dyspepsia, active inflammatory bowel disease, untreated peptic ulcer disease, gastroesophageal reflux disease, and mild asthma.

The 28-item Patient Assessment of Constipation QOL (PAC-QOL) Questionnaire has 4 subscales: worries or concerns, physical discomfort, psychosocial discomfort, and satisfaction. Satisfaction with bowel movements and treatment, physical discomfort, bloated, heaviness, discomfort, or inability to have a bowel movement were prominent negative scores on PAC-QOL in chronic constipation, and the scores were worse in patients with more severe constipation compared with those in patients with constipation-predominant IBS (IBS-C) or normal-transit constipation. Total PAC-QOL scores were not associated with age, sex, or duration of constipation (Bellini 2017; see suggested reading).

symptoms 1 or more times per week, the mean number of missed days of work or school due to gastrointestinal symptoms was 0.8 per month. In patients with chronic constipation without abdominal symptoms, the mean number of missed days was 0.4 per month. In addition, productivity was disrupted 4.9 days per month in IBS-C, 3.2 days per month in chronic constipation with abdominal symptoms, and 1.2 days per month in chronic constipation without abdominal symptoms (Heidelbaugh 2015; see suggested reading).

Health care costs are considerable. Mean annual all-cause and gastrointestinal-related costs for patients with chronic constipation were $11,991 and $4,049, respectively, in the United States, exceeding those for age-matched and sex-matched controls. Health care costs in patients with chronic constipation are associated with outpatient services, including visits or tests for comorbidities (45%) and costs are related to gastrointestinal issues (34%). Costs were higher for patients with abdominal pain or bloating than for those without these symptoms (Cai 2014; see suggested reading).

Economic Burden

In a US population burden-of-disease study of patients with IBS-C and chronic constipation with abdominal

Primary Constipation

Most frequently, chronic constipation is the result of a primary disturbance of bowel function related to diet

Table 10.1   Primary and Secondary Constipation

Type or Cause	Contributing Conditions
Primary Constipation	
Colonic motor dysfunction	Chronic idiopathic constipation: normal-transit constipation and constipation-predominant irritable bowel syndrome
Rectal evacuation disorder	Dyssynergic defecation, rectal mucosal intussusception, descending perineum syndrome, rectal mucosal prolapse, and rectocele
Slow-transit constipation, including megacolon	Colonic inertia, Hirschsprung disease, Chagas disease, chronic idiopathic megacolon, and megacolon with multiple endocrine neoplasia type 2B
Secondary Constipation	
Medications	Opioids, calcium channel blockers, α_2-adrenergic agonists, tricyclic antidepressants, serotonin receptor antagonists, dopaminergic drugs, anticholinergic drugs, neuroleptics, and chemotherapeutic agents
Electrolyte imbalance	Hypercalcemia, hypokalemia
Hormonal changes	Hypothyroidism, pregnancy
Psychiatric disorders	Depression, eating disorders
Neurologic disorders	Parkinson disease, multiple sclerosis, spinal cord injury
Aging	Immobility, comorbid conditions
Generalized myopathy	Progressive systemic sclerosis, amyloidosis
Organic disease of gastrointestinal tract	Colorectal cancer or polyps

Modified from Camilleri M, Ford AC, Mawe GM, Dinning PG, Rao SS, Chey WD, et al. Chronic constipation. Nat Rev Dis Primers. 2017 Dec 14;3:17095; used with permission.

(eg, insufficient fiber intake), lifestyle (eg, sedentary lifestyle), or a disorder of colonic propulsion or rectal emptying. There are 3 types of primary chronic constipation: normal-transit constipation, rectal evacuation disorders (including dyssynergic defecation), and slow-transit constipation (Table 10.1).

Normal-Transit Constipation

In referral gastroenterology practices, approximately 65% of patients with chronic constipation have normal-transit constipation (also known as functional constipation) (Box 10.1). These patients have no identifiable structural or biochemical cause of constipation and no evidence of either slow colonic transit or dyssynergic defecation. This group overlaps with IBS-C.

Rectal Evacuation Disorders

Approximately 30% of patients with primary chronic constipation have rectal evacuation disorders as a result of incoordination of abdominal and pelvic floor muscles to evacuate stools. This incoordination results most frequently from functional disorders and rarely from anatomical defects.

Dyssynergic defecation (see Figure 3.5) is the most prevalent rectal evacuation disorder and is due to incoordination in the pelvic floor and anal sphincter muscles such as paradoxical contraction, inadequate anal relaxation, or impaired rectal or abdominal propulsive forces manifested as a highly negative rectoanal pressure differential (eg, ≥ 30 mm Hg). These are acquired, behavioral disorders of defecation that result typically from faulty toilet habits, painful defecation, obstetric or back injury, or brain-gut dysfunction. The faulty toilet habits may originate in childhood, from either behavioral problems or parent-child conflicts, and persist into adulthood. Because of failed evacuation, slow transit may be documented on formal measurement in approximately 60% of patients with dyssynergic defecation. Rectal hyposensitivity is found in 60% of patients with dyssynergia and likely reflects an enlarged rectum due to stool retention.

In patients with chronic constipation, puborectalis tenderness elicited on digital rectal examination is

Rome IV Diagnostic Criteria for Normal-Transit Constipation

Diagnosis of normal-transit constipation requires presence of the following criteria for the past 3 months with symptom onset >6 months before diagnosis

Presence of ≥2 of the following criteria:

Straining during >25% of defecations

Bristol Stool Form types 1-2 for >25% of defecations

Sensation of incomplete evacuation for >25% of defecations

Sensation of anorectal obstruction or blockage for >25% of defecations

Manual maneuvers to facilitate >25% of defecations (eg, digital evacuation or support of the pelvic floor)

<3 spontaneous bowel movements per week

Without the use of laxatives, loose stools rarely present Insufficient criteria for irritable bowel syndrome

From Camilleri M, Ford AC, Mawe GM, Dinning PG, Rao SS, Chey WD, et al. Chronic constipation. Nat Rev Dis Primers. 2017 Dec 14;3:17095; used with permission.

Slow-Transit Constipation

Approximately 5% of patients with chronic constipation have slow-transit constipation (also termed colonic inertia or chronic colonic pseudo-obstruction). It manifests as delayed transit of stool in the colon, particularly delayed emptying of the reservoir regions of the ascending and transverse colon. These patients have reduced frequency or even absence of propulsive HAPCs, reduced mass movements of stool, and poor postprandial increase in colonic motility or retrograde propulsion of content to the transverse colon. Slow-transit constipation is associated with disturbances of extrinsic parasympathetic or enteric neural control, including loss of or abnormal morphologic features of interstitial cells of Cajal in the resected colon. A small minority of patients with slow-transit constipation have chronic megacolon, which is associated with a large diameter, reduced colonic compliance, and reduced tone and compliance responses to the acetylcholinesterase inhibitor neostigmine. Chronic megacolon in adults may result from defects in neuroblast migration and differentiation during fetal development, or it may be a manifestation of syndromes such as multiple endocrine neoplasia type 2B (see Chapter 1, "Genetics and Molecular Aspects of Gastrointestinal Motility Disorders").

suggestive of pelvic floor myofascial pain. A Mayo Clinic case-control study found that patients with this finding are approximately 2 times as likely to have dyssynergic defecation as patients with normal or slow-transit constipation. Other clinical features that identify pelvic floor myofascial pain are increased resting anal sphincter tone, paradoxical contraction of the puborectalis on simulated evacuation and on anorectal manometry, higher maximum resting sphincter pressure (102.9 mm Hg vs 90.7 mm Hg; $P<.01$), and lower rectoanal pressure gradient (–39.4 mm Hg vs –24.7 mm Hg) compared with constipation controls (Neurogastroenterol Motil. 2020 Jul;32[7]:e13845).

Structural disorders may impede rectal evacuation. These include rectocele (usually anterior and associated with multiparity and perineal injury), descending perineum syndrome (DPS), and mucosal intussusception. These disorders may also result from prolonged and excessive straining over several years, weakening of pelvic floor muscles, pudendal neuropathy, and anterior bulging of the rectal wall.

Secondary Constipation

Chronic constipation may be secondary (Table 10.1) to medications (eg, opioids or antihypertensive agents), to organic diseases including systemic or neurologic diseases (eg, hypothyroidism or Parkinson disease), or to a local abnormality in the colon (eg, colon cancer or diverticular stricture).

Descending Perineum Syndrome

There are only a few large series of patients with this syndrome. Among 39 patients with the diagnosis at Mayo Clinic (38 female; mean [SD] age 53.6 [14] years), the main manifestations were constipation (97%), incomplete evacuation (92%), excessive straining (97%), digital rectal evacuation (38%), and fecal incontinence (15%) (Harewood 1999; see suggested reading).

Table 10.2   Results of Anorectal and Evacuation Tests in Descending Perineum Syndrome

Test	Result, Mean (SD)
Mean anal sphincter pressure	
At rest	54 (26) mm Hg
During squeeze	96 (35) mm Hg
Added weight required to empty balloon from rectum[a]	492 (132) g (N <200 g)
Rectal evacuation of radiolabeled Veegum/30 s	61% (24%) (N >54%)
Increase in rectoanal angle from rest to straining during defecation	14.0° (11°) (N >14°)
Perineal descent	4.4 (1) cm (N <4 cm)

Abbreviation: N, normal.

[a] This test applies only to patients unable to expel the balloon from the rectum.

From Harewood GC, Coulie B, Camilleri M, Rath-Harvey D, Pemberton JH. Descending perineum syndrome: audit of clinical and laboratory features and outcome of pelvic floor retraining. Am J Gastroenterol. 1999 Jan;94(1):126-30; used with permission.

The most frequent associations (Table 10.2) of DPS (Figure 10.9) are female sex, multiparity with vaginal delivery (55% of Mayo Clinic series), hysterectomy or cystocele or rectocele repair (74% of Mayo Clinic series), and aging (sometimes with sarcopenia).

Another Mayo Clinic series identified DPS in 23 of 300 consecutive patients evaluated for constipation by a single gastroenterologist from 2007 to 2019. These patients were older, had significantly more births (including more vaginal deliveries [84.2% vs 31.2% in patients without DPS]), more instrumental or traumatic vaginal deliveries, more hysterectomies, more rectoceles on proctography (86.7% vs 28.6% in those without DPS), lower squeeze anal sphincter pressures, and lower rectal sensation than patients without DPS who had constipation. On univariate logistic regression, history of vaginal delivery, hysterectomy, and Ehlers-Danlos syndrome increased the odds for development of DPS. Vaginal delivery was confirmed as a risk factor on multivariate analysis. Estimated perineal descent on DRE was more in patients with DPS (mean 3.4 cm) than in the controls without DPS who had constipation (mean 2.1 cm), whereas puborectalis tenderness, increased resting anal sphincter tone, and paradoxical contraction of puborectalis during straining were each 2 to 4 times more prevalent in the non-DPS group than in the DPS group. Defecating proctography, performed in a similar number of patients with DPS and non-DPS constipation, identified greater maximal descent of the rectoanal junction below the pubococcygeal line (median, 7.5 cm vs 2.7 cm) and 3-fold likelihoods of rectocele and cystocele in patients with DPS compared with constipated controls (Wang 2020; see suggested reading).

When DPS, rectocele, or rectal mucosal prolapse occur in younger patients or in the absence of multiple vaginal deliveries, the most common association

Figure 10.9   Descending Perineum Syndrome

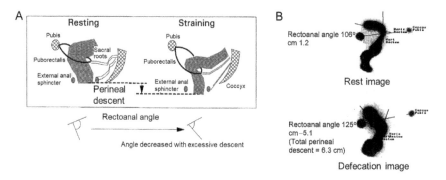

A, Spatial relationship between the different anatomical structures constituting the pelvic floor during resting and straining in descending perineum syndrome. Descent of the perineum is associated with a failure of the rectoanal angle to open, or a paradoxical narrowing of the angle (which provides further obstruction to the defecation process), and stretching of the sacral roots and pudendal nerve. B, Scintigraphic evaluation of rectoanal angle and perineal descent. Despite opening of the rectoanal angle, the defecation dynamics are impaired by the excessive perineal descent.

(From Harewood GC, Coulie B, Camilleri M, Rath-Harvey D, Pemberton JH. Descending perineum syndrome: audit of clinical and laboratory features and outcome of pelvic floor retraining. Am J Gastroenterol. 1999 Jan;94(1):126-30; used with permission.)

Figure 10.10   Descending Perineum Associated With Ehlers-Danlos Syndrome

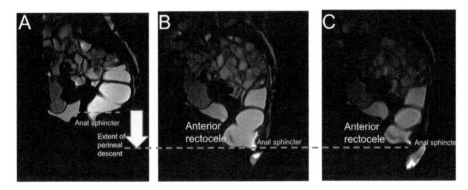

Magnetic resonance imaging defecography in 3 different settings: during anal squeeze (A), during straining (B), and post-evacuation (C) phases. There is evidence of approximately 5 cm perineal descent and anterior rectocele compared with the rectal and perineum appearance during the anal squeeze phase.

(From Vijayvargiya P, Camilleri M, Cima RR. COL1A1 mutations presenting as descending perineum syndrome in a young patient with hypermobility syndrome. Mayo Clin Proc. 2018 Mar;93(3):386-91; used with permission.)

is Ehlers-Danlos syndrome (hypermobility syndrome) (Figures 10.10 and 10.11). Figures 10.12 and 2.31 show DPS on MRI defecography.

Neurologic testing (electromyography) is rarely used for patients with constipation or obstructed defecation and may be more helpful for patients with incontinence. In the absence of neurologic signs in the lower extremities, anal sphincter or puborectalis denervation is most likely the result of pelvic (usually obstetric) injury or of stretch

Figure 10.11   Uterine Descent Causing Obstruction of the Rectum on Magnetic Resonance Defecography in a 38-Year-Old Patient With Hypermobility Syndrome

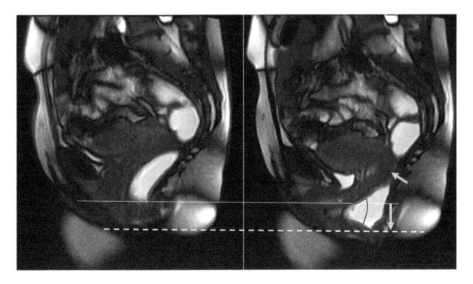

Patient presented with constipation. Findings show anatomy at rest (left) and during straining (right). Findings included excessive pelvic floor descent to 7.7 cm, 2.5 cm anterior rectocele (blue outline; right), small cystocele with the bladder base descending 3.1 cm below the pubococcygeal line (solid line), and cervix descending to 2.4 cm below (dashed line) the pubococcygeal line (lower arrow). During defecation, the cervix and vaginal vault descended inferiorly, posteriorly, and to the right and appeared to prohibit emptying of the upper rectum and lower sigmoid (upper arrow).

Figure 10.12   Magnetic Resonance Proctograms of Patient With Descending Perineum Syndrome

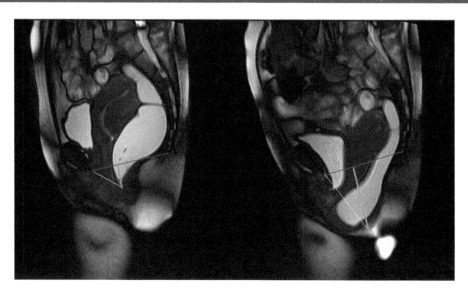

Images were obtained at rest (left) and strain (right). Left, Rest image shows a 1.2-cm descent of rectoanal junction (RAJ). Right, During simulated evacuation, there is 6.4-cm descent of the RAJ below the pubococcygeal line (PCL). Red line delineates PCL; white line delineates RAJ; thick blue line measures descent of the RAJ below PCL.

(From Wang XJ, Chedid V, Vijayvargiya P, Camilleri M. Clinical features and associations of descending perineum syndrome in 300 adults with constipation in gastroenterology referral practice. Dig Dis Sci. 2020 Jul 14. [Epub ahead of print]; used with permission.)

neuropathy of the pudendal nerve by chronic, long-standing straining.

Investigation of Severe Constipation

Among patients evaluated for chronic constipation in tertiary-referral care, approximately 5% have severe, intractable, slow-transit constipation without evidence of a rectal evacuation disorder. Transit can be measured with wireless motility capsule, radiopaque markers, or scintigraphy (see Figures 2.16, 2.17A, 2.18, 2.20, and 2.21). About 30% of patients with chronic constipation have evacuation disorders (see Figures 2.27 and 2.28; Figure 10.13). About 60% of patients with rectal evacuation disorders have evidence of slow colonic transit due to the disorder of defecation. The remaining patients (about 65%) have normal-transit constipation without evacuation disorder. Table 10.3 lists methods for measuring colonic transit.

In these patients, evaluation of the physiologic functions of the colon, pelvic floor, and anal sphincters and also evaluation of psychologic status aid in the rational choice of treatment (Camilleri 2017; see

suggested reading). In dyssynergic defecation type I, intrarectal pressure increases appropriately, but the anal sphincter paradoxically contracts. In dyssynergic defecation type II, intrarectal pressure does not increase, and the anal sphincter paradoxically contracts. In dyssynergic defecation type III, intrarectal pressure increases, but the anal sphincter has no or inadequate relaxation. In dyssynergic defecation type IV, intrarectal pressure and anal sphincter relaxation are absent or inadequate (see Figure 2.27).

Anorectal and Pelvic Floor Tests

Digital Rectal Examination

Digital rectal examination (DRE) is mandatory to exclude a rectal mass or other mechanical obstruction (such as anal stenosis, rectal prolapse, or intussusception). The key elements of the DRE in patients with chronic constipation are as follows:

1. Failure of perineal descent by more than 1.5 cm on inspection and palpation: indicates decreased

Figure 10.13   Rectal Gas Volume (RGV) by Computed Tomography (CT) Identifies Evacuation Disorders With Constipation

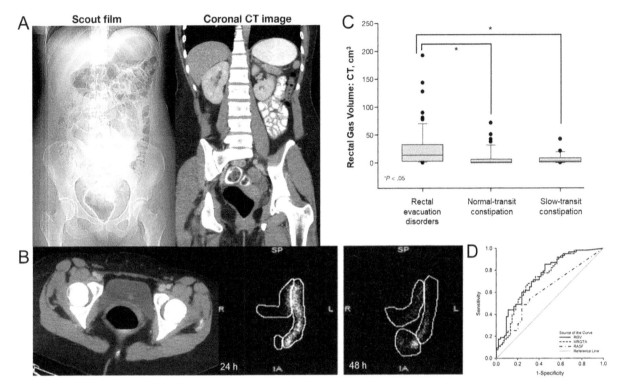

A and B, Images from a 28-year-old woman with rectal evacuation disorder (RED), as shown by gas in the rectum in the abdominal scout film (A, left, yellow outline), coronal (A, right) and transaxial (B, left) scintigraphic images, and the retained isotope in the left colon at 24 hours (B, middle) and in the rectum at 48 hours (B, right). C, RGV (median, interquartile range) on abdominal scout film in patients with REDs, normal-transit constipation, and slow-transit constipation. D, Receiver operating characteristics curve of RGV, maximal rectal gas transaxial area (MRGTA), and area of rectal gas (vertical) on 2-dimensional abdominal scout film (RASF) to identify a RED. RASF of 9 cm^2 had a positive predictive value of 68.8% for identifying constipated patients with RED. The 2 approaches of measured RGV and RASF have similar performance characteristics. IA indicates inferior; L, left; R, right; SP, superior.

(A-C, From Park SY, Khemani D, Nelson AD, Eckert D, Camilleri M. Rectal gas volume measured by computerized tomography identifies evacuation disorders in patients with constipation. Clin Gastroenterol Hepatol. 2017 Apr;15(4):543-52; used with permission. D, From Park SY, Khemani D, Acosta A, Eckert D, Camilleri M. Rectal gas volume: defining cut-offs for screening for evacuation disorders in patients with constipation. Neurogastroenterol Motil. 2017 Jul;29(7):e13044.)

Table 10.3   Measurements of Colonic Transit

Transit Measurement	Method Details	Comment
Radiopaque marker	Ingestion of 24 markers on each of 3 successive days and abdominal radiography on day 4	Easy, repeatable, generally safe, inexpensive, reliable, and highly applicable in evaluating constipated patients in clinical practice
	Ingest 20 markers; radiograph day 5: abnormal if >5 retained	
Radioscintigraphy	Delayed release capsule	4 regions and stool used to determine geometric center at 24 h, 48 h (max score 5); best validated method
	Radiolabel liquid phase of ingested meal	6 regions and stool used to determine geometric center at 24 h, 48 h, 72 h (max score 7)
Wireless motility capsule	Recording of pH, temperature, and pressure profile from oral intake to excretion in stool	Provides reliable measurement of whole gut, small bowel, colonic, and combined SBTT and CTT

Abbreviations: CTT, colonic transit time; max, maximum; SBTT, small bowel transit time.

anal sphincter relaxation during stimulated defecation

2. Excessive perineal descent more than 4 cm on inspection and palpation suggestive of DPS

3. Contraction of the puborectalis or anal sphincter during stimulated defecation: may be associated with tenderness on palpation of these muscles through the posterior and lateral aspects of the anal canal and lower rectum, and the associated tenderness leads to the diagnosis of pelvic floor tension myalgia syndrome

4. Inability to contract abdominal wall musculature sufficiently during straining, resulting in insufficient force to push examining finger out of the rectum

Examination in the squatting position may be required to identify rectal mucosal prolapse.

The DRE has a sensitivity of 75% to 93% and specificity of 59% to 87% for diagnosing dyssynergic defecation. Thus, the DRE is useful for selecting patients for further testing, including anorectal manometry, balloon expulsion, and defecography. In addition, if constipation is not improved with fiber supplements (at least 12 g per day), over-the-counter laxatives (eg, osmotic laxatives or colonic stimulants), or prosecretory agents, anorectal structure or function testing is required. Because 60% of patients with rectal evacuation disorder can have delayed colonic transit, evaluation of the anorectum and pelvic floor is recommended as a first step in investigation (see Figure 2.29), particularly if plain abdominal radiography shows gas retained in the rectum above the pelvic floor (Figure 10.12).

Methods for anorectal function testing are listed in Table 10.4. At least 4 reproducible types of dyssynergia are recognized on the basis of anorectal manometry and provide information to physical medicine therapists providing patient-specific treatments. Clinical correlation (including findings in the medical history and on DRE) is essential.

Balloon Expulsion Test

Although the balloon expulsion test does not distinguish between functional and structural causes of disordered defecation, additional testing, such as defecography, is usually restricted to older patients in whom such structural disorders are more likely. Although 60 seconds is regarded as the threshold for abnormal balloon expulsion time, recent data suggest this value is associated with 93% specificity, 39% sensitivity, 70% positive

Test	Method or Measurement of Interest	Abnormal[a]
Balloon expulsion	Deflated balloon is placed in the rectum, inflated to 50 mL, and time taken to expulsion in seated position is recorded by patient with a stopwatch	>60 s expulsion time is abnormal; weight-based expulsion abnormal if >200 g added to achieve expulsion
High-resolution manometry	Resting anal sphincter tone	>110 mm Hg
	Squeeze sphincter pressure	>240 mm Hg
	Residual anal pressure, % anal relaxation	Pressure >100 mm Hg, <7%
	Rectoanal pressure differential	≥ −50 mm Hg
	Intrarectal pressure on straining	<50 mm Hg reflects poor expulsive forces or incoordination
Rectal sensation	Larger balloon: first sensation, urge, pain	>20, >60, >120 mL may signify reduced sensitivity or rectal enlargement (eg, due to prolonged stool retention)
Rectal gas	Surface area or volume of gas in rectum on pelvic radiography or computed tomography	>900 mm^2 has ~70% sensitivity for rectal evacuation disorder

Table 10.4   Anorectal Function Tests

[a] Normal range differs by age and sex.

Figure 10.14   Barium Defecography in a 43-Year-Old Woman With 2 Children Born by Vaginal Delivery

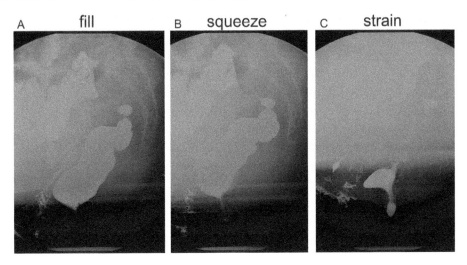

The patient presented with constipation (A) and sensation of a shelf-blocking defecation at squeeze (B), shown to be due to a significant anterior rectocele, best appreciated on straining (C).

predictive value, and 78.4% negative predictive value. Expulsion time of more than 22 seconds is associated with 78% specificity, 70% sensitivity, 52% positive predictive value, and 88% negative predictive value. Thus, a balloon expulsion time longer than 22 seconds may support the diagnosis in patients suspected of having rectal evacuation disorder on the basis of history, rectal examination, and other features on anorectal manometry, such as high resting anal sphincter pressure and rectoanal pressure differential of 30 mm Hg or more.

Defecography

Contrast defecograpy (with barium) or functional magnetic resonance imaging (magnetic resonance defecography) (Figure 10.14; see Figure 2.31) acquires information about anorectal function (dyssynergic defecation) and anatomy (anal stenosis, enterocele, intussusception, rectal prolapse, and rectocele). Age and sex affect normal anorectal functions (Figure 10.15). Surgically remediable conditions are identified in only a few patients: whole-thickness intussusception with complete outlet obstruction or an extremely large rectocele. Clinically relevant rectoceles are those that fill preferentially during attempts at defecation instead of

expulsion of the barium or magnetic resonance image contrast through the anus. Defecography can identify failure of the puborectalis muscle to relax. Magnetic resonance defecography is particularly helpful for DPS, complementing clinical evaluation, as in elderly and patients with hypermobility such as Ehlers-Danlos syndrome.

Figure 10.15   Effects of Age and Sex on Pelvic Floor Function

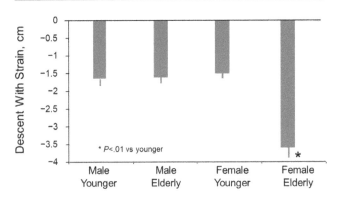

Descent while straining was measured as the descent of the rectoanal angle relative to the pubococcygeal line.

(Data from Bannister JJ, Abouzekry L, Read NW. Effect of aging on anorectal function. Gut. 1987 Mar;28(3):353-7.)

Colonic Manometry

Conventional and high-resolution colonic manometry measure phasic pressure activity that reflects colonic contraction (Figures 10.16 and 10.17; see Figure 2.25). Colonic myopathy is documented in children and is rare in adults unless associated with megacolon; myopathy results in low-amplitude contractions. Colonic neuropathy is characterized by absence of colonic response to a 1,000-kcal liquid meal, to intravenous neostigmine 1 mg, or intraluminal bisacodyl 10 mg (a stimulant laxative). For colonic neuropathy or myopathy, failed medical therapy for constipation and failure of correction of disordered defecation with biofeedback are indications for colectomy. Colonic manometry is performed at few specialized motility centers.

Colonic barostat measurements are sometimes incorporated with manometry and are essential for diagnosis of megacolon (see Figure 1.10) if the radiologic features are inconclusive. An algorithm for the diagnosis and management of chronic constipation is provided in Figure 10.18.

Treatment

First-line Therapies

First-line therapies for chronic constipation are listed in Table 10.5.

Constipation Unresponsive to First-line Treatments

When fiber or osmotic laxatives are ineffective (Figure 10.19, an evacuation disorder or a secondary cause (medication or colonic inertia) should be investigated.

Slow-transit constipation requires aggressive medical or surgical treatment; pelvic floor dysfunction dyssynergia responds to biofeedback management in about 75% of patients (Figures 10.20 and 10.21).

Many patients with constipation have normal colonic transit and can be treated symptomatically. Patients with spinal cord injuries or other neurologic disorders require a dedicated bowel regimen that often includes rectal

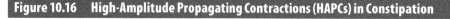

Figure 10.16   High-Amplitude Propagating Contractions (HAPCs) in Constipation

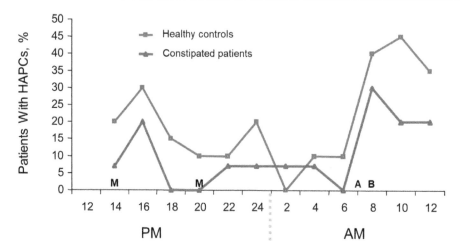

Daily distribution of mass movements (expressed as hourly percentage) in patients (red line) and controls (blue line). Incidence increased after meals and on awakening in the morning and decreased during the night. A indicates awakening; B, breakfast; M, standard meal.

(Modified from Bassotti G, Gaburri M, Imbimbo BP, Rossi L, Farroni F, Pelli MA, et al. Colonic mass movements in idiopathic chronic constipation. Gut. 1988 Sep;29(9):1173-9; used with permission.)

Figure 10.17   **Postprandial High-Amplitude Propagating Contractions (HAPCs) in Constipation**

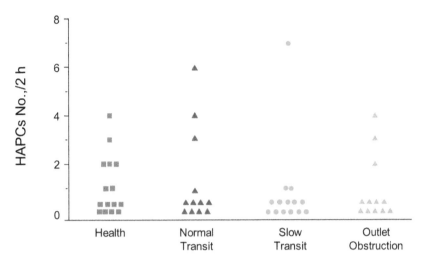

HAPCs were defined as contraction of more than 75 mm Hg propagated over at least 10 cm. Postprandial HAPCs were reduced in all patients (except 1) with slow-transit constipation; some patients with outlet obstruction defecation and normal-transit constipation also had reduced HAPCs postprandially.

(From O'Brien MD, Camilleri M, von der Ohe MR, Phillips SF, Pemberton JH, Prather CM, et al. Motility and tone of the left colon in constipation: a role in clinical practice? Am J Gastroenterol. 1996 Dec;91(12):2532-8; used with permission.)

stimulation, enema therapy, and carefully timed laxative therapy.

The spectrum of treatments for constipation includes bulk, osmotic, prokinetic, secretory, and stimulant laxatives and, in some countries, prucalopride, a serotonin-4 receptor agonist (Table 10.6, Figures 10.22 through 10.35).

Network Meta-analysis of Treatments for Constipation

Given that there are no head-to-head comparative trials among pharmacologic treatments for constipation, network meta-analysis was used to compare different treatments. Network meta-analyses combine the effect sizes for all possible comparisons (direct and indirect) simultaneously. A multivariate meta-regression model was used to conduct analysis with the network suite in Stata v.14.0 (StataCorp). The results of such an analysis for drugs used in chronic constipation are shown in Figures 10.36 and 10.37.

The network analysis included 21 eligible randomized clinical trials involving 9,189 patients (9 randomized clinical trials with prucalopride, 3 lubiprostone, 3 linaclotide, 2 tegaserod, 1 each velusetrag, elobixibat, bisacodyl, and sodium picosulphate). Bisacodyl, sodium picosulphate, prucalopride, and velusetrag were superior to placebo for the end point of 3 or more complete spontaneous bowel movements per week. No drug was superior for improving the primary end points. Bisacodyl appeared superior to the other drugs for the secondary end point of change from baseline in the number of spontaneous bowel movements per week. The analysis concluded that current drugs for chronic idiopathic constipation have similar efficacy.

When Medical Therapy Fails

If an optimal 3- to 6-month trial of medical therapy fails, laparoscopic colectomy with ileorectostomy should be considered if there is no associated

Figure 10.18   Diagnosis and Management Algorithm for Chronic Constipation

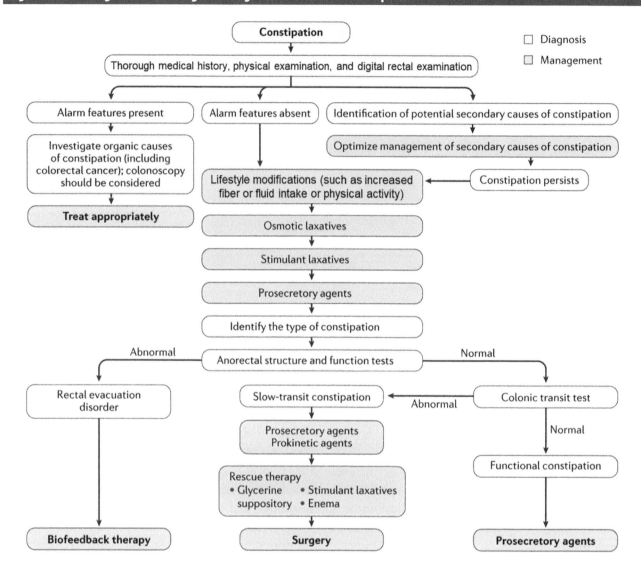

(From Camilleri M, Ford AC, Mawe GM, Dinning PG, Rao SS, Chey WD, et al. Chronic constipation. Nat Rev Dis Primers. 2017 Dec 14;3:17095; as modified from Tse Y, Armstrong D, Andrews CN, Bitton A, Bressler B, Marshall J, et al. Treatment algorithm for chronic idiopathic constipation and constipation-predominant irritable bowel syndrome derived from a Canadian national survey and needs assessment on choices of therapeutic agents. Can J Gastroenterol Hepatol. 2017;2017:8612189.)

Table 10.5   First-line Therapies for Chronic Constipation

Lifestyle Modifications	Mechanism of Action
Increase fluid intake	May help if there is evidence of dehydration
Ingest high-fiber diet	High water-holding capacity of gel-forming soluble fiber (eg, psyllium) resists dehydration and carries water to colon to loosen stool consistency Recommended intake of fiber is at least 25-30 g per day; 12.5 g fiber per day (wheat bran) does not improve symptoms associated with constipation. Systematic reviews support the intake of soluble fibers (eg, pectins, gums, mucilages, and storage polysaccharides present in oat bran, barley, nuts, seeds, beans, lentils, peas, some fruits and vegetables, and psyllium fiber supplements)
Increase physical activity	Positive effect on overall gastrointestinal symptoms and well-being, may help in inactive elderly

Data from Camilleri M, Ford AC, Mawe GM, Dinning PG, Rao SS, Chey WD, et al. Chronic constipation. Nat Rev Dis Primers. 2017 Dec 14;3:17095.

Figure 10.19   Success of Dietary Fiber in Chronic Constipation

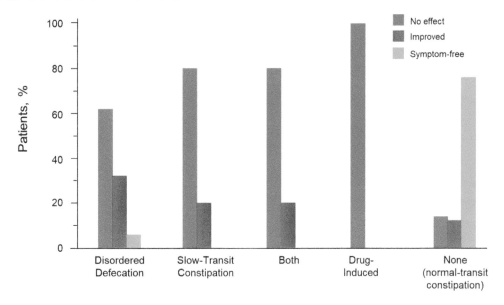

If patients do not respond to dietary fiber, the most likely causes are disordered defecation, slow-transit constipation, or drug-induced constipation.

(From Voderholzer WA, Schatke W, Muhldorfer BE, Klauser AG, Birkner B, Muller-Lissner SA. Clinical response to dietary fiber treatment of chronic constipation. Am J Gastroenterol. 1997 Jan;92(1):95-8; used with permission.)

Figure 10.20   Biofeedback Is Superior to Laxatives for Normal-Transit Constipation Due to Pelvic Floor Dyssynergia

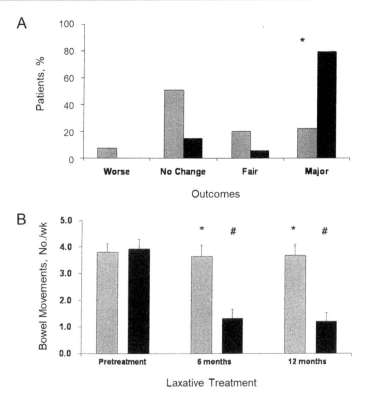

A, Proportion of laxative-treated patients (gray bars) and biofeedback-treated patients (black bars) reporting different treatment outcomes at 6 months. *Differences between groups were significant at $P<.001$. B, Average number of bowel movements per week accompanied by straining in laxative-treated patients (gray bars) and biofeedback-treated patients (black bars). T bars show standard errors. *Indicates significant difference ($P<.01$) between groups at 6 months or 12 months; # indicates a significant ($P<.01$) change from pretreatment within the biofeedback group.

(From Chiarioni G, Whitehead WE, Pezza V, Morelli A, Bassotti G. Biofeedback is superior to laxatives for normal transit constipation due to pelvic floor dyssynergia. Gastroenterology. 2006 Mar;130(3):657-64; used with permission.)

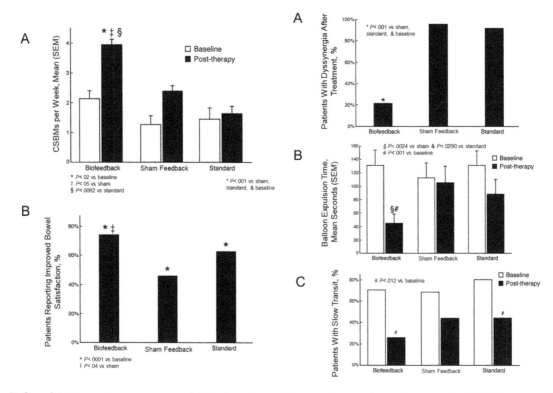

Left, Results for subjective outcome measures. A, Number of complete spontaneous bowel movements (CSBMs) per week in each of the 3 treatment groups before and after treatment. B, Percentage of patients who reported improved global bowel satisfaction and a visual analog scale with each treatment. SEM indicates standard error of the mean. Right, Results for the physiologic outcome measures. A, Proportion of patients who exhibited a dyssynergic pattern on anorectal manometry after each treatment. B, Effect of each treatment on the balloon expulsion time. C, Percentage of patients with slow transit in the colon before and after each treatment.

(From Rao SS, Seaton K, Miller M, Brown K, Nygaard I, Stumbo P, et al. Randomized controlled trial of biofeedback, sham feedback, and standard therapy for dyssynergic defecation. Clin Gastroenterol Hepatol. 2007 Mar;5(3):331-8; used with permission.)

Table 10.6   Therapies for Constipation

Drug Class	Agent	Dose	Comment
Fiber	Dietary or supplemental fiber	Minimum 20 g dietary fiber or equivalent per day	RCT showed 12.5 g/d was insufficient
Osmotic laxative	Magnesium salts	500 mg up to 4/d	Avoid with chronic renal insufficiency
	PEG 3350	17 g in 240 mL daily or twice daily	
	Lactulose	15-30 mL (10-20 g) daily	Bloating/gas AE
Prosecretory	Lubiprostone	24 µg/d	Ingestion with meal reduces nausea (otherwise 24% AE)
	Linaclotide	72, 145, or 290 µg/d	Titrate dose
	Plecanatide	3 mg/d	
Colon motor stimulants	Bisacodyl	5-10 mg/d orally or 10 mg suppository	May induce cramping
	Senna (anthraquinone)	8.6 mg/d	Theoretical risk of myenteric plexus damage
	Prucalopride (serotonin-4 agonist)	2 mg/d; 1 mg/d in >65 y	Not approved in United States
IBAT inhibitor	Elobixibat	15 mg/d (range, 5-15 mg/d)	Approved in Japan

Abbreviations: AE, adverse event; IBAT, ileal bile acid transport; PEG, polyethylene glycol; RCT, randomized clinical trial.

Figure 10.22   Effect of Polyethylene Glycol, 14.6 g Twice a Day, in 250 mL Water-Electrolyte (PMF-100) on Bowel Frequency in Chronic Constipation

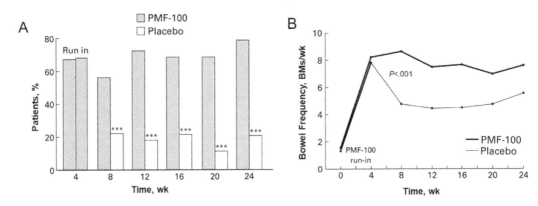

A, Percentage of patients with complete remission of constipation symptoms, consisting of more than 3 bowel movements per week, no use of laxatives, no straining at defecation, feeling of complete evacuation, and no hard or pellety stools during PMF-100 and placebo treatment. ***$P<.001$. B, Bowel frequency during the 24-week therapy with PMF-100 and placebo. After the run-in period, bowel frequency was significantly higher in the PMF-100 group throughout the study. Adverse effects included nausea and epigastric pain. BM indicates bowel movement.

(From Corazziari E, Badiali D, Bazzocchi G, Bassotti G, Roselli P, Mastropaolo G, et al. Long term efficacy, safety, and tolerability of low daily doses of isosmotic polyethylene glycol electrolyte balanced solution (PMF-100) in the treatment of functional chronic constipation. Gut. 2000 Apr;46(4):522-6; used with permission.)

Figure 10.23   Effect of Bisacodyl on Colonic Transit

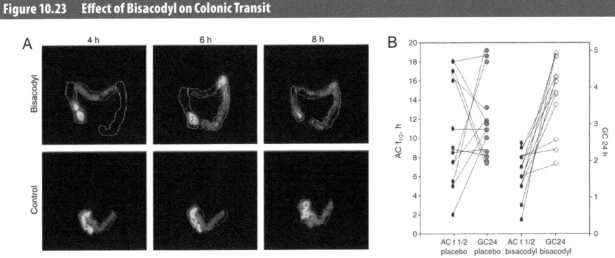

A, Colonic transit scintiscans at 4, 6, and 8 hours in patients receiving bisacodyl or placebo. Intensity of image reflects the concentration of counts in each region. Variable regions of interest are drawn around isotope in ascending, transverse, and descending regions. Bisacodyl accelerates ascending colon emptying compared with placebo. B, Effect of bisacodyl on ascending colon emptying time for half of radioactive meal (AC $t_{1/2}$) and on overall colonic transit at 24 hours (geometric center of colon isotope at 24 hours, GC 24 h). The bisacodyl group had significantly accelerated ascending colon emptying compared with the placebo group ($P=.03$). In response to placebo, the progression from ascending colon to overall transit at 24 hours is highly variable; in contrast, there is a consistent progression for ascending colon to overall colonic transit in the bisacodyl group in all but 3 participants. Thus, although overall colonic GC was not significant in bisacodyl vs placebo ($P=.19$), 9 of the 12 participants had substantial progression from ascending to overall colonic transit. GC indicates geometric center.

(From Manabe N, Cremonini F, Camilleri M, Sandborn WJ, Burton DD. Effects of bisacodyl on ascending colon emptying and overall colonic transit in healthy volunteers. Aliment Pharmacol Ther. 2009 Nov 1;30(9):930-6; used with permission.)

Figure 10.24   Oral Bisacodyl Is Effective and Well-Tolerated in Chronic Constipation

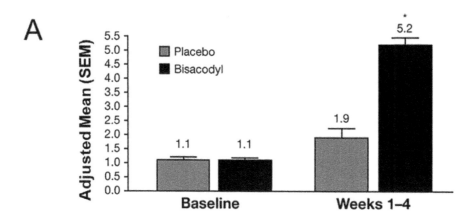

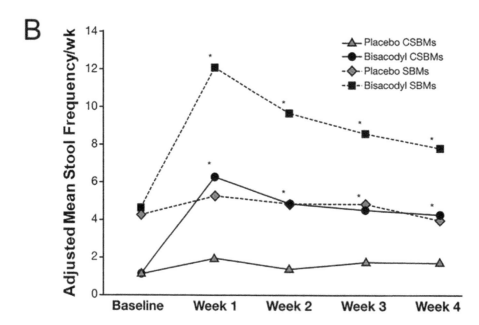

A, Adjusted mean number of complete spontaneous bowel movements (CSBMs) per week over 4-week treatment period. The number of CSBMs per week with bisacodyl was significantly higher than with placebo, and the number in the 2 groups at baseline was similar. B, CSBMs and SBMs per week during 4-week treatment period. The number for both stool frequencies increased every week with bisacodyl compared with number with placebo. *$P<.0001$.

(From Kamm MA, Mueller-Lissner S, Wald A, Richter E, Swallow R, Gessner U. Oral bisacodyl is effective and well-tolerated in patients with chronic constipation. Clin Gastroenterol Hepatol. 2011 Jul;9(7):577-83; used with permission.)

Figure 10.25   Chloride Channels: Actions in Gastroenterology

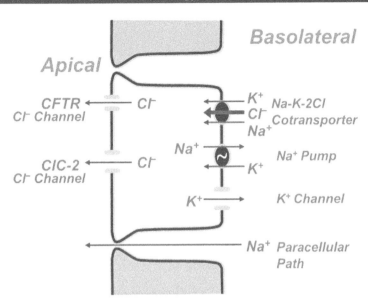

Schematic model of Cl⁻ transport in intestinal epithelial cells. At the basolateral membrane, Cl⁻ enters the cell from blood across the Na⁺-K⁺-2Cl cotransporter. Na⁺ is expelled by the Na⁺ pump, and K⁺ leaves via a K⁺ channel. Na⁺ is shown crossing the cell layer via a paracellular pathway, but Na⁺ channels also exist (not shown). Both cystic fibrosis transmembrane regulator (CFTR) and ClC-2 Cl⁻ channels are present on the apical membrane and can allow Cl⁻ to exit the cell. Cl⁻ indicates chloride; ClC-2, chloride type 2 channel; K⁺, potassium; Na⁺, sodium; 2Cl, 2 chloride atoms.

(From Cuppoletti J, Malinowska DH, Tewari KP, Li QJ, Sherry AM, Patchen ML, et al. SPI-0211 activates T84 cell chloride transport and recombinant human ClC-2 chloride currents. Am J Physiol Cell Physiol. 2004 Nov;287(5):C1173-83; as adapted from Pilewski JM, Frizzell RA. Role of CFTR in airway disease. Physiol Rev. 1999 Jan;79(1 Suppl):S215-55; used with permission.)

Figure 10.26   Effect of Lubiprostone, 24 µg Twice Daily, in Constipation

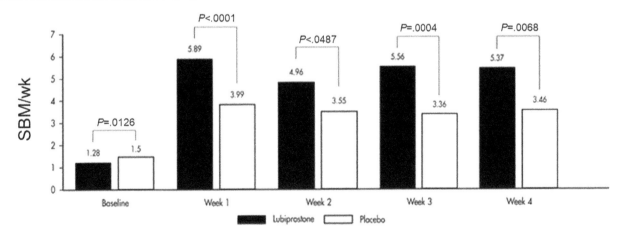

Frequency of spontaneous bowel movements (SBM) at baseline and weeks 1, 2, 3, and 4 (intention-to-treat population with missing values imputed by the last observation carried forward technique). SBM frequency calculated as the number of SBMs divided by the number of days, multiplied by 7. *P* values were based on van Elteren tests adjusted for pooled center. With use of a final mixed model testing for overall treatment effect, the frequency of SBMs at week 1 was significantly greater among those randomized to lubiprostone (*P*<.0001). The discontinuation rate due to adverse events was 12.6%.

(From Barish CF, Drossman D, Johanson JF, Ueno R. Efficacy and safety of lubiprostone in patients with chronic constipation. Dig Dis Sci. 2010 Apr;55(4):1090-7; used with permission.)

Figure 10.27   Known Mammalian Guanylate Cyclase C (GC-C) Agonists

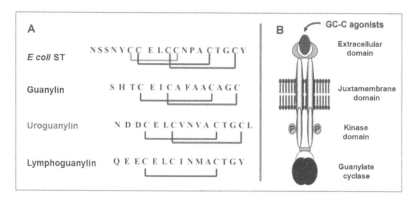

A, Amino acid sequences (indicated by separate initials in the amino acid chains) of the different endogenous GC-C agonists and the heat-stable enterotoxin of *Escherichia coli* (*E coli*) that also binds to the GC-C receptor. B, Binding of the agonist to the GC-C receptor. Two drugs, linaclotide and plecanatide, mimic endogenous GC-C ligands. ST indicates heat-stable enterotoxin.

Figure 10.28   Effects of Guanylate Cyclase-C (GC-C) Agonists

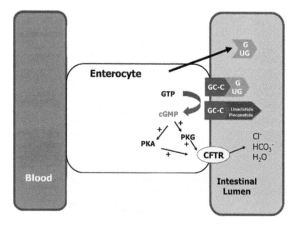

The natural peptide hormones guanylin (G) and uroguanylin (UG) are secreted by enterocytes into the intestinal lumen, probably in response to high sodium levels in the intestinal lumen. Linaclotide has an amino acid sequence similar to that of the guanylin peptides and also acts as agonist of the intestinal GC-C, which is a transmembrane protein located in the epithelial wall. Activation of the GC-C induces the intracellular transformation from guanosine triphosphate (GTP) into the second messenger cyclic guanosine monophosphate (cGMP). Cyclic GMP activates the protein kinase G (PKG) and the protein kinase A (PKA), which both activate the cystic fibrosis transmembrane conductance regulator (CFTR). Activation of the CFTR induces the secretion of chloride (Cl^-), bicarbonate (HCO_3^-), and water into the intestinal lumen.

obstructed defecation or generalized gastrointestinal dysmotility. The decision to proceed to surgery is facilitated in the presence of megacolon and megarectum or if colonic manometry shows evidence of inertia, that is, failure of the colon to respond to a 1,000-kcal meal or intravenous neostigmine 1 mg. Complications after surgery include small bowel obstruction (11%) and fecal soiling, particularly at night, during the first postoperative year. Frequency of defecation is about 3 to 8 per day during the first year, but it decreases to 1 to 3 per day from the second year after surgery.

Patients who have a combined evacuation and transit or motility disorder should first pursue pelvic floor retraining (biofeedback and muscle relaxation) and relaxation and address any psychologic issues and dietary and lifestyle modifications. If symptoms are intractable despite biofeedback and optimized medical therapy, colectomy and ileorectostomy could be considered as long as the evacuation disorder is resolved and optimized medical therapy is unsuccessful. Surgical procedures for pelvic floor dysfunction (internal anal sphincter or puborectalis muscle division) or injections with botulinum toxin have achieved only mediocre success and have been largely abandoned.

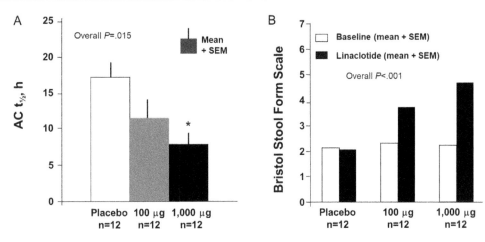

A, Effect of linaclotide on AC emptying t$_{1/2}$ in patients with irritable bowel syndrome with constipation (IBS-C). Overall, *P*=.015; *Pairwise comparison, *P*=.004 vs placebo. B, Effect of linaclotide on stool consistency in patients with IBS-C. Baseline data are from 11 patients in the 1,000-μg group because 1 patient did not have any bowel movements at baseline. Overall, *P*<.001; both pairwise comparisons for 100-μg and 1,000-μg groups vs placebo, *P*<.05.

(From Andresen V, Camilleri M, Busciglio IA, Grudell A, Burton D, McKinzie S, et al. Effect of 5 days linaclotide on transit and bowel function in females with constipation-predominant irritable bowel syndrome. Gastroenterology. 2007 Sep;133(3):761-8; used with permission.)

Figure 10.30   Linaclotide for Chronic Constipation

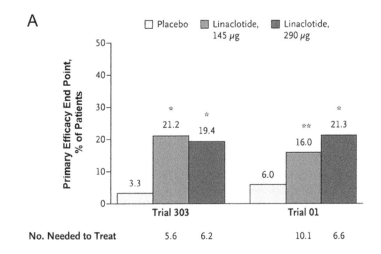

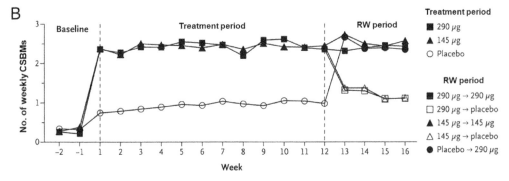

A, Estimated number needed to treat. Primary efficacy end point was 3 or more complete spontaneous bowel movements (CSBMs) per week and increase of 1 or more CSBMs from baseline for at least 9 weeks of 12 weeks of treatment. *P≤.001 vs placebo; **P<.01 vs placebo. B, Number of weekly complete spontaneous bowel movements (CSBMs). Most common adverse event was diarrhea (16%). RW indicates randomized withdrawal.

(From Lembo AJ, Schneier HA, Shiff SJ, Kurtz CB, MacDougall JE, Jia XD, et al. Two randomized trials of linaclotide for chronic constipation. N Engl J Med. 2011 Aug 11;365(6):527-36; used with permission.)

Figure 10.31　Effect of Plecanatide for Chronic Idiopathic Constipation

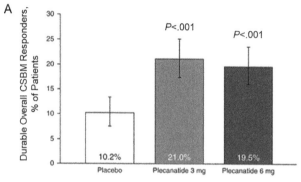

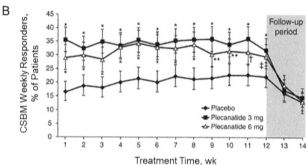

A, Percentage of patients in each treatment group assessed as a durable overall complete spontaneous bowel movement (CSBM) responder in the intention-to-treat population, the primary efficacy end point. Durable overall CSBM responders were defined as patients who fulfilled both 3 or more CSBMs per week and an increase of 1 or more CSBM from baseline, in the same week, for 9 or more of the 12 treatment weeks, including 3 or more of the last 4 weeks of treatment. Error bars represent 95% confidence intervals. B, Weekly evolution of the percentage of CSBM responders in the intention-to-treat population. Values are least square means; bars represent 95% CIs. *P=.001, **P=.003, †P=.005, ‡P=.011 vs placebo.

(From Miner PB Jr, Koltun WD, Wiener GJ, De La Portilla M, Prieto B, Shailubhai K, et al. A randomized phase III clinical trial of plecanatide, a uroguanylin analog, in patients with chronic idiopathic constipation. Am J Gastroenterol. 2017 Apr;112(4):613-21; used with permission.)

Specific Treatments for Secondary Constipation

Specific treatments are approved for opioid-induced constipation: the secretory agent lubiprostone and the orally administered, peripherally active μ-opiate receptor antagonists methyl naltrexone, naloxegol, and

Figure 10.32　Effect of Prucalopride on Colonic Transit in Functional Constipation

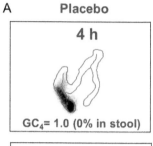 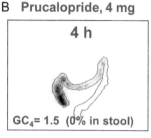

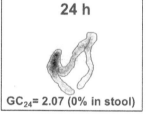 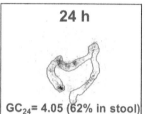

Two sets of scintigraphic images obtained from 2 study patients: 1 receiving placebo (A) and the other receiving 4 mg prucalopride (B). Top images are 4-hour scans and bottom images are 24-hour scans for each patient. Prucalopride accelerates movement of the radioisotope through the colon both at 4 and 24 hours in comparison with placebo. GC indicates geometric center at 4 (GC$_4$) and 24 (GC$_{24}$) hours. The higher GC value implies more rapid colonic transit, and a value of 4.1 indicates that most of the isotope has already been excreted.

(From Bouras EP, Camilleri M, Burton DD, Thomforde G, McKinzie S, Zinsmeister AR. Prucalopride accelerates gastrointestinal and colonic transit in patients with constipation without a rectal evacuation disorder. Gastroenterology. 2001 Feb;120(2):354-60; used with permission.)

naldemedine. Selection of patients for this treatment should be based on insufficient response to first-line treatments (lifestyle modification and over-the-counter preparations) and a score of 30 or more on the bowel function index, a clinician assessment tool to appraise severity and responsiveness to current treatment (Ueberall 2011; see suggested reading). It includes ease of defecation, feeling of incomplete bowel evacuation, and personal judgment of constipation. Each variable is rated by the patient from 0 to 100 on the basis of the experience in 7 days.

An experimental treatment for constipation in Parkinson disease is ENT-01, an oral inhibitor of α-synuclein aggregation, which relieved constipation (frequency and consistency of stool) and had beneficial effects on neurologic manifestations.

Figure 10.33   Effect of Prucalopride in Chronic Constipation

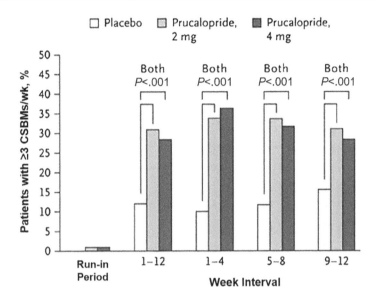

The primary efficacy end point in the intention-to-treat population was the proportion of patients having an average of 3 or more complete spontaneous bowel movements (CSBMs) per week.

(From Camilleri M, Kerstens R, Rykx A, Vandeplassche L. A placebo-controlled trial of prucalopride for severe chronic constipation. N Engl J Med. 2008 May 29;358(22):2344-54; used with permission.)

Figure 10.34   Effect of Elobixibat (A3309) on Colonic Transit in Functional Constipation

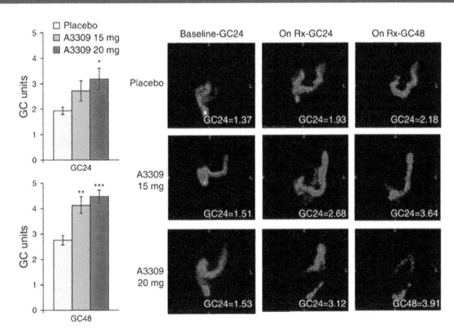

Colonic transit was accelerated. GC indicates geometric center; Rx, therapy. *P<.05, **P<.01, ***P<.001.

(From Wong BS, Camilleri M, McKinzie S, Burton D, Graffner H, Zinsmeister AR. Effects of A3309, an ileal bile acid transporter inhibitor, on colonic transit and symptoms in females with functional constipation. Am J Gastroenterol. 2011 Dec;106(12):2154-64; used with permission.)

Figure 10.35   Effects of Elobixibat on Change From Baseline in the Frequency of Spontaneous Bowel Movements (SBMs) (A) and Complete Spontaneous Bowel Movements (CSBMs) (B) in Chronic Constipation

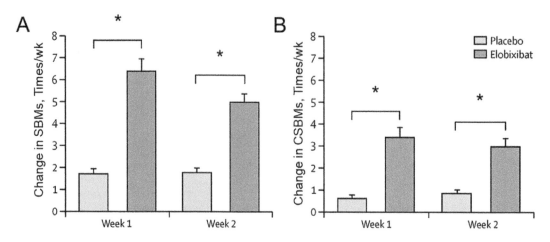

Comparison of elobixibat and placebo on changes from baseline in the frequency of SBM and CSBM. Data are least-squares mean (SE). Change in the frequency of SBMs during week 1 of treatment was the primary end point. *P<.0001.

(From Nakajima A, Seki M, Taniguchi S, Ohta A, Gillberg PG, Mattsson JP, et al. Safety and efficacy of elobixibat for chronic constipation: results from a randomised, double-blind, placebo-controlled, phase 3 trial and an open-label, single-arm, phase 3 trial. Lancet Gastroenterol Hepatol. 2018 Aug;3(8):537-47; used with permission.)

Figure 10.36   Network Diagram of the Numbers of Patients and Numbers of Trials With Different Drugs and Placebo in the Analysis

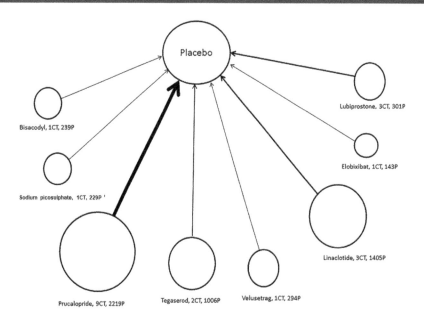

CT indicates clinical trial; P, patients.

(From Nelson AD, Camilleri M, Chirapongsathorn S, Vijayvargiya P, Valentin N, Shin A, et al. Comparison of efficacy of pharmacological treatments for chronic idiopathic constipation: a systematic review and network meta-analysis. Gut. 2017 Sep;66(9):1611-22; used with permission.)

Figure 10.37 Pooled Relative Risk (95% CIs) (for Network Meta-analysis) for Primary End Points: Responders With 3 or More CSBM/week (A) or Increase Over Baseline by 1 or More CSBM/week (B)

A Responders with ≥3 CSBM/week

Responders with ≥3 CSBM per week for the drugs for CIC

	Bisacodyl	Sodium picosulphate	Prucalopride	Tegaserod	Velusetrag	Linaclotide
Placebo	**2.46 (1.14 to 5.31)**	**2.83 (1.27 to 6.31)**	**1.84 (1.40 to 2.43)**	1.47 (0.7 to 3.12)	**4.86 (1.58 to 14.99)**	1.96 (0.8 to 4.81)
Bisacodyl		1.15 (0.38 to 3.49)	0.75 (0.33 to 1.69)	0.59 (0.20 to 1.75)	1.97 (0.51 to 7.72)	0.79 (0.24 to 2.60)
Sodium picosulphate			0.65 (0.28 to 1.52)	0.52 (0.17 to 1.56)	1.72 (0.43 to 6.84)	0.69 (0.21 to 2.31)
Prucalopride				0.80 (0.36 to 1.78)	2.64 (0.83 to 8.41)	1.06 (0.41 to 2.72)
Tegaserod					3.30 (0.85 to 12.79)	1.33 (0.41 to 4.30)
Velusetrag						0.40 (0.09 to 1.70)
Linaclotide						

B Responders with increase over baseline by ≥1 CSBM/week

Responders with ≥1 CSBM per week for the drugs for CIC

	Bisacodyl	Sodium picosulphate	Prucalopride	Tegaserod	Velusetrag	Linaclotide	Elobixibat
Placebo	**2.04 (1.3 to 3.19)**	**2.03 (1.27 to 3.23)**	**1.54 (1.30 to 1.83)**	1.33 (0.97 to 1.83)	**3.1 (1.61 to 5.95)**	**1.72 (1.0 to 2.96)**	**1.97 (1.09 to 3.55)**
Bisacodyl		0.99 (0.52 to 1.9)	0.76 (0.47 to 1.22)	0.65 (0.38 to 1.13)	1.52 (0.69 to 3.35)	0.84 (0.42 to 1.71)	0.96 (0.46 to 2.02)
Sodium picosulphate			0.76 (0.46 to 1.25)	0.66 (0.37 to 1.16)	1.53 (0.69 to 3.41)	0.85 (0.42 to 1.74)	0.97 (0.46 to 2.06)
Prucalopride				0.86 (0.60 to 1.23)	**2.01 (1.02 to 3.93)**	1.11 (0.63 to 1.97)	1.27 (0.69 to 2.35)
Tegaserod					**2.33 (1.13 to 4.80)**	1.29 (0.69 to 2.42)	1.48 (0.76 to 2.89)
Velusetrag						0.56 (0.24 to 1.30)	0.64 (0.26 to 1.53)
Linaclotide							1.14 (0.51 to 2.55)
Elobixibat							

Significant relative risk ratios and 95% CIs are in bold. CIC indicates chronic idiopathic constipation; CSBM, complete spontaneous bowel movement.

(From Nelson AD, Camilleri M, Chirapongsathorn S, Vijayvargiya P, Valentin N, Shin A, et al. Comparison of efficacy of pharmacological treatments for chronic idiopathic constipation: a systematic review and network meta-analysis. Gut. 2017 Sep;66(9):1611-22; used with permission.)

Suggested Reading

Bellini M, Usai-Satta P, Bove A, Bocchini R, Galeazzi F, Battaglia E, et al; ChroCoDiTE Study Group, AIGO. Chronic constipation diagnosis and treatment evaluation: the "CHRO.CO.DI.T.E." study. BMC Gastroenterol. 2017 Jan 14;17(1):11.

Bharucha AE, Rao SS. An update on anorectal disorders for gastroenterologists. Gastroenterology. 2014 Jan;146(1):37–45 e2. Epub 2013 Nov 12.

Cai Q, Buono JL, Spalding WM, Sarocco P, Tan H, Stephenson JJ, et al. Healthcare costs among patients with chronic constipation: a retrospective claims analysis in a commercially insured population. J Med Econ. 2014 Feb;17(2):148–58. Epub 2013 Nov 15.

Camilleri M, Ford AC, Mawe GM, Dinning PG, Rao SS, Chey WD, et al. Chronic constipation. Nat Rev Dis Primers. 2017 Dec 14;3:17095. Epub 2017 Dec 15.

Harewood GC, Coulie B, Camilleri M, Rath-Harvey D, Pemberton JH. Descending perineum syndrome: audit of clinical and laboratory features and outcome of pelvic floor retraining. Am J Gastroenterol. 1999 Jan;94(1):126–30.

Heidelbaugh JJ, Stelwagon M, Miller SA, Shea EP, Chey WD. The spectrum of constipation-predominant irritable bowel syndrome and chronic idiopathic constipation: US survey assessing symptoms, care seeking, and disease burden. Am J Gastroenterol. 2015 Apr;110(4):580–7. Epub 2015 Mar 17.

Lembo A, Camilleri M. Chronic constipation. N Engl J Med. 2003 Oct 2;349(14):1360–8. Epub 2003 Oct 03.

Liu A, Chedid V, Wang XJ, Vijayvargiya P, Camilleri M. Clinical presentation and characteristics of pelvic floor myofascial pain in patients presenting with constipation. Neurogastroenterol Motil. 2020 Jul;32(7):e13845. Epub 2020 Apr 13.

Ueberall MA, Müller-Lissner S, Buschmann-Kramm C, Bosse B. The Bowel Function Index for evaluating constipation in pain patients: definition of a reference range for a nonconstipated population of pain patients. J Int Med Res. 2011;39(1):41–50.

Wang XJ, Chedid V, Vijayvargiya P, Camilleri M. Clinical features and associations of descending perineum syndrome in 300 adults with constipation in gastroenterology referral practice. Dig Dis Sci. 2020 Jul 14. Epub ahead of print.

Irritable Bowel Syndrome: Peripheral Mechanisms, Biomarkers, and Management[a]

Introduction

Several peripheral mechanisms result in symptoms of irritable bowel syndrome (IBS). They include abnormal colonic transit and rectal stool evacuation; intraluminal irritants such as short-chain fatty acids (SCFA), bile acids (BA), or gluten; microbiome changes; enteroendocrine cell products; and genetic susceptibility. Irritants can increase mucosal permeability, cause immune activation, activate local reflexes to alter intestinal motility or secretion, and induce visceral hypersensitivity and pain. IBS management is based on predominant symptom relief rather than targeting specific mechanisms. However, biomarkers are being identified and introduced into practice, such as colonic transit and fecal BA excretion and should lead to individualized, specific treatments of IBS.

Epidemiology and Symptoms

IBS is currently diagnosed on the basis of symptom criteria and exclusion of organic diseases. It affects 10% to 20% of adults in most countries (Figure 11.1) and has enormous direct health care costs and indirect costs through absenteeism from work.

The symptoms of IBS are recurrent abdominal pain or discomfort at least 3 days per month in the past 3 months associated with 2 or more of the following: improvement with defecation, onset associated with a change in frequency of stool, and onset associated with a change in form (appearance) of stool.

Pathophysiology and Mechanisms

The predominant pathophysiologic mechanisms in IBS are abnormalities in smooth muscle function in the gut, visceral hypersensitivity, and central nervous system hypervigilance. Hypersensitivity may result from brain dysfunction or abnormal interaction with the peripheral afferents in IBS. Hypersensitivity and central dysfunction are important mechanisms in about 50% of patients with IBS according to multiple series (see Chapter 12, "Visceral Sensation"). There has been a renaissance in views of IBS: Symptoms possibly are manifestations of several peripheral mechanisms that perturb motor and sensory functions. These mechanisms are summarized in Table 11.1 and are discussed briefly in the next section (Figure 11.2).

Abnormal Colonic Transit and Disorders of Evacuation

There is considerable overlap of symptoms of IBS-C (constipation-predominant IBS) and chronic constipation. Several treatments of functional or chronic idiopathic constipation are also efficacious in IBS-C, such as secretagogues (lubiprostone, linaclotide

---

[a] Portions previously published in Camilleri M. Management options for irritable bowel syndrome. Mayo Clin Proc. 2018 Dec;93(12):1858-72; used with permission of Mayo Foundation for Medical Education and Research.

Figure 11.1   Global Prevalence of Irritable Bowel Syndrome (IBS)

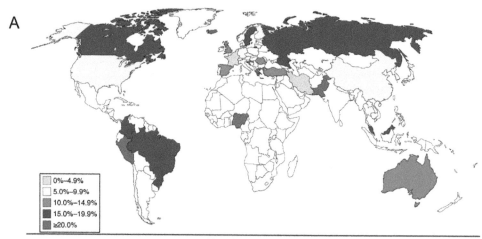

A

0%–4.9%
5.0%–9.9%
10.0%–14.9%
15.0%–19.9%
≥20.0%

B

	No. of Studies	No. of Patients	Pooled Prevalence, %	95% CI
All studies	80	260,960	11.2	9.8-12.8
North European	21	72,031	12.0	9.0-15.0
Southeast European	19	55,545	7.0	5.0-9.0
North American	10	52,790	11.8	7.4-17.2
South European	9	36,577	15.0	11.0-20.0
Middle Eastern	8	32,374	7.5	3.5-12.8
South Asian	4	5,857	17.0	5.0-33.0
South American	4	1,272	21.0	18.0-25.0
Australasian	3	3,739	14.0	13.0-15.0
African	2	775	19.0	2.0-46.0

A, Prevalence of IBS by country. B, Pooled prevalence of IBS by geographic location. IBS indicates irritable bowel syndrome.

(Modified from Lovell RM, Ford AC. Global prevalence of and risk factors for irritable bowel syndrome: a meta-analysis. Clin Gastroenterol Hepatol. 2012 Jul;10(7):712-21; used with permission.)

and plecanatide) and the serotonin-receptor agonist tegaserod, which were approved for both chronic idiopathic constipation and IBS-C. They relieve constipation and associated pain and bloating. About 25% (range, 5%-46% in different studies) of patients with IBS-C have slow colonic transit.

Symptoms of rectal evacuation disorders (see Chapter 10, "Chronic Constipation") overlap those of IBS-C: constipation, straining, sense of incomplete rectal evacuation, bloating, and left-sided abdominal pain relieved with bowel movement. Moreover, treatment of the evacuation disorder relieves the IBS-C symptoms (see Chapter 10, "Chronic Constipation").

Diarrhea-predominant IBS (IBS-D) is associated with acceleration of colonic transit in 15% to 45% of patients (see Figure 9.23 and Figure 11.3).

Several disorders that mimic IBS-D require exclusion. Examples include food allergy or intolerance, disaccharidase deficiencies (most frequently lactase and less frequently sucrose-isomaltase deficiencies [Figure 11.4] or fructose malabsorption), celiac disease, gluten intolerance without celiac disease, microscopic colitis, and idiopathic BA malabsorption. A systematic review of several studies from all over the world showed that about 30% of patients with IBS-D or functional diarrhea have evidence of BA diarrhea (Valentin 2016; see suggested reading).

The relevance of colonic transit is emphasized by evidence that prokinetic or secretagogue agents that substantially alter colonic transit in pharmacodynamics studies are also efficacious in relief of symptoms in phase 2b or 3 randomized controlled trials (Table 11.2).

Table 11.1   Peripheral Factors in the Biology of IBS

Peripheral Mechanism	Pathophysiology	Examples of Factors Involved	Comments and Clinical Correlates
Colonic motility	Accelerated or delayed colonic transit; may be secondary to secretory mechanism	Neuromuscular dysfunction, enteroendocrine cell products (eg, 5-HT, granins); organic acids (BAs, SCFAs), genetic predisposition: BA synthesis (Klothoβ), *GUCY2C* mutation	Up to 45% of IBS-D, 20% of IBS-C
Colonic motor and sensory response to feeding	Neurally (eg, vagally) mediated induction of colonic HAPCs, increased ileocolonic transit, increased rectal sensitivity	Fat content of meal, high caloric content	Contributes to postprandial pain, urgency, diarrhea
Small bowel and colonic sensing and responses	Activation of local secretory or motor reflexes and sensory mechanisms	Food stimulation of enteroendocrine cell products, organic acids (BAs, SCFAs)	Typically associated with diarrhea, bloating, pain
Rectal evacuation disorder	Failure of rectal emptying with reflex inhibition of colonic motor function	Anismus, pelvic floor dyssynergia, descending perineum syndrome	Typical IBS-C symptoms + incomplete evacuation and straining reversed with pelvic floor Rx
Small bowel mucosal permeability	Increased permeability, altered expression (mRNA, protein) of tight junction proteins	Prior gastroenteritis, atopy, food intolerance (eg, gluten,? FODMAP), stress	Typically associated with IBS-D, may increase fluid secretion or activate sensory mechanism
Colonic mucosal permeability	Increased permeability, altered expression (mRNA, protein) of tight junction proteins	Malabsorbed CHO or fats increase SCFA, BA malabsorption (25% IBS-D), immune activation, genetic predisposition: immune activation (eg, TLR9, TNFSF15), BA synthesis (Klothoβ)	Typically associated with IBS-D, may increase fluid secretion or activate sensory mechanism
Mucosal immune activation	Increased permeability, activation of submucosal secretory reflexes and sensory mechanisms	Prior gastroenteritis, mast cells, T lymphocytes, circulating cytokines	Typically associated with IBS-D and abdominal pain
Colonic microbiome	Production of SCFAs with effects on motor, secretory, and sensory functions	Increased Firmicutes or ratio of Firmicutes to Bacteroidetes, modified by antibiotics, or probiotics, BAs influence microbial species	Associated abdominal bloating, pain, diarrhea

Abbreviations: BA, bile acid; CHO, carbohydrate; FODMAP, fructose oligosaccharide, disaccharide, monosaccharide, and polyol; HAPC, high-amplitude propagated contraction; 5-HT, 5-hydroxytryptamine (serotonin); IBS, irritable bowel syndrome; IBS-C, constipation-predominant IBS; IBS-D, diarrhea-predominant IBS; Rx, therapy; SCFA, short-chain fatty acid; TLR9, toll-like receptor 9; TNFSF15, tumor necrosis factor superfamily 15.

Modified from Camilleri M. Peripheral mechanisms in irritable bowel syndrome. N Engl J Med. 2012 Oct 25;367(17):1626-35; used with permission.

The Irritated Bowel in IBS

Luminal and mucosal factors activate immune, motor, and sensory mechanisms in the small bowel or colon. Such irritation leads to the pathophysiology of IBS and may be associated with immune activation or inflammatory response (Figure 11.5).

Irritated Bowel: Luminal Factors

Prominent Colorectal Responses to Feeding

Pain after eating meals containing fat and at least 500 kcal may be associated in IBS-D with induction of repeated high-amplitude propagated contractions that induce colonic mass movements. Motor and sensory dysfunctions may converge to induce IBS symptoms.

Malabsorbed or Maldigested Nutrients

Malabsorbed sugars, such as lactose, fructose, and sorbitol, may mimic IBS, and prevalence differs by ethnic groups and races: lactose malabsorption is common in Asians and Africans and rare in Norwegians presenting with IBS; fructose and sorbitol malabsorption occur in patients with IBS from Denmark but not in those from the Netherlands. Functional variants in the sucrase-isomaltase gene (including a common sucroase-isomaltase variant [15Phe]) result in defective disaccharidase enzyme activity and are associated with an increased risk of IBS (Figure 11.4).

In contrast to malabsorption, abnormal digestion of complex carbohydrates results in increased fecal SCFAs (<6 carbon atoms) in IBS-D. With mild fat malabsorption or rapid small bowel transit, SCFAs or medium-chain (6 to 12 carbon atoms) fatty acids reach the right colon. In healthy volunteers, 2% to 20% (average, 10%) of dietary starch is not absorbed in the small bowel and is metabolized by colonic bacteria to produce SCFAs, which can stimulate SCFA receptor 2 (also called free fatty acid receptor 2 or G protein–coupled receptor 43) on enteroendocrine cells and mucosal mast cells in the intestine. These release serotonin and stimulate colonic transit and motility, including high-amplitude propagated contractions. The SCFA propionate also induces transepithelial ion and fluid transport in the distal colon.

Fermentable oligosaccharides, disaccharides, monosaccharides, and polyols (FODMAP) are poorly absorbed in the small bowel, and their metabolism by the colonic microbiota contributes to nutrient-induced symptoms.

Gluten Intolerance

Celiac disease is no more prevalent in IBS than in controls. In a randomized trial (Vazquez-Roque 2013; see suggested reading) of gluten-containing versus gluten-free diets in patients with IBS-D, patients with IBS but not celiac disease who were carriers of HLA-DQ2 or HLA-DQ8 genotypes (which predispose to celiac disease) were more likely to respond (reduced stool frequency) to gluten withdrawal than were noncarriers. Gluten resulted in increased bowel permeability and reduced tight junction protein expression in bowel mucosa.

Increased Intracolonic BA

In a systematic literature analysis (Valentin 2016; see suggested reading), the estimated prevalence of BA malabsorption was approximately 30% in patients with IBS-D. This finding was based on selenium-75–homocholic acid taurine (^{75}SeHCAT) retention at 7 days of less than 15%, fasting serum 7α-hydroxy-4-cholesten-3-one (a BA precursor) value of more than 52.5 ng/mL, or 48-hour total fecal BA excretion (>2,337

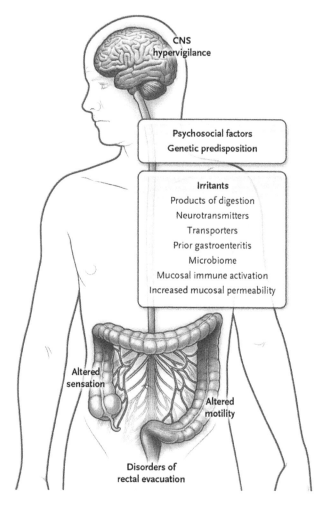

Figure 11.2   Mechanisms Underlying Irritable Bowel Syndrome

CNS hypervigilance

Psychosocial factors
Genetic predisposition

Irritants
Products of digestion
Neurotransmitters
Transporters
Prior gastroenteritis
Microbiome
Mucosal immune activation
Increased mucosal permeability

Altered sensation

Altered motility

Disorders of rectal evacuation

Various peripheral mechanisms initiate perturbation of gastrointestinal motor and sensory functions and lead to symptoms. Identification of the peripheral irritants provides an opportunity to prevent or reverse symptoms. CNS indicates central nervous system.

(From Camilleri M. Peripheral mechanisms in irritable bowel syndrome. N Engl J Med. 2012 Oct 25;367(17):1626-35; used with permission.)

Figure 11.3   Detection Rates of Abnormal Transit With Radiopaque Marker in Diarrhea and Constipation

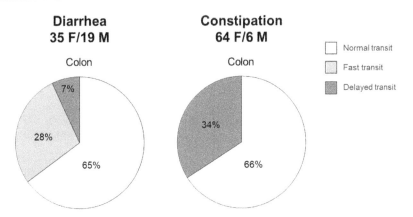

(Modified from Sadik R, Stotzer PO, Simren M, Abrahamsson H. Gastrointestinal transit abnormalities are frequently detected in patients with unexplained GI symptoms at a tertiary centre. Neurogastroenterol Motil. 2008 Mar;20(3):197-205; used with permission.)

µmol/48 h). Even among patients with IBS-D who do not have overtly increased fecal BA excretion, there is a suggestive correlation between fecal BA levels and colonic transit. In fact, different parameters of fecal BA excretion are associated with accelerated colonic transit or increased fecal weight (>400 g/48 h): total fecal BA more than 1,000 µmol/48 h plus primary BAs (cholic acid plus chenodeoxycholic acid) more than 4% (normal, <0.4%) or primary BAs in a 48-hour collection of more than 10%.

Figure 11.4   Properties of Sucrase-Isomaltase (SI) Mutants and Common Coding Polymorphisms

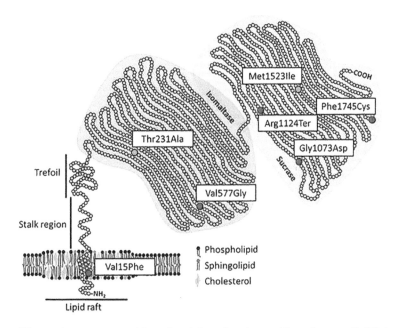

Schematic representation of SI protein structure and functional domains, the position of congenital SI deficiency (CSID) mutations, and common coding variants, color-coded according to their functional effects (red=damaging, green=benign). Although rare, CSID mutations with known defective disaccharidase (SI) properties occur more often in patients with irritable bowel syndrome (IBS) than in controls (P=.074; odds ratio=1.84). A common SI variant (15Phe), which shows reduced enzymatic activity in vitro, is strongly associated with increased risk of IBS.

(Modified from Henstrom M, Diekmann L, Bonfiglio F, Hadizadeh F, Kuech EM, von Kockritz-Blickwede M, et al. Functional variants in the sucrase-isomaltase gene associate with increased risk of irritable bowel syndrome. Gut. 2018 Feb;67(2):263-70; Open Access article distributed under the Creative Commons Attribution Non Commercial (CC BY-NC 4.0) license [http://creativecommons.org/licenses/by-nc/4.0/].)

Table 11.2 Evidence of Clinical Efficacy Predicted by Colonic Transit Measured by Scintigraphy

Drug Class	Pharmacodynamics (Intestine or Colon)	Clinical Efficacy: Phase 2b or 3 Studies
5-HT$_3$ antagonist, alosetron	1 mg twice daily delayed colonic transit diarrhea in IBS-D	2b, 3 studies in thousands of patients with non-IBS-C or IBS-D: adequate relief of pain and discomfort of IBS, bowel dysfunction (including diarrhea), and urgency
5-HT$_4$ agonist, tegaserod	2 mg twice daily accelerated small bowel and colonic transit in health and IBS-C (without evacuation disorder)	2b, 3 studies in several thousands of patients with IBS-C and chronic constipation experienced relief of pain and discomfort of IBS and bowel dysfunction
5-HT$_4$ agonist, prucalopride	Increases small bowel and colon transit in health and patients with chronic constipation	2b, 3 studies in thousands of patients with chronic constipation: BM frequency and satisfaction with bowel function both improved
5-HT$_4$ agonist, velusetrag	Dose-related increase in small bowel and colon transit in health	2b dose-ranging study in 401 patients with chronic constipation increased BM frequency and proportion with adequate relief
5-HT$_4$ agonist, YKP10811	Accelerates colonic transit and improves stool consistency in chronic constipation	ClinicalTrials.gov: NCT01989234; study completed, no posted results
Bisacodyl	Accelerates colon transit in health	Relief of constipation after acute administration and for chronic constipation
Recombinant human NT-3	NT-3 accelerates colonic transit in chronic constipation	NT-3, administered TTW, increased stool frequency, accelerated colon transit, and improved symptoms of chronic constipation
Cl-C2 channel activator, lubiprostone	Accelerates small bowel and colonic transit in healthy controls	Several phase 3 in several hundred patients with chronic constipation and IBS-C: efficacious in relief of pain and bowel dysfunction
Guanylate cyclase-C agonist, linaclotide	Accelerated ascending colonic transit and induced looser bowel function in 36 women with IBS-C	Several 2a, 2b, and 3 studies in patients with chronic constipation or IBS-C (several hundred): increased BM frequency, relief of bloating and abdominal discomfort
GLP-1 analog, ROSE010	Accelerated colonic transit at 48 hours	Relieved severity of pain attacks and enhanced satisfaction score in IBS
Ileal bile acid transport inhibitor, elobixibat	Accelerates colonic transit and loosens stool consistency in functional constipation patients	2b study showed improved stool frequency and constipation-related symptoms in idiopathic chronic constipation
Bile acid sequestrant, colesevelam	Retards ascending colon emptying	Improves stool consistency in IBS-D with high fecal bile acid excretion (phase 4 study)
Combination probiotic, VSL-III	Retards colonic transit in IBS-D, improves flatulence and bloating in IBS-D	Meta-analyses demonstrate symptom relief of multiple symptoms in IBS: global IBS, abdominal pain, bloating, and flatulence scores
κ-Opioid agonist, asimadoline	No significant effect on colonic transit in healthy volunteers	On-demand dosing not effective in reducing severity of abdominal pain in 100 patients with IBS; in 2b, dose-ranging study in 596 patients with IBS: post-hoc analysis showed benefit in moderate pain in IBS-D and IBS-Alt
CCK$_1$ antagonist, dexloxiglumide	Slower AC emptying with no effect on overall colonic transit in IBS-C	Two initial 2b or 3 trials: not efficacious in IBS-C; a randomized withdrawal design trial showed longer time to loss of therapeutic response for dexloxiglumide
CRH$_1$ antagonist, pexacerafont	No effect on colonic transit and bowel function in IBS-D	2b study showed GW876008 had no significant difference from placebo in the global improvement scale, daily self-assessment of IBS pain or discomfort, or individual lower GI symptoms
β$_3$-Adrenergic agonist, solabegron	No significant effect on GI or colonic transit	2b study showed no significant change in bowel symptoms, although a significant effect on adequate relief of IBS pain and discomfort

Abbreviations: AC, ascending colon; BM, bowel movement; CCK$_1$, cholecystokinin; Cl-C2, chloride channel type 2; CRH$_1$, corticotropin-releasing hormone; 5-HT, 5-hydroxytryptamine (serotonin); GI, gastrointestinal; GLP, glucagon-like peptide; IBS, irritable bowel syndrome; IBS-Alt, alternating IBS; IBS C, constipation-predominant IBS; IBS-D, diarrhea-predominant IBS; NT, neurotrophin; TTW, 3 times weekly.

Modified from Camilleri M. Scintigraphic biomarkers for colonic dysmotility. Clin Pharmacol Ther. 2010 Jun;87(6):748-53; used with permission.

Excess intracolonic BAs in IBS-D result from reduced feedback inhibition of hepatocyte synthesis of BAs by fibroblast growth factor 19 (FGF19) from ileal enterocytes (Figure 11.6). FGF19 binds to fibroblast growth factor receptor 4 (FGFR4) and Klothoβ (KLB) on the hepatocyte cell membrane, an action that suppresses the rate-limiting enzyme for BA synthesis, cytochrome P450 7A1 isozyme. Excess BA synthesis overcomes ileal absorption capacity, the result of which is increased concentrations of BAs in the colon and diarrhea.

Microbiota and Organic Acids

The precise role of the microbiome in IBS is still under investigation. An abundance in the fecal microbiome of Firmicutes, with or without decrease in the abundance of Bacteroidetes in the fecal microbiome, has been a consistent finding that is associated with colonic transit and levels of depression in IBS. Changes in mucosa-associated microbiota include increases in *Bacteroides* and Clostridia organisms and decreases in *Bifidobacterium* organisms in IBS-D. However, a systematic review and meta-analysis of 24 studies from 22 articles in the literature on the microbiome in IBS concluded that specific bacteria were associated with microbiomes of patients with IBS (increased *Lactobacillaciae*, *Bacteroides*, and *Enterobacteriaceae* and decreased *Bifidobacterium* and *Faecalibacterium*) compared with controls. However, whether these microbes are a product or cause of IBS could not be determined. Moreover, there were no consistent differences in the microbiomes of patients with IBS-C and those with IBS-D (Pittayanon 2019; see suggested reading).

Modifications in the microbiome with the non-absorbed antibiotic rifaximin or probiotic mixtures to relieve IBS symptoms, particularly a probiotic mixture, retarded colonic transit in patients with IBS-D, whereas rifaximin actually accelerated colonic transit.

Microbial interactions with intraluminal factors lead to changes in colonic functions, which may result from effects of organic acids (such as SCFAs) or the dihydroxylation of primary BAs to the secondary BAs (deoxycholic and lithocholic acid), of which deoxycholic acid is pro-secretory. A larger proportion of primary BAs (chenodeoxycholic acid and cholic acid) in stool of patients with IBS-D may also result from rapid colonic transit.

The primary or secondary BAs with at least 2 α-hydroxyl groups (chenodeoxycholic [3, 7], cholic [3, 7, 12], and deoxycholic [3, 12] acid) induce intestinal or colonic secretion. In addition, chenodeoxycholic acid induces high-amplitude propagated contractions in healthy humans and accelerates colonic transit in IBS-C. Conversely, the BA sequestrant colesevelam retards ascending colon transit in IBS-D, and the effect is correlated with the level of BA synthesis. Bacterial dehydroxylation of chenodeoxycholic acid results in production of lithocholic acid, which is not secretory, but lithocholic acid stimulates TGR5 receptors in the colon and could, thereby, stimulate motility and potentially accelerate transit.

BAs may also modify the microbial content of the colon. In rats, administration of cholic acid results in cecal microbiota that reflect the increased ratio of Firmicutes to Bacteroidetes observed in IBS.

Irritated Bowel: Enteroendocrine Signals Arising in the Mucosa

Enteroendocrine cells release several peptides and amines, such as serotonin, on exposure to dietary amines or tastants, or their metabolites, and BAs. Levels of plasma serotonin are higher in IBS-D and lower in IBS-C (Figure 11.7). Serotonin has a multitude of stimulatory effects on motor, secretory, and sensory functions. Selective serotonergic agonists and antagonists have a substantial effect on the treatment of different IBS phenotypes.

Enteroendocrine cells store and release chromogranins (Cg) and secretogranins, which promote the sorting and release from enteroendocrine cells of other peptide hormones and antimicrobial peptides. Faster colonic transit in IBS is associated with higher levels of fecal CgA, secretogranin II, and secretogranin III but lower levels of CgB. Other diarrheal diseases, such as lymphocytic colitis and celiac disease, also increase fecal Cg. The CgA cells (such as enteroendocrine cells) also express free fatty acid receptor 2s that respond to SCFAs, with release of bioactive peptides or amines. Thus, enteroendocrine cells and their products such as serotonin interact with or stimulate enterocytes, intrinsic primary afferent and submucosal neurons, and goblet cells (Figure 11.8).

Figure 11.5   Immune Responses, Increased Permeability, and Pain in Irritable Bowel Syndrome (IBS)

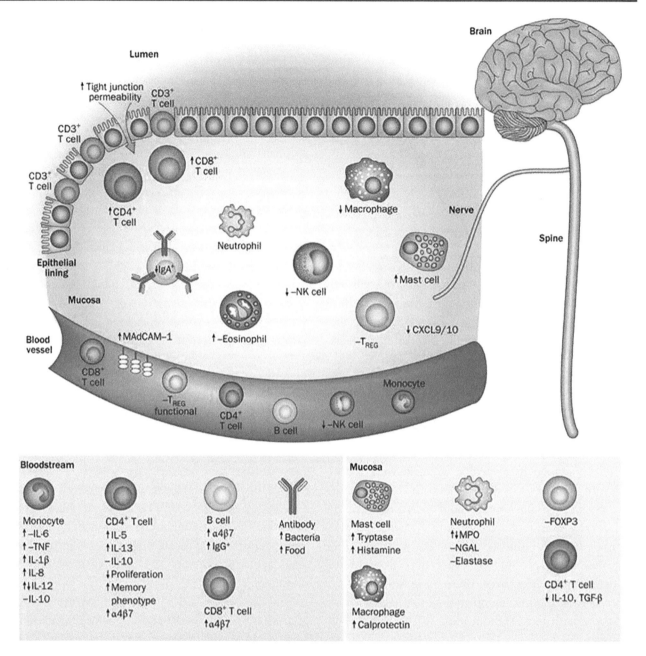

Increases in innate immune activity in the intestinal mucosa and blood are found in subpopulations of patients with IBS. IBS may also be associated with an activated adaptive immune response: increased T cells and altered B-cell activity and antibody production. Levels of mast-cell mediators (eg, histamine, tryptase, and trypsin) in colonic and jejunal biopsy supernatants are higher in both constipation- and diarrhea-dominant IBS. CXCL indicates CXC-chemokine ligand; IL, interleukin; MAdCAM–1, mucosal addressin cellular adhesion molecule 1; MPO, myeloperoxidase; NGAL, neutrophil gelatinase-associated lipocalin; NK, nuclear killer; TGF-β, transforming growth factor β; TNF, tumor necrosis factor; T_{REG}, T-regulatory cell.

(From Ohman L, Simren M. Pathogenesis of IBS: role of inflammation, immunity and neuroimmune interactions. Nat Rev Gastroenterol Hepatol. 2010 Mar;7(3):163-73; used with permission.)

Figure 11.6 Serum C4 Levels Show Increased Bile Acid Synthesis (A) and the Reciprocal Relationship of C4 and FGF19 Shows Reduced FGF19 in IBS-D (B)

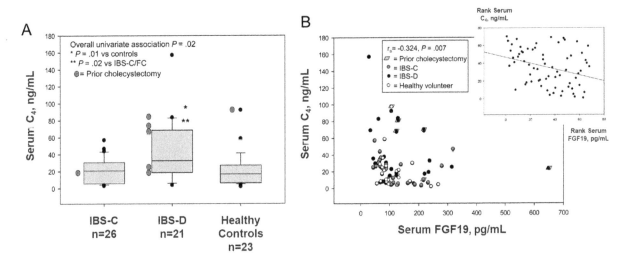

FC indicates functional constipation; FGF19, fibroblast growth factor 19; IBS, irritable bowel syndrome; IBS-C, constipation-predominant IBS; IBS-D, diarrhea-predominant IBS.

(Modified from Wong BS, Camilleri M, Carlson P, McKinzie S, Busciglio I, Bondar O, et al. Increased bile acid biosynthesis is associated with irritable bowel syndrome with diarrhea. Clin Gastroenterol Hepatol. 2012 Sep;10(9):1009-15; used with permission.)

Consequences of Irritation of the Colon

Immune Activation, Minimal Inflammation

There is evidence of immune activation in blood and intestinal or colonic mucosa (Figure 11.5).

Increased T lymphocytes in rectal mucosa and host mucosal immune response to microbial pathogens in subgroups of patients with IBS (possibly associated with genetic susceptibility) are associated with increased intestinal permeability.

Increased Mucosal Permeability

The intestinal barrier is made up of several components (Figure 11.9). In the lumen, bacteria and antigens are degraded by endogenous chemicals, particularly bile, gastric acid, and pancreatic juice. Commensal bacteria produce antimicrobial substances to inhibit the colonization by pathogens. In the microclimate on the luminal side of epithelial cells, the unstirred water layer, glycocalyx, and mucus layer prevent bacterial adhesion, and secretory immunoglobulin A from immunocytes in the lamina propria also attack the pathogens within the microclimate. Epithelial cells, connected by junctional complexes, allow transport of luminal content, but they also react to noxious stimuli by secretion of chloride and antimicrobial peptides. In the lamina propria, the innate and acquired immunity cells secrete immunoglobulin and cytokines, and the endocrine and enteric nervous systems complete the barrier by inducing intestinal propulsive motility to rid the intestine of the pathogen.

There are several measures of human intestinal or colonic permeability (Table 11.3), including urine excretion of probe molecules after oral ingestion in vivo (Table 11.4), barrier protein expression in mucosal biopsies, probe molecule flux, transepithelial resistance of mucosal biopsies in vitro, and responses of Caco-2 monolayers or rodent mucosa to fecal supernatants (Table 11.5). The results obtained from these tests need to be interpreted with caution.

Increased intestinal and colonic permeability and low-grade inflammation in children with IBS are associated with cow's milk allergy, prior nonspecific infection, atopic disease (rhinoconjunctivitis, rhinitis, eczema), stress, and dietary fat intake. Effects of stress on intestinal permeability are in part mediated by mast cells in response to corticotrophin-releasing hormone,

Figure 11.7   Serotonin Levels in Circulation in IBS: Increased in IBS-D and Decreased in IBS-C

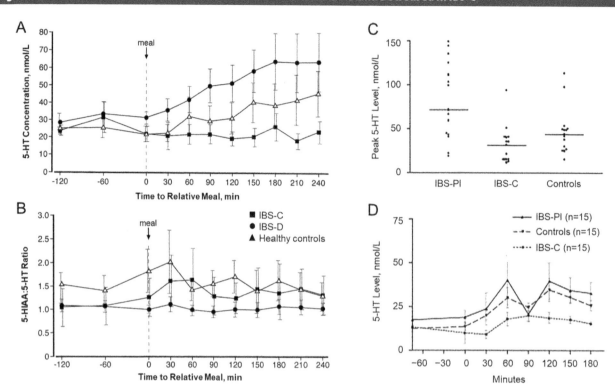

A, Circulating levels of 5-HT. B, Ratio of 5-HIAA (metabolite of 5-HT) to 5-HT. C, Peak levels of 5- HT in IBS- PI, IBS- C, and controls. D, Fasting and postprandial profiles of plasma 5- HT levels in IBS- PI, IBS- C, and controls. 5- HIAA indicates 5- hydroxyindoleacetic acid; 5- HT, 5- hydroxytryptamine (serotonin); IBS, irritable bowel syndrome; IBS- C, constipation- predominant IBS; IBS- D, diarrhea- predominant IBS; IBS- PI, postinfectious IBS.

(A and B, Modified from Atkinson W, Lockhart S, Whorwell PJ, Keevil B, Houghton LA. Altered 5-hydroxytryptamine signaling in patients with constipation- and diarrhea-predominant irritable bowel syndrome. Gastroenterology. 2006 Jan;130(1):34-43; used with permission. C, From Dunlop SP, Coleman NS, Blackshaw E, Perkins AC, Singh G, Marsden CA, et al. Abnormalities of 5-hydroxytryptamine metabolism in irritable bowel syndrome. Clin Gastroenterol Hepatol. 2005 Apr;3(4):349-57; used with permission.)

and stress induced by cold pain increased jejunal permeability in female, but not in male, healthy volunteers.

High-fat diet administration in human participants increased serum lipopolysaccharide (from gut-derived endotoxemia) and may contribute to the immune activation found in some patients with IBS. Parallel findings have been found in animals administered emulsified fats. Increased mucosal permeability with IBS may conceivably enhance mucosal immune activation and activate local reflexes, effects stimulating secretion and visceral sensation.

Soluble Mediators in IBS

Several chemical and molecular factors have potentially important roles in IBS, particularly IBS-D. These include organic acids (particularly BAs and SCFAs),

mucosal barrier proteins, mast cell products (such as histamine, proteases, and tryptase), enteroendocrine cell products, and mucosal mRNAs, proteins, and micro-RNAs. The locations of the mediators are summarized in Table 11.6.

Soluble mediators identified in stool or mucosal biopsies, summarized in Table 11.7, provide further support for the role of peripheral mechanisms in IBS. The mechanisms of action and possible therapeutic roles of different microRNAs involved in IBS are summarized in Table 11.8.

Genetic Factors in IBS

Genetic factors affecting inflammation, BA synthesis, expression of bioactive neuropeptides, and intestinal

Figure 11.8 Interactions of Enteroendocrine Cells With Other Pivotal Cells

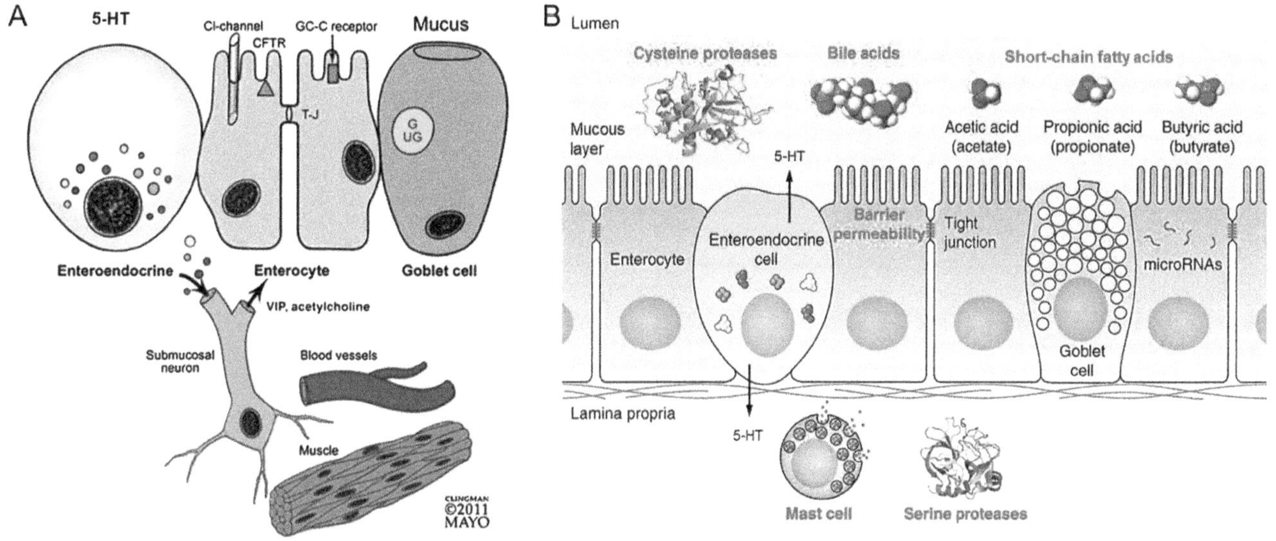

A, Three important cell types are involved in the response to intraluminal factors and may result in diarrhea. The enteroendocrine cells serve a sensory function, secreting different transmitters into the lamina propria, and stimulating afferent neurons, which may activate vasoactive intestinal peptide (VIP)- and acetylcholine-induced secretion either by direct effects on the enterocyte or by indirect effects on submucosal secretomotor neurons. Both VIPergic and cholinergic secretomotoneurons are activated by cholinergic interneurons. Acetylcholine released from interneurons activates both types of secretomotoneurons via nicotinic receptors. B, The goblet cells discharge mucus in response to intraluminal stimuli and, with it, the endogenous peptides guanylin and uroguanylin, which bind to the guanylate cyclase-C receptor on the luminal domain of enterocytes to cause guanylate cyclase production in the enterocyte and, ultimately, chloride secretion through chloride channels or the cystic fibrosis transmembrane regulator. The intraluminal factors also can induce changes in tight junction permeability. Intraluminal chemicals and molecules such as organic acids, proteases, and products of digestion interact with all these mechanisms. 5-HT indicates 5-hydroxytryptamine (serotonin); CFTR, cystic fibrosis transmembrane regulator; Cl, chloride; G, guanylin; GC-C, guanylate cyclase-C; T-J, tight junction; UG, uroguanylin.

(A, From Camilleri M, Nullens S, Nelsen T. Enteroendocrine and neuronal mechanisms in pathophysiology of acute infectious diarrhea. Dig Dis Sci. 2012 Jan;57(1):19-27; used with permission Mayo Foundation for Medical Education and Research. B, From Camilleri M, Oduyebo I, Halawi H. Chemical and molecular factors in irritable bowel syndrome: current knowledge, challenges, and unanswered questions. Am J Physiol Gastrointest Liver Physiol. 2016 Nov 1;311(5):G777-84.)

secretion are associated with symptoms or biomarkers of IBS.

Genetic Susceptibility to Immune Activation

The most convincing evidence of genetic susceptibility to immune activation in IBS is the experience with patients with post-infectious IBS in Walkerton, Ontario, Canada, that showed an association with susceptibility loci in TLR9 (Villani 2010; see suggested reading). Colonic transit in patients with IBS was univariately associated with 4 inflammation susceptibility genes that included 2 variants in *TLR9*, *CDH1*, and *IL6* in the 172 participants (142 patients and 30 healthy controls).

In a multinational Swedish, United States, and United Kingdom, study of 30 genetic susceptibility loci associated with epithelial transport, barrier function, bacterial recognition, autophagy, prostaglandin production, and TH_{17} lymphocyte differentiation, there was a noteworthy association between *TNFSF15* (tumor necrosis factor superfamily member 15 gene) and IBS phenotype (Zucchelli 2011; see suggested reading). However, in a Mayo Clinic study of 172 patients (Camilleri 2011; see suggested reading), there was no univariate association of the *TNFSF15* gene variant with colonic transit.

Figure 11.9   Multiple Components of the Intestinal Barrier

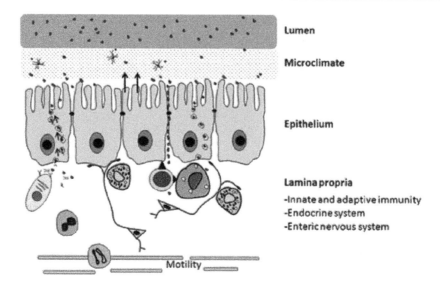

The lumen is where the degradation of bacteria and antigens by bile, gastric acid, and pancreatic juice occurs. Commensal bacteria inhibit the colonization of pathogens by production of antimicrobial substances. The microclimate is the unstirred water layer, glycocalyx, and mucous layer preventing bacterial adhesion by immunoglobulin A secretion. The epithelium is where the epithelial cells, connected by junctional complexes, have the ability to transport luminal content but also react to noxious stimuli by secretion of chloride and antimicrobial peptides. The lamina propria consists of innate and acquired immunity cells secreting immunoglobulins and cytokines and the endocrine and enteric nervous system. Intestinal propulsive motility is important to function of the barrier.

(From Keita AV, Soderholm JD. The intestinal barrier and its regulation by neuroimmune factors. Neurogastroenterol Motil. 2010 Jul;22(7):718-33; used with permission.)

BA Synthesis and Receptor

Genetic variation in the KLB gene (*Arg728Gln*) results in impaired KLB protein synthesis. This impairment prevents binding of FGF19 (in portal circulation after synthesis by ileal enterocytes) to the combined KLB-FGFR4 receptor on the hepatocyte and, consequently, reduces inhibition of hepatocyte synthesis of BAs. The result is increased BAs reaching the bowel and induction of diarrhea. In fact, variation in the gene for KLB is associated with IBS-D and accelerated colonic transit.

A second gene variant related to BA effects is in the G-protein–coupled bile acid receptor 1 (also known as TGR5) located on myenteric, cholinergic, and nitrergic neurons in the colon and proximal small bowel. A variation in the G-protein–coupled bile acid receptor is univariately associated with symptom phenotype, colonic transit, and gas sensation ratings in IBS.

Neurotransmitters or Cytokines

The receptor for neuropeptide S (NPS), NPSR$_1$, is expressed by gastrointestinal enteroendocrine cells, influences synthesis of several neuropeptides, and is involved in inflammation, anxiety, and nociception. Genetic variations in 3 single nucleotide polymorphisms of the *NPSR$_1$* gene are associated with colonic transit in IBS.

The endocannabinoid anandamide is synthesized in the postsynaptic neuron and acts on presynaptic receptors that influence release of neurotransmitters; for example, anandamide inhibits release of

Table 11.3   Inferences Obtained From Specific Methods Used to Evaluate Mucosal Permeability

Method	Barrier Function In Vivo	Barrier Function In Vitro	Neuroimmune Function	TJ Morphology
Cell monolayers, eg, Caco-2/HT29	−	+	−	−
Using chambers with human mucosa	−	+	−	−
Urine excretion of oral probes	+	−	−	−
Human fecal or biopsy supernatant applied to animal tissue	+	−	+/−	+/−
ZO-1 immunohistochemistry	−	−	−	+
mRNA expression of TJ proteins	−	−	−	−
Duodenal mucosal impedance	+	−	−	−
Laser confocal endomicroscopy	+	−	+	−
Serum bacterial lipopolysaccharide	+	−	−	−

Abbreviations: TJ, tight junction; ZO, zonula occludens; +, method addresses that function; −, method does not address that function; +/−, the method tests a component of the barrier (+) or does not (−).

Modified from Camilleri M, Lasch K, Zhou W. Irritable bowel syndrome: methods, mechanisms, and pathophysiology: the confluence of increased permeability, inflammation, and pain in irritable bowel syndrome. Am J Physiol Gastrointest Liver Physiol. 2012 Oct;303(7):G775-85.

norepinephrine. Anandamide is inactivated by the enzyme fatty acid amide hydrolase (FAAH). A single nucleotide polymorphismin the human FAAH gene (*C385A*) reduces FAAH expression. This reduction would be expected to lead to increased anandamide in the synaptic space and more presynaptic inhibition of norepinephrine release. By inhibiting release of norepinephrine, which would retard transit, the increase in anadamide in the synaptic space should accelerate colonic transit. In fact, FAAH CA/AA is associated with the phenotypes IBS-D or IBS-alternating bowel function and with accelerated colonic transit in IBS-D.

The gene for the cannabinoid receptor type 1 is *CNR1*. There are noteworthy associations of *CNR1* rs806378 genotype with IBS phenotype, colonic transit in IBS-D, and sensation of gas but not pain.

The gene controlling the serotonin reuptake transporter (SLC6A4 or solute carrier family 6 member 4) protein is *5-HTTLPR*. There are important variations in the short ("s") and long ("l") alleles in the long polymorphic repeat section of the gene; there is a preponderance of "s" in Asians and "l" in Europeans. There is an association with the IBS phenotype in some, but not all, ethnicities. In Japanese patients, "s" allele (associated with reduced SLC6A4 protein function and therefore reduced serotonin reuptake) is associated with higher ratings of rectal pain sensation and increased activation of regional cerebral blood flow during painful colorectal distentions.

Table 11.4   Summary of Studies With In Vivo Measurements of Intestinal Permeability (IP) in Humans With IBS

Author (Year)	Method	No. of IBS Patients/ Controls	IP of IBS Patients (% Above Normal or LMR)	Comments
Strobel et al (1984)	Cellobiose/M	15 IBS/10 controls	Mean ratio: 0.024 (normal 0.037)	Nonbiopsied volunteers as controls
Lobley et al (1990)	Raffinose/ L-Arabinose	62 IBS/40 controls	Mean ratio: 0.016 (normal 0.015)	No significant difference in IP between IBS and controls
Barau and Dupont (1990)	L/M	17 IBS/39 controls (children)	47% IBS vs 0% controls above normal (normal was <0.0245)	Threshold of normal defined by a control group of non-IBS children
Vogelsang et al (1995)	L/M	40 symptomatic/ 30 controls	30% of symptomatic patients above normal (>0.030)	Patients with nonspecific GI symptoms
Dainese et al (1999)	L/M	33 IBS/0 controls	12% IBS above normal (>0.025)	IP normal in 88% of patients
Berstad et al (2000)	^{51}Cr-EDTA	18 IBS/0 controls	Excretion: 0.07% in IBS	IBS patients (abdo pain and/or diarrhea) used as controls in IBD study
Spiller et al (2000)	L/M	10 PI-IBS/21 acute *Campylobacter* enteritis, 12 controls	50% IBS vs 12 controls; mean L:M ratio: 0.060; range: 0.008-0.22 (normal <0.03)	Increased IP in subset of PI-IBS compared with asymptomatic controls
Tibble et al (2002)	L/R	339 IBS, 263 organic disease	Mean ratio: 0.028; range: 0.005-0.216 (normal <0.05)	SB IP close to normal in IBS
Marshall et al (2004)	L/M	132 IBS/86 controls	35.6% IBS vs 18.6% controls above normal (>0.020 L:M)	After outbreak of acute gastroenteritis, small bowel IP was slightly elevated in IBS (no difference between PI-IBS and non–PI-IBS)
Dunlop et al (2006)	^{51}Cr-EDTA	15 IBS-D + 15 IBS-C/15 controls and 15 PI-IBS + 15 non-PI-IBS/12 controls	Excretion %: In proximal small bowel: 0.19% IBS-D, 0.085% IBS-C, 0.07% controls. In small bowel: 0.43% PI-IBS, 0.84% non–PI-IBS, 0.27% controls	2 studies: 1 comparing IBS-D and IBS-C vs controls; and the other comparing PI-IBS and non–PI-IBS with IBS-D vs controls. There may be subtle differences in IP between IBS subgroups
Shulman et al (2008)	L/M and S/L	109 Children with IBS or functional abdo pain/66 controls	Increased SB and colonic permeability	No correlation between GI permeability and pain-related symptom or stool form
Park et al (2009)	PEG 3,350/400 ratio by HPLC	38 IBS (all subtypes), 12 healthy controls	Increased in whole IBS group	No relationship of increased permeability and positive L breath test
Zhou et al (2009)	L/M	54 IBS-D/22 controls	Increased LMR in 39% of patients	Relationship to increased abdo pain and visceral and thermal sensitivity
Kerckhoffs et al (2010)	PEG	14 IBS (all subtypes)/15 healthy controls	No difference between IBS and healthy	NSAIDs increase permeability more in IBS than healthy controls
Zhou et al (2010)	L/M	19 IBS-D/10 controls	Increased in 42% of patients	

Table 11.4   Continued

Author (Year)	Method	No. of IBS Patients/ Controls	IP of IBS Patients (% Above Normal or LMR)	Comments
Rao et al (2011)	L/M	12 IBS-D, 12 healthy, and 10 inactive or treated ulcerative or microscopic colitis	Increased urine M excretion at 0-2 h and 2-8 h, and L excretion at 8-24 h in IBS-D	Demonstrated validity of individual sugar excretion as well as LMR
Gecse et al (2012)	^{51}Cr-EDTA	18 IBS-D and 12 IBS-C, 13 inactive UC, 10 healthy	Decreased in proximal SB of IBS-C; increased in colon of IBS-D patients	Elevated gut permeability is localized to the colon both in IBS-D and in inactive UC patients
Vazquez-Roque et al (2013)	L/M	45 patients with IBS-D: trial of ± gluten diets	GCD increased SB permeability (based on mannitol and LMR); no increase in colon permeability	GCD significantly decreased expression of ZO-1, claudin-1, occludin in rectosigmoid mucosa; all effects of gluten were greater in HLA-DQ2/8 positive patients
Del Valle-Pinero et al (2013)	4 probes: S, sucrose, M, L	20 IBS and 39 matched healthy controls	Colonic permeability significantly lower in IBS than in healthy controls, shown by lower S excretion in IBS than in controls	IBS subgroups not specified
Turcotte et al (2013)	Confocal laser endomicroscopy	18 healthy controls and 16 IBS patients	Median epithelial gap densities for control and IBS patients were 6 and 32 gaps per 1,000 epithelial cells, respectively	Median difference in gap density between IBS and controls was 26 (95% CI, 12-39) gaps/1,000 cell; small effects of age and sex
Fritscher-Ravens et al (2014)	Confocal laser endomicroscopy	36 IBS patients with suspected food intolerance	Positive results in 22/36: increased number of intraepithelial lymphocytes, formation of epithelial leaks/gaps, and intervillous spaces widened	Diluted food antigens administered directly to the duodenal mucosa; however, no correlation with conventional histology
Mujagic et al (2014)	Sucrose excretion and LRR in 0-5-h urine; 00-24 and 5-24-h S:erythritol ratio	34 IBS-D, 21 IBS-C, 30 IBS-M, 6 IBS-U, 94 healthy controls	0-5-h LRR only different in IBS-D vs healthy controls; no other differences in gastroduodenal or colonic permeability	Analysis adjusted for age, sex, BMI, anxiety or depression, smoking, alcohol intake, and use of medication
Peters et al (2017)	L/^{13}C-M, mucosal impedance, serum LPS	19 IBS-C and 18 healthy volunteers	Normal SB and colonic permeability in IBS-C	Concordant results (normal) using duodenal mucosal impedance, ex vivo barrier measurements and colonic mucosal expression of occludin, ZO-1, 2, 3 and claudin genes
Edogawa et al (2018)	L/^{13}C-M	9 healthy volunteers	Increased L SB permeability by indomethacin, recovered to baseline 4-6 weeks later	Only women had decreased fecal microbial diversity, including an increase in *Prevotella* abundance, after indomethacin Inflammatory parameters and markers of bacterial translocation (IL-6 and LPS) were significantly higher in IBS-D with increased permeability of SB

(continued)

Table 11.4 Continued

Author (Year)	Method	No. of IBS Patients/ Controls	IP of IBS Patients (% Above Normal or LMR)	Comments
Linsalata et al (2018)	Urinary sucrose, L:M over 5 h, circulating biomarkers	39 IBS-D and 20 healthy volunteers	2 distinct IBS-D subtypes identified, 1 with increased L, sucrose excretion, and I-FABP and DAO levels, suggesting increased permeability of SB	

Abbreviations: abdo, abdominal; BMI, body mass index; ^{13}C-M, [^{13}C]mannitol; ^{51}Cr-EDTA, chromium-labeled ethylenediam in etetraacetic acid; DAO, diamine oxidase; GCD, gluten-containing diet; GI, gastrointestinal; HLA-DQ2/8, human leukocyte antigen DQ2 or DQ8; HPLC, high-performance liquid chromotography; IBD, irritable bowel disease; IBS, irritable bowel syndrome; IBS-C, constipation-predominant IBS; IBS-D, diarrhea-predominant IBS; IBS-M, IBS with mixed bowel function; IBS-U, unsubtyped IBS; I-FABP, intestinal fatty acid-binding protein; IL, interleukin; L, lactulose; LMR, lactulose-to-mannitol ratio; LPS, lipopolysaccharide; LRR, lactulose-to-rhamnose ratio; M, mannitol; NSAIDs, nonsteroidal anti-inflammatory drugs; PEG, polyethylene glycol; PI-IBS, postinfectious IBS; R, rhamnose; S, sucralose; SB, small bowel; UC, ulcerative colitis; ZO-1, zonula occludens-1.

From Camilleri M, Lyle BJ, Madsen KL, Sonnenburg J, Verbeke K, Wu GD. Role for diet in normal gut barrier function: developing guidance within the framework of food-labeling regulations. Am J Physiol Gastrointest Liver Physiol. 2019 Jul 1;317(1):G17-39. Open access article licensed under Creative Commons Attribution CC-BY 4.0 (https://creativecommons.org/licenses/by/4.0/deed.en_US). Full reference citations can be found in the original source.

Intestinal Secretion Associated With Guanylate Cycle-C Secretory Pathway

GUCY2C is the gene for the guanylate cyclase-C receptor, which induces chloride secretion from enterocytes. In a Norwegian family with a rare form of familial diarrhea diagnosed as IBS-D, there was a dominantly inherited, fully penetrant disease due to a heterozygous base substitution, c.2519G→T, in exon 22 of chromosome 12, *GUCY2C*. This functional, missense mutation encodes for increased guanylate cyclase-C receptor and increased intracellular cyclic guanosine monophosphate, which induces enterocyte secretion.

Clinical and Therapeutic Implications of Peripheral Mechanisms in IBS

Evidence of peripheral mechanisms in IBS has led to advances beyond the concept that IBS is an idiopathic bowel dysfunction resulting from stress or brain dysfunction. After first-line management with simple education, psychotherapy, and symptomatic remedies, clinical evaluation in nonresponders should include further testing:

1. Fecal tests (eg, calprotectin, lactoferrin) or colonoscopy and biopsies to exclude inflammatory bowel disease, cancer and microscopic colitis

2. Tests of colonic transit and rectal evacuation in patients with IBS-C

3. Tests to assess carbohydrate or fat maldigestion, increased BA synthesis (fasting serum 7αC4) or loss (48-hour fecal BAs), and, possibly, dietary intolerance (eg, gluten) in patients with IBS-D

Biomarkers (Figure 11.10) can identify different potential mechanisms causing the IBS phenotype and help to select individualized therapy, such as dietary recommendations (eg, gluten or FODMAP exclusion), biofeedback retraining for defecation disorders, BA sequestrants and serotonin type 3 antagonists for diarrhea and urgency, prokinetics or secretagogues for predominant constipation, and possibly probiotics, nonabsorbed antibiotics, or anti-inflammatory agents, for immune activation or increased mucosal permeability.

Current Treatments

Dietary Modifications

Many patients believe their IBS symptoms are due to food sensitivity, and this belief is partly supported by effects of food ingestion on colonic function (gastrocolonic response), association of symptoms with high FODMAP content in the diet, or specific sugars in patients with diverse disaccharidase deficiencies.

Table 11.5   In Vitro Effects of Soluble Factors on Barrier Function and Tissue Expression in IBS

Author (Year)	Method	IBS Group(s)	Permeability	Comments
Gesce et al (2008)	FSN applied to murine colonic strips mounted in Ussing chambers; FITC-dextran transfer	All IBS subtypes, n=52; 25 HCs	Increased with IBS-D supernatants, no difference with IBS-C	FSN also rapidly increased phosphorylation of myosin light chain and delayed redistribution of ZO-1 in colonocytes
Piche et al (2009)	Colonic biopsies in Ussing chambers; fluorescein-5-(and-6)-sulfonic acid as probe and ZO-1 and occludin expression	All IBS subtypes, n=51; 14 HCs	Increased FITC paracellular permeability in all IBS subtypes; reduced ZO-1 expression	No difference in occludin expression; increase in FITC-dextran in Caco-2 cell monolayer correlated with pain score
Lee et al (2010)	Colonic biopsies in Ussing chambers; horseradish peroxidase as probe	20 IBS-D, 30 HCs	Increased in IBS-D compared with controls	Increased permeability decreased with mast cell tryptase inhibitor, nafamostat
Bertiaux-Vandaele et al (2011)	Colonic mucosal biopsies and ZO-1, occludin, and claudin-1 expression	50 IBS (-C, -D, -A, or -U), 31 HCs	Occludin and claudin-1 expression decreased in IBS-D but not in IBS-C or IBS-A	Occludin (r=0.40) and claudin-1 (r=0.46) expression significantly correlated with duration of symptoms
Vivinus-Nébot et al (2012)	Colonic biopsies mounted in Ussing chambers; fluorescein-5-(and-6)-sulfonic acid	34 IBS, all subtypes; 15 HCs	Increased in all IBS subtypes	Also higher number of mast cells and spontaneous release of tryptase; worse in IBS with allergic factors
Vivinus-Nébot et al (2014)	Cecal biopsies: Ussing chambers, FITC-sulfonic acid as probe, and mRNA expression of TJ proteins (ZO-1, α-catenin, and occludin)	49 inactive IBD (IBS), 51 IBS, 27 HCs	Increased permeability and lower expression of ZO-1 and α-catenin in both inactive IBD and in IBS	Persistent increase in TNF-α in colonic mucosa may contribute to the epithelial barrier defects in quiescent (inactive) IBD, but not in IBS
Peters et al (2017)	Transmucosal resistance and FITC–dextran flux (4 kDa)	19 IBS-C patients and 18 HC	No differences	Results consistent with in vivo permeability measurements
Wu et al (2017)	H&E and semiquantitative immunohistochemistry for phosphorylated MLC, MLC kinase, claudins-2, -8, and -15	27 IBS-D +/− gluten diet	Increased MLC phosphorylation and colonocyte expression of the paracellular Na+ channel claudin-15 by GCD	Small intestine MLC phosphorylation increased by GCD correlated with increased intestinal permeability

Abbreviations: FITC, fluorescein isothiocyanate; FSN, fecal supernatant; GCD, gluten-containing diet; HC, healthy control; H&E, hematoxylin-eosin; IBD, inflammatory bowel disease; IBS, irritable bowel syndrome; IBS-A, IBS with alternating constipation and diarrhea; IBS-C, constipation-predominant IBS; IBS-D, diarrhea-predominant IBS; IBS-U, unsubtyped IBS; MLC, myosin II regulatory light chain; TJ, tight junction; TNF-α, tumor necrosis factor α; ZO-1, zonula occludens-1.

From Camilleri M, Lyle BJ, Madsen KL, Sonnenburg J, Verbeke K, Wu GD. Role for diet in normal gut barrier function: developing guidance within the framework of food-labeling regulations. Am J Physiol Gastrointest Liver Physiol. 2019 Jul 1;317(1):G17-39. Open access article licensed under Creative Commons Attribution CC-BY 4.0 (https://creativecommons.org/licenses/by/4.0/deed.en_US). Full reference citations can be found in the original source.

These observations provide a rationale for dietary modifications, although the quality of published trials of dietary interventions in IBS is generally weak, and more evidence is needed. Current evidence based on sham-controlled trials is discussed briefly here.

Elimination Diets

One study of food elimination found that symptoms improved substantially at 12 weeks. Immunoglobin G antibody titers increased 3-fold over background for the items selected for elimination. Reintroducing the eliminated foods resulted in substantial worsening of symptoms in approximately 25% of patients (Atkinson 2004; see suggested reading).

Increased Dietary Fiber

In the largest trial of increased dietary fiber in 275 patients with IBS (all subtypes) in a primary care setting, the IBS symptom severity score was reduced with psyllium compared with placebo at 12 weeks. Adverse event rates were not different between the psyllium and placebo groups (Bijkerk 2009; see suggested reading). In a systematic review and meta-analysis of fiber in 14 randomized controlled trials (including 906 patients),

Table 11.6	Summary of Location of Soluble Mediators in IBS			
Location	Secretion/ Absorption	Barrier	Inflammation	Sensation
Lumen	Bile acids; short-chain fatty acids	Bile acids	Bacterial proteases/toxins	
Mucosa	Ion channel expression	Tight junction expression; microRNA expression		MicroRNA expression; neurotransmitters
Lamina propria		Serine proteases	Mast cells; serine proteases	

Abbreviation: IBS, irritable bowel syndrome.

Modified from Camilleri M, Oduyebo I, Halawi H. Chemical and molecular factors in irritable bowel syndrome: current knowledge, challenges, and unanswered questions. Am J Physiol Gastrointest Liver Physiol. 2016 Nov 1;311(5):G777-84.

beneficial effect was limited to psyllium (based on evaluation on 499 patients in 7 studies; number needed to treat [NNT] of 7) (Moayyedi 2014; see suggested reading).

Low FODMAP Diet

FODMAPs are poorly absorbed sugars, fructans, or sugar alcohols present in many commonly consumed foods (such as stone fruits and legumes), lactose-containing foods, and artificial sweeteners. The clinical benefits of a low FODMAP diet remain indeterminate and may not be superior to a sensible National Institute of Clinical Excellence diet or supplementing a prebiotic, yoga, or gut-directed hypnotherapy.

Gluten-Free Diet

In the absence of celiac disease, those carrying the HLA DQ2/8 genotypes may benefit from a gluten-free diet and the benefit is partly explained by reduction in fructans in the gluten-free diet.

Exercise

Yoga reduces severity of IBS and somatic symptoms, and walking improves overall gastrointestinal symptoms, negative affect, and anxiety.

Alternative and Herbal Treatments

Prebiotics and Probiotics

Prebiotics include food ingredients such as fructo-oligosaccharides or inulin that can promote the growth or activity of gut bacteria. Probiotics are live or attenuated microorganisms that can affect the composition of intestinal microorganisms and may have anti-inflammatory and antinociceptive properties. Trials of prebiotics in IBS found considerable improvement in bloating from altered microbial fermentation of foods; no benefit for global symptoms, abdominal pain, visceral sensation, or quality of life; and variable effect on bowel function. In a meta-analysis of probiotics in IBS, the NNT was 7, and the greatest effect was on abdominal pain, bloating, and flatulence (Ford 2014; see suggested reading).

Herbal Therapies

Iberogast, an herbal mixture with antispasmodic and secretory effects, improves global symptoms and abdominal pain scores. The benefits of Chinese herbal medicines in IBS are inconsistent.

Pharmacologic Treatments

Current pharmacologic treatments of IBS are summarized in Table 11.9.

Medications for Pain

Pain medications are discussed in Chapter 12, "Visceral Sensation."

Central Neuromodulators

This class of medications addresses psychologic disorders in IBS that may aggravate perception of gut

Table 11.7   Summary of Published Literature on the Role of Soluble Mediators in IBS

Author (Year)	Supernatant of Stool or Mucosal Biopsies	Patient Group	Receptor/Mechanism of Action	Biologic Effect
Annahazi et al (2013)	Cysteine proteases (CPA) from FSN	Sum of 2 cohorts; 26 IBS-D, 44 IBS-C, 56 HCs	CPA increased in IBS-C vs HCs and IBS-D	Level of CPA correlated with pain Increased visceral hypersensitivity in PAR$_2$-deficient and normal mice infused with FSN from high CPA IBS-C vs normal CPA IBS-C and HCs
			Decreased occludin in mice and T84 cells after repeated infusion of FSN from IBS-C vs HCs and in colonic mucosal biopsies in 8 IBS-C vs 6 HCs	Increased intestinal permeability in PAR$_2$ knockout mice and T84 cells infused with FSN from high CPA IBS-C vs normal CPA IBS-C and HCs
Valdez Morales et al (2013)	Serine protease from mucosal biopsies	10 IBS-D, 5 IBS-C, 12 HC	Activation of PAR$_2$ receptors	Increased hyperexcitability in DRG neurons from wild-type mice vs PAR$_2$-deficient mice in IBS-D vs IBS-C and HCs
	CPA from mucosal biopsies		CPA receptor	Increased hyperexcitability in DRG neurons from mice in IBS-D
Buhner et al (2009)	Serine protease (tryptase), histamine, and 5-HT from mucosal biopsies	7 IBS-D, 4 IBS-C, 5 HCs	Serine protease, serotonin, and histamine receptors	Activation of submucosal neurons in surgical specimen of human colon, mediated by H$_1$-H$_3$, 5-HT$_3$, and serine protease receptors
Piche et al (2009)	Mucosal biopsies	17 IBS-D, 19 IBS-C, 15 IBS-A, 14 HCs	Decreased ZO-1 mRNA expression in Caco-2 cells incubated with IBS SUP (all subtypes)	Increased intestinal permeability in Caco-2 cells incubated with SUP of 39 IBS patients (15 IBS-C, 14 IBS-D, 14 IBS-A) vs 14 HCs
			Decreased ZO-1 expression in colonic biopsies of 21 IBS vs 12 HCs	Increased permeability in colonic biopsies of 12 IBS (3 IBS-C, 4 IBS-D, 5 IBS-A) vs 5 HCs
Gesce et al (2008)	Serine proteases from FSN	24 IBS-D, 18 IBS-C, 10 IBS-A, 17 UC, 23 INF, 25 HC	Activation of PAR$_2$ receptors	Increased visceral hypersensitivity in wild-type mice vs PAR$_2$-deficient mice
			Increased phosphorylation of myosin light chain; internalization of ZO-1	Increased permeability in wild-type mice vs PAR$_2$-deficient mice
Wang et al (2016)		22 IBS-D, 17 HC	PAR$_2$-mediated increase BDNF expression in Caco-2 cells and mice; p38 MAPK phosphorylation in Caco-2 cells	Increased visceral hypersensitivity in mice
Cenac et al (2015)	Serine proteases from mucosal biopsies	20 IBS-D, 10 IBS-C, 10 IBS-mixed, 11 HCs	PAR$_2$-mediated increase of 5,6-EET in DRG neurons from mice and increased stimulation of transient receptor potential vanilloid-4 in mice treated with SUP of IBS-D vs HCs	Increased visceral hypersensitivity in mice exposed to SUP of IBS-D patients
Han et al (2012)	Reactive oxygen species from mucosal biopsies	14 PI IBS-D, 12 HCs	Activation of PAR$_2$ receptors on mast cells in rats	Mast cell activation in rats with production of histamine

Abbreviations: BDNF, brain-derived neurotrophic factor; CPA, cysteine proteases; DRG, dorsal root ganglion; EET, epoxyeicosatrienoic acid; 5-HT, 5-hydroxytryptamine (serotonin); FSN, fecal supernatant; H, histamine; HC, healthy control; IBS, irritable bowel syndrome; IBS-A, alternating pattern irritable bowel syndrome; IBS-C, constipation-predominant IBS; IBS-D, diarrhea-predominant IBS; INF, infectious acute diarrhea; MAPK, mitogen-activated protein kinase; PAR$_2$, protease-activated receptors; PI, postinfectious; SUP, supernatant; UC, ulcerative colitis; ZO-1, zonula occludens-1.

Modified from Camilleri M, Oduyebo I, Halawi H. Chemical and molecular factors in irritable bowel syndrome: current knowledge, challenges, and unanswered questions. Am J Physiol Gastrointest Liver Physiol. 2016 Nov 1;311(5):G777-84. Full reference citations can be found in the original source.

Table 11.8   Summary of the Mechanisms of Action and Possible Therapeutic Roles of Different MicroRNAs Involved in IBS

Author (Year)	MicroRNA	Target	Population Studied	Results	Suggested Mechanism	Potential Clinical Applicability
Liao et al (2016)	miRNA-24	Serotonin reuptake transporter	10 IBS patients and 10 healthy patients; IBS mouse model	miRNA-24 upregulated in IBS patients and intestinal mucosa of mice	miRNA-24 inhibits SERT expression and aggravates IBS	miRNA-24 inhibitor
Zhou et al (2015)	miRNA-29	NFKB-repressing factor (NKRF) and claudin-1 genes	183 IBS and 36 HCs	Increased levels of miRNA-29 and reduced levels of NKRF and claudin-1 in patients with IBS-D	miRNA-29 targets and reduces claudins and NKRF, an effect that increases intestinal permeability	miRNA-29 inhibitors for IBS with increased permeability
			Mir-29 knock-out mice	Decreased intestinal hyperpermeability in Mir-29 knockout mice		
Zhou et al (2010)	miRNA-29	Glutamine synthetase gene (GLUL)	19 IBS-D and 10 HCs	Increased miRNA-29a in IBS-D patients with increased intestinal permeability (42% of IBS-D patients)	miRNA-29a increases membrane permeability by decreasing GLUL gene expression and glutamine level	miRNA-29 inhibitor and glutamine for IBS with increased intestinal permeability
Fourie et al (2014)	miRNA-150 and miRNA-342-3p	Multiple targets including telomerase-related proteins dyskerin and prosurvival protein kinase AKT2	5 patients with IBS-D, 5 patients with IBS-C, 2 patients with IBS-M, and 31 HCs	Increased level of miRNA-150 and miRNA-342-3p in IBS	Inflammatory, pain, and motility pathways	Possible role as biomarkers
Zhou et al (2016)	miRNA-199	Transient receptor potential vanilloid type 1 signaling	45 IBS-D and 40 HCs	Decreased colonic miRNA-199 correlates with visceral pain in patients with IBS-D	miRNA-199a decreases visceral pain via inhibition of TRPV1 signaling	miRNA-199 precursors for pain in IBS
			Visceral hyper-sensitivity rat models	Reduced miRNA-199a in rat DRG and colon tissue associated with visceral hypersensitivity		
Kapeller et al (2008)	miRNA-510	5-HT$_3$ receptor type 3 subunit gene (HTR3E)	98 IBS-D, 99 IBS-C, and 100 HCs (United Kingdom); 119 IBS-D and 195 HCs (Germany)	HTR3E variant c. *76G>A, associated with female IBS-D	Variant of HTR3E reduces binding and inhibitory effect of miRNA-510, thus increasing expression of 5-HT3E protein in IBS-D	Unclear clinical impact of miRNA-510 in IBS

Abbreviations: DRG, dorsal root ganglia; 5-HT, 5-hydroxytryptamine (serotonin); HC, healthy control; IBS, irritable bowel syndrome; IBS-C, constipation-predominant IBS; IBS-D, diarrhea-predominant IBS; IBS-M, IBS with mixed bowel function; NFKB, nuclear factor-κB; NKRF, NFKB-repressing factor.

Modified from Camilleri M, Oduyebo I, Halawi H. Chemical and molecular factors in irritable bowel syndrome: current knowledge, challenges, and unanswered questions. Am J Physiol Gastrointest Liver Physiol. 2016 Nov 1;311(5):G777-84. Full reference citations can be found in the original source.

Figure 11.10   Biomarkers in and Mechanisms in Irritable Bowel Syndrome

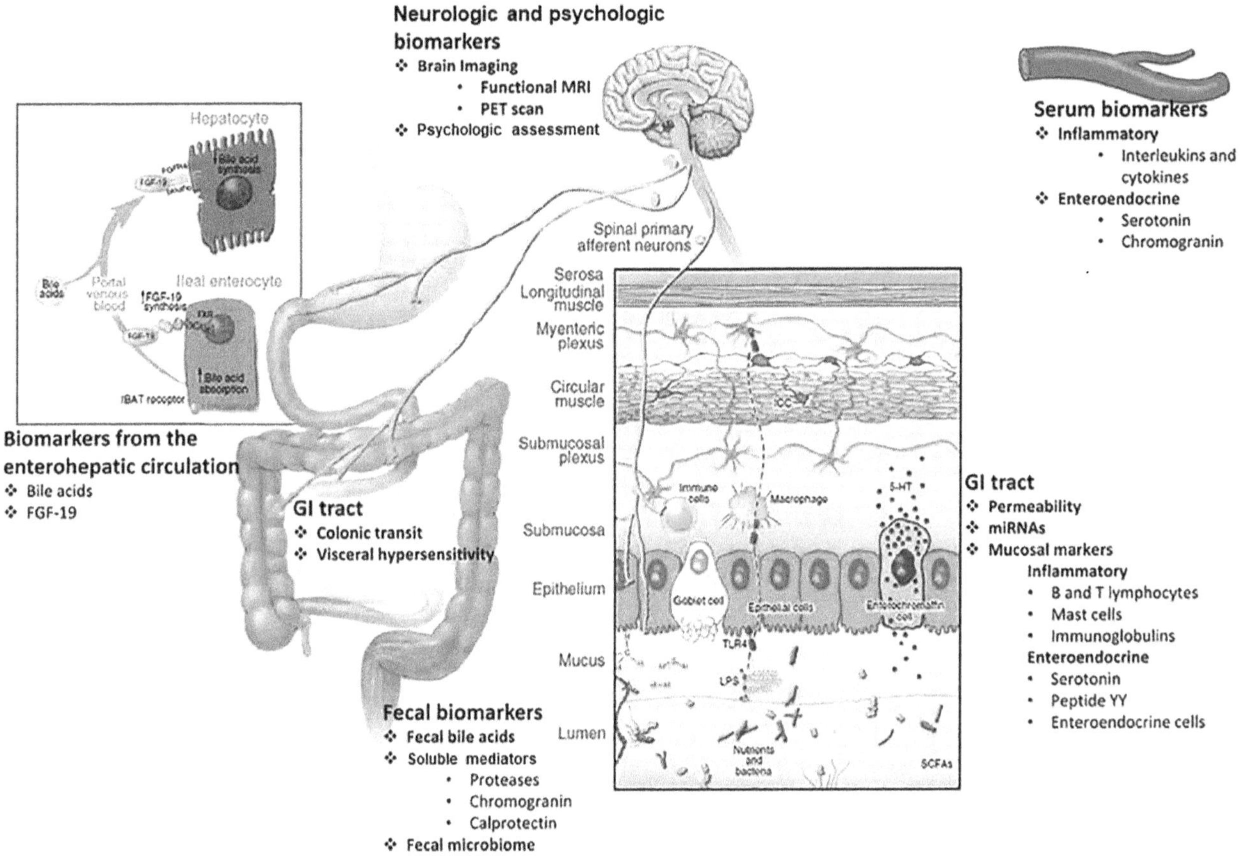

These diverse biomarkers are documented in detail in Tables 11.5 through 11.7 and 11.11. FGF-19 indicates fibroblast growth factor 19; 5-HT, 5-hydroxytryptamine; GI, gastrointestinal; IBAT, ileal bile acid transporter; ICC, interstitial cells of Cajal; LPS, lipopolysaccharide; MRI, magnetic resonance imaging; PET, positron emission tomography; SCFAs, short-chain fatty acids; TLR4, toll-like receptor 4.

(Modified from Camilleri M. Review article: biomarkers and personalised therapy in functional lower gastrointestinal disorders. Aliment Pharmacol Ther. 2015 Oct;42(7):818-28.)

and somatic pain. In addition, antidepressants alter intestinal transit: tricyclic antidepressants (TCAs) slow transit and selective serotonin reuptake inhibitors accelerate transit. Therefore, TCAs are preferred in IBS-D, and selective serotonin reuptake inhibitors are preferred in IBS-C. These neuromodulators may have several beneficial effects in IBS, including reduced activation of pain centers in the brain and peripheral effects such as increased colonic compliance and decreased visceral afferent function.

Systematic reviews and meta-analyses claim an overall symptom effect of antidepressants in IBS with an NNT of 4 (Ford 2014; see suggested reading). However, low-level trial quality raises questions about the accuracy of the reported NNT, and there is no correlation between improvement in IBS symptoms and depression scores.

Adverse effects were notably more common with TCAs. The most frequent adverse effects were drowsiness and dry mouth due to anticholinergic effects. The risks of long-term use of psychotropic drugs for nonpsychiatric indications include higher prevalence of dementia, based on population studies, although a cause-and-effect relationship has not been proved.

Drugs Acting on Peripheral Opioid Receptors

Opioid receptor agonists acting peripherally slow transit at all levels of the digestive tract and increase fluid absorption, and those with central activity also reduce pain.

Table 11.9   Summary of Current Pharmacologic Treatments of IBS

Mode of Action	Therapy	Efficacy	Quality of Data	Adverse Events	Limitations of Data
Smooth muscle relaxants	Antispasmodic drugs	+/−	Low	Dry mouth, dizziness, and blurred vision	No high-quality trials, only a small number of RCTs assessing each individual antispasmodic
	Peppermint oil	+	Moderate	No increase in AEs	Heterogeneity between studies
Secretagogues	Lubiprostone (Cl− channels)	+	Moderate	Nausea more common vs placebo	Only a modest benefit over placebo in published RCTs
	Linaclotide (GC-C agonist)	+	High	Diarrhea more common vs placebo	None
	Plecanatide (GC-C agonist)	+	High	Diarrhea more common vs placebo	None
	Tenapanor (NHE3 antagonist)	+/−	Moderate	Diarrhea more common vs placebo	Awaiting phase 2b/3 trials
Neuromodulators	Antidepressants	+	Moderate	Dry mouth and drowsiness	Few high-quality trials, some atypical trials included
	Neurokinin$_2$ antagonist	Promising in phase 2b RCT	Moderate	No increase in AEs	Awaiting phase 3 trials
	Histamine$_1$ antagonist	Promising in single RCT	Low	No increase in AEs	Awaiting phase 2b trials
	TSPO inhibitor	+/−	Low	Modest efficacy in a single POC trial	Awaiting phase 2b trials
Opioids	Loperamide (peripheral μ agonist)	+/−	Low	Limited data	Few RCTs, with a small number of participants, not all of whom had IBS
	Eluxadoline (peripheral μ and κ agonist and δ antagonist)	+	High	Serious AEs: acute pancreatitis and sphincter of Oddi spasm. Nausea and headache common	Only a modest benefit over placebo in published RCTs. No benefit over placebo in terms of abdominal pain
5-HT$_3$–receptor antagonists: alosetron, ondansetron, ramosetron		+	High	Serious AE with alosetron: ischemic colitis; constipation more common vs placebo	Fewer RCTs of ramosetron and ondansetron. Ondansetron may have no benefit over placebo for abdominal pain
5-HT$_4$ receptor agonists		+/−	High	Diarrhea, cramping, and CV AEs with "old generation" drugs in this class	Data available for tegaserod and mosapride, not for "new generation" drugs in this class: prucalopride, naronapride, velusetrag, YKP10811
Bile acid sequestrants		?	Low	Limited data	No published RCTs
Rifaximin		+	Moderate	No increase in AEs	Modest benefit over placebo in published RCTs, mainly bloating

Abbreviations: AE, adverse event; Cl−, chloride; CV, cardiovascular; 5-HT, 5-hydroxytryptamine (serotonin); GC-C, guanylate cyclase C; IBS, irritable bowel syndrome; NHE3, sodium-hydrogen exchange channel #3; POC, proof of concept; RCT, randomized, controlled trial; TSPO, translocator protein.

Modified from Camilleri M. Management options for irritable bowel syndrome. Mayo Clin Proc. 2018 Dec;93(12):1858-72; used with permission.

Loperamide and diphenoxylate, μ-opioid agonists, are antidiarrheal agents with no convincing evidence of pain relief in IBS and no central effects up to a maximum dose of 16 mg per day for loperamide.

Eluxadoline is a novel κ- and μ-opioid receptor agonist and δ-opioid receptor antagonist that is efficacious for diarrhea or the composite end point of diarrhea and pain in IBS-D at a dosage of 100 mg twice a day, or, if not tolerated, 75 mg twice a day. Rare cases of pancreatitis and sphincter of Oddi spasm have been reported. The medication should not be prescribed for patients with a history of biliary obstruction, cholecystectomy, pancreatitis, severe hepatic impairment, or severe constipation or those who consume more than 3 alcoholic drinks per day.

Medications for Diarrhea

In addition to their effects on pain, opioid agents and antidepressants (TCAs and serotonin norepinepherine reuptake inhibitors) may also relieve diarrhea. (See also Chapter 9, "Chronic Diarrhea".)

Serotonin Type 3 Receptor Antagonists.

Intestinal enterochromaffin cells produce 90% of the body's serotonin, and there are several different classes of serotonin receptors in the brain and gut. Serotonin type 3 receptors are important mediators of visceral pain. Serotonin type 3 receptor antagonists such as alosetron retard colonic transit. Alosetron is an effective agent in IBS-D; it has an NNT of 8 for abdominal pain and an NNT of 4 for global symptoms. Alosetron is approved for women with severe IBS-D in the United States through a US Food and Drug Administration prescribing program. Ramosetron is efficacious and licensed for use in both male and female patients with IBS-D in Japan. Ondansetron appreciably affects stool consistency, urgency, frequency, and bloating but not pain.

Serotonin type 3 antagonists can cause constipation. Alosetron, unlike other drugs in this class, was associated with a superficial, reversible form of ischemic colitis (about 1:800 treated patients) in clinical trials. The mechanism is unclear, with no biological basis, because vascular reactivity, platelet aggregation, and coagulation factors were all normal. Epidemiologic databases show that IBS itself may be associated with an increased prevalence of ischemic colitis.

BA Sequestrants.

No randomized control trials of BA sequestrants in IBS have been reported. In patients with IBS-D and increased fecal BA excretion or [75]SeHCAT retention less than 20% at 7 days, open-label trials of colesevelam, 1,875 mg twice a day for 10 days, or of colestipol, 1 g twice a day for 8 weeks, reported reduction in stool consistency and frequency.

Antibiotics.

Rifaximin is a nonabsorbable antibiotic that has shown improved global symptoms and bloating in IBS and inconsistent effects on stool consistency, frequency of bowel movements, and urgency. Rifaximin induced acceleration of colonic transit at 48 hours in IBS-D, an effect that would not be expected to improve the symptoms of IBS-D. Conversely, acceleration of colonic transit may be a factor to explain reported improvement in IBS-C (bloating, constipation, and straining), which is not an approved indication for this medication. Rifaximin seems to be safe compared with placebo, without increased risk of *Clostridioides difficile* infection.

Medications for Constipation

Medications for constipation are covered extensively in Chapter 10, "Chronic Constipation."

Intestinal Secretagogues

Chloride Channel–Related.

Lubiprostone, a prostaglandin derivative, induces chloride secretion at channels on the apical membrane of enterocytes. The approved dose is 8 μg twice a day for women with IBS-C and 24 μg twice a day for chronic constipation. There are general improvements in abdominal pain scores that parallel efficacy on bowel function. Nausea is experienced by 8% of patients and is generally relatively mild and self-limited.

Linaclotide and plecanatide are minimally absorbed guanylate cyclase C receptor agonists that secrete chloride and bicarbonate (with obligate water and sodium) into the intestinal lumen via the cystic fibrosis transmembrane regulator. They both relieve constipation and considerably improve abdominal discomfort and bloating in IBS-C and may have a separate effect on pain mechanisms via cyclic guanosine monophosphate. The dose can be titrated to achieve benefit without inducing diarrhea; linaclotide is available in 72-, 145-, and 290-μg doses, and plecanatide is available in 3- and 6-mg doses.

Serotonin Type 4 Receptor Agonists.

Tegaserod (back on the market in the United States) relieves overall symptoms of IBS-C and abdominal pain and discomfort, bloating, and constipation. Adverse effects associated with tegaserod are diarrhea, cramping, and rare cardiovascular events, attributed to effects on other serotonin receptors (eg, types 2A and 2B). Restrictions on its use are intended to reduce potential cardiovascular morbidity.

Cognitive Behavioral Therapy and Hypnotherapy

These forms of nonpharmacologic therapy are efficacious, have long-term benefits, and are efficacious in minimal-contact technologic formats (eg, internet, telephone, smartphone applications), in self-help interventions, and with trained nonprofessional mental health providers.

Future Application of Biomarkers and Their Use for Selecting Therapy

Despite all current dietary, pharmacologic, and behavioral treatments, there is still considerable unmet need. New approaches to treatment that target important actionable biomarkers of IBS augur well for the development of treatments that will affect symptoms and the natural history of IBS (Tables 11.10 and 11.11).

In addition, there is much hope that novel, peripherally active visceral analgesics, including opioid agents with no risk of respiratory depression or addiction potential, may address the considerable unmet need of pain in IBS (see Chapter 12, "Visceral Sensation").

Table 11.10   Main Characteristics of Potential Biomarkers and Markers in IBS

Biomarker or Marker	Diagnostic Utility	Predominant Application in IBS-D/IBS-C	Availability[a]	Noninvasive	Cost Efficacy
Serum biomarkers					
Inflammatory (interleukins, cytokines)	Low	IBS-D	Moderate	High	Moderate
Enteroendocrine (serotonin, chromogranin)	Low	IBS-D	Moderate	High	Moderate
Fecal biomarkers					
Fecal bile acids	High	IBS-D	Low	High	High
Soluble mediators (proteases, chromogranin, calprotectin)	Low	IBS-D	Moderate	High	Low
Microbiome	Moderate	IBS-D/IBS-C	Moderate	High	Low
GI tract biomarkers					
Colonic transit	High	IBS-D/IBS-C	Moderate	High	Moderate
Visceral hypersensitivity	Low	IBS-D/IBS-C	Low	Moderate	Low
Permeability	Moderate	IBS-D	Low	Moderate	Moderate
Mucosal biomarkers	Low	IBS-D	Low	Low	Low
miRNAs		IBS-D/IBS-C			
Neurologic and psychologic markers					
Brain imaging	Moderate	IBS (pain)	Low	Low	Low
Psychologic markers	Moderate	IBS	High	Low	Low

Abbreviations: GI, gastrointestinal; IBS, irritable bowel syndrome; IBS-C, constipation-predominant IBS; IBS-D, diarrhea-predominant IBS; miRNA, microRNA.

[a] High = widely available; moderate = available in only specialized clinics; low = available in only referral laboratories or centers.

Table 11.11 IBS Biomarkers as Potential Targets for Specific Therapies

Potential Biomarkers	Therapy														
	5-HT$_4$ agonists	5-HT$_3$ antagonists	Opioid agonists	Bile acid sequestrants	Obeticholic acid	Octreotide	Antibiotics	Low FODMAP	Ketotifen	miRNA inhibitors	miRNA precursors	Glutamine	Anxiolytics	Neuromodulators	Probiotics
Serum biomarkers															
Inflammatory															
Interleukins															+
Cytokines															
Enteroendocrine															
Serotonin						+									
Chromogranin						+									
Fecal biomarkers															
Fecal bile acids				+++	+										
Soluble mediators															
Proteases															
Chromogranin															
Calprotectin															
Microbiome							+	+							+
GI tract biomarkers															
Colonic transit															
Rapid		++	++		++										
Slow	++														
Visceral hypersensitivity			+												
Permeability									+			+			
Mucosal biomarkers															
Mast cells									+						
B and T cells															
miRNAs									+		+				

(continued)

Table 11.11 Continued

Potential Biomarkers	Therapy														
	5-HT₄ agonists	5-HT₃ antagonists	Opioid agonists	Bile acid sequestrants	Obeticholic acid	Octreotide	Antibiotics	Low FODMAP	Ketotifen	miRNA inhibitors	miRNA precursors	Glutamine	Anxiolytics	Neuromodulators	Probiotics
Enteroendocrine					+										
Neurologic and psychologic biomarkers															
Brain imaging													+	+	
Psychologic markers													+	+	

Abbreviations: 5-HT, 5-hydroxytryptamine (serotonin); FODMAP, fermentable oligosaccharides, disaccharides, monosaccharides, and polyols; GI, gastrointestinal; IBS, irritable bowel syndrome; miRNA, microRNA; +, potential effect; ++, effect is likely; +++, effect is highly likely.

From Camilleri M, Halawi H, Oduyebo I. Biomarkers as a diagnostic tool for irritable bowel syndrome: where are we? Expert Rev Gastroenterol Hepatol. 2017 Apr;11(4):303-16; used with permission.

Suggested Reading

Atkinson W, Sheldon TA, Shaath N, Whorwell PJ. Food elimination based on IgG antibodies in irritable bowel syndrome: a randomised controlled trial. Gut. 2004 Oct;53(10):1459–64.

Bijkerk CJ, de Wit NJ, Muris JW, Whorwell PJ, Knottnerus JA, Hoes AW. Soluble or insoluble fibre in irritable bowel syndrome in primary care? Randomised placebo controlled trial. BMJ. 2009 Aug 27;339:b3154.

Camilleri M. Management Options for Irritable Bowel Syndrome. Mayo Clin Proc. 2018 Dec;93(12):1858–72. Epub 2018 Dec 14.

Camilleri M. Peripheral mechanisms in irritable bowel syndrome. N Engl J Med. 2012 Oct 25;367(17):1626–35. Epub 2012 Oct 26.

Camilleri M, Carlson P, McKinzie S, Zucchelli M, D'Amato M, Busciglio I, et al. Genetic susceptibility to inflammation and colonic transit in lower functional gastrointestinal disorders: preliminary analysis. Neurogastroenterol Motil. 2011 Oct;23(10):935–e398. Epub 2011 Jul 14.

Camilleri M, Chedid V. Actionable biomarkers: the key to resolving disorders of gastrointestinal function. Gut. 2020 Oct;69(10):1730–7. Epub 2020 Apr 8.

Camilleri M, Halawi H, Oduyebo I. Biomarkers as a diagnostic tool for irritable bowel syndrome: where are we? Expert Rev Gastroenterol Hepatol. 2017 Apr;11(4):303–16. Epub 2017 Jan 28.

Camilleri M, Oduyebo I, Halawi H. Chemical and molecular factors in irritable bowel syndrome: current knowledge, challenges, and unanswered questions. Am J Physiol Gastrointest Liver Physiol. 2016 Nov 1;311(5):G777–G84. Epub 2016 Nov 03.

Ford AC, Quigley EM, Lacy BE, Lembo AJ, Saito YA, Schiller LR, et al. Effect of antidepressants and psychological therapies, including hypnotherapy, in irritable bowel syndrome: systematic review and meta-analysis. Am J Gastroenterol. 2014 Sep;109(9):1350–65. Epub 2014 Jun 17.

Ford AC, Quigley EM, Lacy BE, Lembo AJ, Saito YA, Schiller LR, et al. Efficacy of prebiotics, probiotics, and synbiotics in irritable bowel syndrome and chronic idiopathic constipation: systematic review and meta-analysis. Am J Gastroenterol. 2014 Oct;109(10):1547–61. Epub 2014 Jul 29.

Moayyedi P, Quigley EM, Lacy BE, Lembo AJ, Saito YA, Schiller LR, et al. The effect of fiber supplementation on irritable bowel syndrome: a systematic review and meta-analysis. Am J Gastroenterol. 2014 Sep;109(9):1367–74. Epub 2014 Jul 29.

Pittayanon R, Lau JT, Yuan Y, Leontiadis GI, Tse F, Surette M, et al. Gut microbiota in patients with irritable bowel syndrome-a systematic review. Gastroenterology. 2019 Jul;157(1):97–108. Epub 2019 Mar 30.

Valentin N, Camilleri M, Altayar O, Vijayvargiya P, Acosta A, Nelson AD, et al. Biomarkers for bile acid diarrhoea in functional bowel disorder with diarrhoea: a systematic review and meta-analysis. Gut. 2016 Dec;65(12):1951–9. Epub 2015 Sep 7.

Vazquez-Roque MI, Camilleri M, Smyrk T, Murray JA, Marietta E, O'Neill J, et al. A controlled trial of gluten-free diet in patients with irritable bowel syndrome-diarrhea: effects on bowel frequency and intestinal function. Gastroenterology. 2013 May;144(5):903–11. Epub 2013 Jan 25.

Villani AC, Lemire M, Thabane M, Belisle A, Geneau G, Garg AX, et al. Genetic risk factors for post-infectious irritable bowel syndrome following a waterborne outbreak of gastroenteritis. Gastroenterology. 2010 Apr;138(4):1502–13. Epub 2010 Jan 4.

Zucchelli M, Camilleri M, Andreasson AN, Bresso F, Dlugosz A, Halfvarson J, et al. Association of TNFSF15 polymorphism with irritable bowel syndrome. Gut. 2011 Dec;60(12):1671–7. Epub 2011 Jun 2.

Introduction

Visceral sensation is one of the important mechanisms that are upregulated, a process resulting in hypersensitivity in functional gastrointestinal (GI) disorders. However, it is also relevant when other mechanisms, such as inflammation or altered motor function, result in signaling the abnormal functions such as stasis or accelerated transit from the gut to the brain. Thus, it is important to understand the physiologic basis of visceral sensation. The factors influencing visceral sensation are the neural pathways and transmitters, viscus compliance and tone, sex, level of attention, and unpleasantness of the sensation.

Physiologic Basis for Visceral Sensation

Brain-Gut Axis

GI functions are controlled by both intrinsic and extrinsic neural pathways. Local stimuli in the gut activate extrinsic afferents, which convey the visceral information to the central nervous system (CNS), from where reflex responses arise and result in alterations in functions such as gastric acid secretion and GI motor activity. The cell bodies of vagal primary afferent neurons are located in vagal (nodose) ganglia, and their processes connect to several central regions from which efferent fibers convey information back to the gut wall, where efferent nerves synapse with neurons from enteric ganglia.

The spinal nerves also contain afferent and efferent fibers. The cell bodies of spinal visceral afferents are located in the dorsal root ganglia. Afferent information from the viscera to the spinal cord also provides input via axon collaterals to the prevertebral and paravertebral ganglia, which reflexly modify gut functions. For example, mechanosensitive afferent neurons with cell bodies in the myenteric plexus (called intestinofugal) function as volume detectors and relay information via axon collaterals to sympathetic neurons of the prevertebral ganglia to reflexly modulate gut functions.

Visceral information is transmitted along several spinal tracts projecting to the CNS, where this information is integrated with information encoded by somatic and visceral vagal afferents (Figure 12.1). Spinal efferent fibers from the cervical, thoracic, and lumbar segments of the spinal cord synapse with postganglionic neurons in the spinal ganglia (celiac, superior and inferior mesenteric ganglia) and provide sympathetic input to the gut along the greater and lesser splanchnic nerves, from which branches reach the gut along the vascular supply.

Symptoms such as abdominal pain, altered bowel function, and affective components of pain, including anxiety and poor coping, are determined by brain networks in the central executive, salience, sensorimotor, emotional arousal, and central autonomic regions. From these networks, descending pathways (eg, originating in the periaqueductal gray) alter autonomic nervous system input to the viscera and potentially modulate ascending afferent information, which would otherwise lead to pain perception.

Increased Pain Perception (Visceral Hypersensitivity) in Irritable Bowel Syndrome

The potential mechanisms causing hypersensitivity in irritable bowel syndrome (IBS) include brain dysfunction, abnormal interaction of the peripheral nervous system and CNS, and aberrant afferent nerve

Figure 12.1   Physiology of Gut Sensation

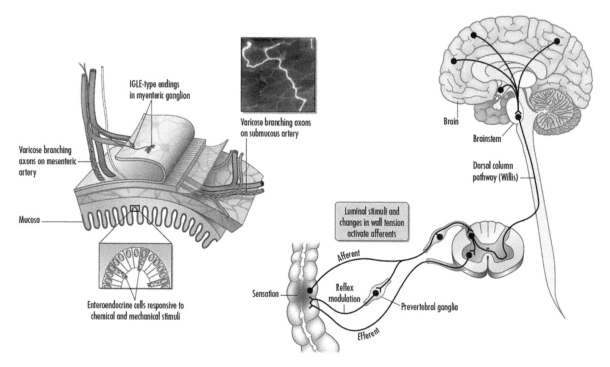

The elements of visceral sensation are enteroendocrine cells (chemical, mechanical), intraganglionic laminar endings (IGLE) (mechanotransduction), reflex responses at the levels of prevertebral ganglia, spinal cord, brainstem, the 3-neuron chain from endorgan to the brain, supraspinal mechanisms involved in perception, autonomic responses (eg, satiety, cardiovascular responses to pain), and the mediators such as 5-hydroxytryptamine (serotonin), substance P, calcitonin gene-related peptide, norepinephrine, κ-opiate, and others.

(Modified from Camilleri M, Boeckxstaens G. Dietary and pharmacological treatment of abdominal pain in IBS. Gut. 2017;66(5):966-74 as adapted from Delgado-Aros S, Camilleri M. Visceral hypersensitivity. J Clin Gastroenterol. 2005;39(5 Suppl 3):S194-210; Lynn PA, Olsson C, Zagorodnyuk V, Costa M, Brookes SJ. Rectal intraganglionic laminar endings are transduction sites of extrinsic mechanoreceptors in the guinea pig rectum. Gastroenterology. 2003;125(3):786-94; and Blackshaw LA, Brookes SJ, Grundy D, Schemann M. Sensory transmission in the gastrointestinal tract. Neurogastroenterol Motil. 2007;19(1 Suppl):1-19; used with permission.)

function. Alterations in afferent function resulting in mechanosensitivity may also result from changes in the compliance or tone of the viscus or from vigorous contractions and the associated movement of intraluminal content (eg, high-amplitude propagated contractions and mass movements).

Visceral hypersensitivity and hyperalgesia are well documented in IBS. Increased perception to distention can be assessed with balloon distention under specified pressures (thresholds or sensation ratings) or with chemical stimuli such as acid or lipids infused into different segments. However, hypersensitivity and CNS dysfunction are not found or documented in all patients with IBS. Across studies, 50% of patients with IBS have hypersensitivity or hyperalgesia. In addition, hypersensitivity is associated with a greater likelihood to report pain.

Control of Gut Sensation and Visceral Hypersensitivity

Afferents from the gut convey sensory information through 3 neurons to the highest centers in the CNS, where the input is coordinated and integrated and results in reflex secretory and motor responses and conscious perception. There are afferent synapses in the dorsal horn of the spinal cord and in the brainstem or thalamus.

In general, vagal and sacral afferents encode nonnoxious GI sensations, such as satiety and nausea. In contrast, spinal afferents encode visceral pain (Figure 12.2).

Sensory signal transduction in the viscera starts by local mechanical or chemical stimuli releasing

Figure 12.2   Visceral Sensation: Parasympathetic and Spinal Afferents Activated

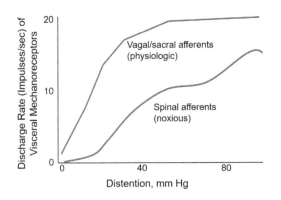

Afferent Discharge Rate (y Axis) According to Pressure Increases (x Axis).

(Data from Sengupta JN, Kauvar D, Goyal RK. Characteristics of vagal esophageal tension-sensitive afferent fibers in the opossum. J Neurophysiol. 1989;61(5):1001-10; Ozaki N, Sengupta JN, Gebhart GF. Mechanosensitive properties of gastric vagal afferent fibers in the rat. J Neurophysiol. 1999;82(5):2210-20; and Sengupta JN, Gebhart GF. Characterization of mechanosensitive pelvic nerve afferent fibers innervating the colon of the rat. J Neurophysiol. 1994 Jun;71(6):2046-60.)

transmitters such as serotonin or cholecystokinin from activated mucosal endocrine cells. These transmitters activate specific receptors, such as serotonin type 3 receptors in intrinsic primary afferent neurons (IPANs) and extrinsic afferent terminals. For pain transduction in spinal afferents, the main transmitters include substance P and calcitonin gene-related peptide.

There are specialized sensory structures in the wall of the gut. For example, in the rectum, there are intraganglionic laminar endings, which serve the function of proprioceptors (stretch or tension receptors). Pacinian corpuscles (similar to those in skin) are located in the mesentery. Nerve fiber terminals of intrinsic afferent nerves respond to the chemical and other neurotransmitters released from enteroendocrine cells to activate the afferent signal. The sensory elements, stimulus, and response and function of chemosensitivity and mechanosensitivity in the enteric nervous system and extrinsic afferents are summarized in Table 12.1.

There are 5 morphologic types of extrinsic sensory neurons to the gut (Figure 12.3).

Splanchnic and pelvic pathways in the colon contribute to mechanosensation in the lower gut (Figure 12.4).

Visceral Hypersensitivity

In addition to the activation of motor and sensory reflexes, visceral sensory input may project to the conscious brain when they exceed peripheral control mechanisms, including the downregulation of ascending spinal pathways by signaling from the periaqueductal gray. Visceral hypersensitivity may result from peripheral or central sensitization mechanisms.

Peripheral Sensitization of Primary Afferents

IPANs in the gut are activated by noxious stimuli that elicit protective reflexes, such as diarrhea in the presence of bacterial products or parasitic infections. In the presence of perturbations such as inflammation of the gut, the properties of IPANs are modified. The modifications lead to abnormal cell signaling that initiates afferent signals that may lead to conscious perception or to altered motor and secretory reflexes. Pro-inflammatory substances released in the presence of tissue damage and inflammation (eg, bradykinin, tachykinins, neural growth factors, prostaglandins, adenosine triphosphate, vanilloid compounds, and serine proteases) modulate visceral sensation by acting on the intrinsic and extrinsic afferent nerves.

Several local (axonal, prevertebral, or spinal) reflexes protect the CNS and consciousness from thousands of motor, secretory, and absorptive functions that occur autonomously within the gut. Descending modulation from higher centers also serves to maintain these homeostatic responses.

Central Sensitization

Spinal afferents respond over a wide range of stimuli, including a subset that respond only to noxious stimuli; these are termed *silent-* or *high-threshold nociceptors.* However, when peripheral nerve endings are injured and inflamed of or noxious stimulation is repetitive, they can respond to lower-intensity stimuli. This phenomenon is called *central sensitization.*

Table 12.1   Sensory Transmission in ENS and Extrinsic Afferents

Sensory Modality	Sensory Elements	Stimulus	Response and Function
Chemosensitivity	EC and other enteroendocrine cells	Luminal chemicals, toxins, nutrients	Release of 5-HT and other mediators to modulate ENS Modulation of vagal activity to regulate physiologic behavior, nausea, and vomiting
	Enteric neurons S neurons AH neurons	Inflammation SCF, glycine, pH SCF, glycine, pH	Modulate ENS activity Activation Activation and inhibition (SCF)
	Vagal and spinal sensory neurons	Acid, SCF, ischemia, inflammation, and injury	Modulation of reflex activity, nociception, cytoprotection
Mechanosensitivity	EC cell	Mucosal deformation	Release of 5-HT to modulate ENS Modulation of vagal activity
	ICC	Stretch	Interaction with muscle or nerves
	Muscle	Tone	Increased tone to support neuron deformation (ENS and extrinsics)
	Enteric neurons S neurons AH neurons	Neuron deformation Slow accommodation Rapid accommodation	Modulate ENS activity Activation Activation (process deformation) or inhibition (soma deformation)
	Vagal sensory neurons	Neuron deformation (low threshold)	Modulation of reflex activity, eating behavior, pain, immune functions. Crosstalk with ENS
	Spinal sensory neurons	Neuron deformation (low and high threshold)	Modulation of reflex activity, nociception, blood flow Crosstalk with ENS

Abbreviations: AH, after hyperpolarization; EC, enterochromaffin cell; ENS, enteric nervous system; 5-HT, 5-hydroxytryptamine (serotonin); ICC, interstitial cells of Cajal; SCF, short-chain fatty acid.

From Blackshaw LA, Brookes SJ, Grundy D, Schemann M. Sensory transmission in the gastrointestinal tract. Neurogastroenterol Motil. 2007;19(1 Suppl):1-19; used with permission.

Descending projections from brainstem nuclei (eg, periaqueductal gray) to the spinal cord enhance or reduce the excitability of dorsal horn neurons, which are the locus of entry of afferent signals from the viscera. These descending projections include opioidergic and adrenergic descending pain inhibitory pathways. Conversely, hypervigilance or focused attention on sensations arising from the GI tract may activate pain facilitatory pathways involving substance P, other tachykinins, and N-methyl-D-aspartate receptors and lead to central sensitization. The balance between ascending signals and descending modulation determines the degree of central projection of visceral signals and, therefore, the level of conscious perception (sensation) and autonomic responsiveness. The conscious perception and autonomic responses are also altered by the degree of vigilance, the limbic system, and brainstem reflexes. The level of attention modulates central

stimulation, as shown in the context of somatic pain (Figure 12.5).

Definitions of Visceral Sensation Parameters

Compliance is measured with an intraluminal polyethylene balloon and is the volume response (y-axis) to an imposed pressure (x-axis). Compliance curves are sigmoid in shape. They have an initial reflex relaxation (change in wall tension without volume change), and this is followed by a linear relationship that reflects partly the elasticity of the viscus wall and by a final plateau phase (see Figure 10.4). It is best to use polyethylene infinitely compliant balloons rather than latex balloons.

Figure 12.3   Five Morphologic Types of Extrinsic Sensory Neurons to the Gut

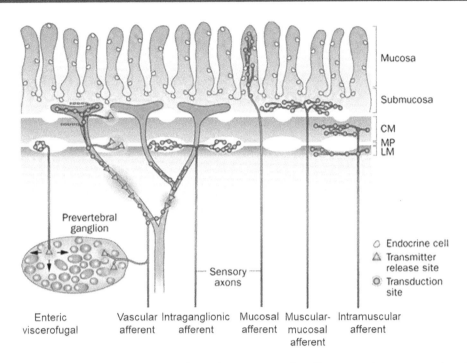

Enteric viscerofugal neurons are included for the sake of completeness. Vascular afferents are the most complex afferents; they have both intramural and extramural perivascular axons and collaterals in enteric ganglia, mucosa, muscularis externa, and prevertebral ganglia. Intraganglionic axons provide intraganglionic laminar endings, mostly in myenteric ganglia. Mucosal afferents innervate the subepithelial mucosa. Muscular–mucosal afferents have endings deep in the mucosa, close to the muscularis mucosae, and intramuscular afferents have nerve endings within longitudinal or circular muscle layers. CM indicates circular muscle; LM, longitudinal muscle; MP, myenteric plexus.

(From Brookes SJ, Spencer NJ, Costa M, Zagorodnyuk VP. Extrinsic primary afferent signalling in the gut. Nat Rev Gastroenterol Hepatol. 2013;10(5):286-96; used with permission.)

The latter have an intrinsic compliance that has to be factored into the measured compliance (eg, subtraction of each latex balloon's compliance) because it may be a significant confounder. Perception data may be affected by changes in organ compliance. When the compliance is unchanged but the sensation is reduced by a medication, the implication is that the medication has altered afferent function. Conversely, if the drug alters viscus compliance, an alteration of perception threshold may not be due to change in afferent nerve function. The first component, or initial cushion, is characterized by no change in volume despite increase in pressure. This cushion can be altered by pharmacologic agents. The second linear portion of the compliance curve partly reflects the elasticity of the viscus and may rarely be altered by diseases associated with replacement fibrosis (scleroderma, radiation) or by drugs.

Hypersensitivity refers to increased sensation of stimuli estimated in practice with measurement of threshold pressures for first sensation, gas, urgency, or pain (Figure 12.6) and increased scores of symptoms (including pain or gas sensation ratings) in response to standard stimuli. Hypersensitivity tends to be more closely associated with IBS-D (diarrhea-predominant IBS), whereas rectal hyposensitivity has been associated with IBS-C (constipation-predominant IBS) (Figure 12.7). The thresholds for sensation may be confounded by change in the compliance of the rectum due to stool retention in IBS-C or associated rectal evacuation disorder.

Hypersensitivity may alter and normalize over time, despite persistence of symptoms suggestive of increased sensation (Figure 12.8).

The prevalence of hypersensitivity in patients with IBS differs markedly across studies (Table 12.2) and the accuracy of rectal sensation thresholds has been assessed with receiver operating characteristic curves (Figure 12.9). Some studies have shown that about

Figure 12.4   Splanchnic (A) and Pelvic (B) Pathways in the Colon and the Channels Contributing to Mechanosensation in the Lower Gut

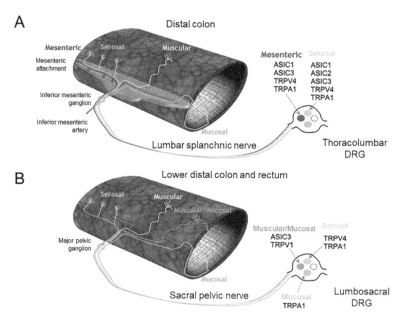

These pathways innervate the distal colon and rectum. In total, 5 different classes of mechanosensitive afferents have been characterized, 3 of which (serosal, muscular, mucosal) are in both pathways. Mesenteric afferents are specific to the splanchnic pathway, and muscular and mucosal afferents are specific to the pelvic pathways. A, In the splanchnic pathway, ASIC1, ASIC3, TRPV4, and TRPA1 contribute to mesenteric mechanoreceptor function, and ASIC1, ASIC2, ASIC3, TRPV4, and TRPA1 all contribute to serosal mechanoreceptor function. B, In the pelvic pathway, ASIC3 and TRPV1 contribute to muscular and mucosal mechanoreceptor function, and TRPV4 and TRPA1 contribute to serosal mechanoreceptor function. In addition, TRPA1 contributes to mucosal mechanoreceptor function. ASIC indicates acid-sensing ion channel; DRG, dorsal root ganglia; TRP, transient potential receptor.

(From Brierley SM. Molecular basis of mechanosensitivity. Auton Neurosci. 2010;153(1-2):58-68; used with permission.)

---

one-third of patients with IBS have increased pain sensation but not urge perception (Figure 12.10). Among 119 patients at Mayo Clinic (Camilleri 2008; see suggested reading), 21% of patients with IBS had increased rectal pain sensations: 7.6% hypersensitive (first threshold for pain <13 mm Hg). The proportion with reduced rectal sensation was 16.5% (Table 12.3).

These differences may reflect diverse levels of psychologic disturbance in different patient cohorts. In fact, the level of sensation is strongly influenced by the tendency to report pain in IBS, and acute stress modifies sensation reported in response to colonic distentions (Figure 12.11). In fact, experimental induction of psychosensory modulation influences colonic sensation, even in healthy volunteers (Figure 12.12).

In addition to hypersensitivity, there is also hyperalgesia in patients with IBS (Figure 12.13).

Hyperalgesia refers to increased pain sensation in response to a stimulus; allodynia refers to the change in

appreciation of pain in response to a stimulus that was not previously perceived as being painful. Peripheral sensitization involves the surrounding uninjured tissue in secondary hyperalgesia or allodynia and results from an increase in the excitability and receptive fields of spinal neurons, which are a reflection of the recruitment and amplification of both non-nociceptive and nociceptive inputs from the adjacent healthy tissue.

Activation of Afferent Discharges by Stretch and Tension

Mechanoreceptors initiate, convey, or perceive the distending stimulus. These mechanoreceptors are either in series or in parallel with muscle fibers. The in-parallel mechanoreceptors respond to stimuli that elongate

Figure 12.5   Nonvisceral Pain Perception: Role of Attention in Activating Primary Somatosensory Cortex

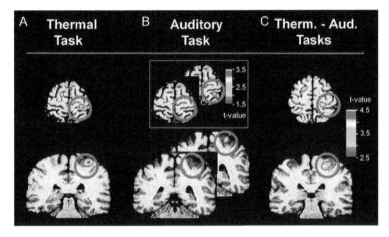

Pain-related activity when attention is directed to the painful heat stimulus (A) or to an auditory stimulus (B) is determined by subtracting positron emission tomography (PET) data recorded when a warm stimulus (32°-38°C) was presented from those recorded when a painfully hot stimulus (46.5°-48.5°C) was presented during each attentional state. Differences in pain-related activity during the 2 attentional conditions are determined (C) by subtracting PET data recorded during the auditory task from that recorded during the heat-discrimination task (using only painful stimulus trials: 46.5°-48.5°C). PET data, averaged across 9 patients, are illustrated against magnetic resonance imaging from 1 patient. Horizontal and coronal slices through S1 are centered at the activation peaks. Red circles surround the region of S1. There was a substantial activation of S1 when patients attended to the painful stimulus (A), but there was no noteworthy activation when patients attended to the auditory stimulus (B). However, there was a less than meaningful activation in S1 during the auditory task (inset). The direct comparison of pain in the 2 attentional conditions (C) shows a meaningful difference in pain-related S1 activity during the 2 attentional states. S1 activation is highly modulated by cognitive factors that alter pain perception, including attention (heat > hearing) and previous experience.

(From Bushnell MC, Duncan GH, Hofbauer RK, Ha B, Chen JI, Carrier B. Pain perception: is there a role for primary somatosensory cortex? Proc Natl Acad Sci USA. 1999;96(14):7705-9; Copyright (1999) National Academy of Sciences USA, used with permission.)

Figure 12.6   Rectal Hypersensitivity in IBS: Onset of Pain at Different Volumes of Balloon Inflation

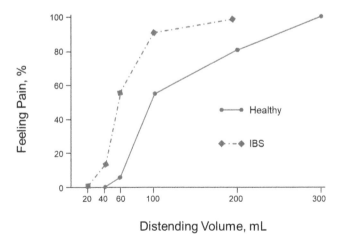

IBS indicates irritable bowel syndrome.

(From Ritchie J. Pain from distension of the pelvic colon by inflating a balloon in the irritable colon syndrome. Gut. 1973;14(2):125-32; used with permission.)

the viscus wall, whereas in-series mechanoreceptors respond to stimuli that increase the tension within the viscus wall. Thus, different stimuli (distention, relaxation, and contraction of smooth muscle) activate receptors, in series or in parallel, depending on the state of contraction, relaxation, or tension within the viscus (Figure 12.14).

Measurement of Visceral Sensations

In humans, 2 types of measurements are used to assess visceral sensation in vivo: standardized symptom-based questionnaires (visual analog scale or adjectival scale) to determine thresholds or severity of symptoms in response to mechanical stimuli, typically viscus distention (Figure 12.15), or changes in cerebral blood flow induced by stimuli (eg, mechanical or electrical)

Figure 12.7   Comparison of Rectal Sensory Thresholds (Measured in Milliliters of Balloon Distention) for IBS-D, IBS-C, and Normal Controls (N)

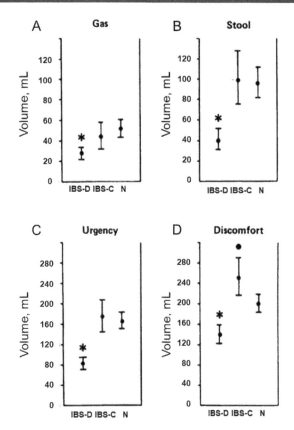

There are differences in hypersensitivity (lower volume of balloon distention to experience the sensation) between IBS-D and IBS-C. Values show hypersensitivity to gas (A), stool (B), and urgency (C) in IBS-D and hyposensitivity (higher volume of balloon distention to experience the sensation) to discomfort (D) in IBS-C. IBS indicates irritable bowel syndrome; IBS-C, constipation-predominant irritable bowel syndrome; IBS-D, diarrhea-predominant irritable bowel syndrome. *P<.001 for IBS-D vs IBS-C and controls; •P<.05 for IBS-C vs controls.

(From Prior A, Maxton DG, Whorwell PJ. Anorectal manometry in irritable bowel syndrome: differences between diarrhoea and constipation predominant subjects. Gut. 1990;31(4):458-62; used with permission.)

(Figures 12.16 and 12.17). Imaging methods (eg, positron emission tomography, functional magnetic resonance imaging [fMRI], single-photon emission computed tomography) and sophisticated analyses of connectivity between centers in the brain are required to measure brain activity on the basis of levels of blood flow or oxygenation. There are sex-related differences in brain centers activated by gut stimuli (Figures 12.18 and 12.19). The changes in cerebral functions range

from 2% to 5%, requiring specialized techniques, such as statistical parametric mapping. This low signal-to-noise ratio renders interpretation difficult. A detailed appraisal of cerebral measurements in visceral sensation studies is shown in the section on Measurements of Cerebral Blood Flow below.

Methods to Measure Sensory Thresholds

Methods to measure thresholds for different sensations have used ascending method of limits, with increasing pressure or volume delivered sequentially, distentions until the patient perceives first sensation, or other symptoms such as urgency in the rectum and gas and discomfort or pain in the colon. After the threshold is identified, a computer method randomly delivers a pressure or volume stimulus, which is either above or below the previously identified threshold; this is called the tracking method. In the random staircase method, the stimulus paradigm applies the stimulus either of greater or lower intensity to avoid response bias.

The definitions of threshold differ between studies, including sensation (eg, discomfort) of 3 on a 0 to 5 scale or the mean pressure at which a certain sensation (eg, pain) is reported. There are differences in sensation thresholds in published literature (Table 12.4).

Sensory Ratings From Distentions Using Pressure-Based Mechanical Stimuli

To avoid potential response bias, 3 to 5 pressure-based mechanical stimuli are applied in random order and sensation is tested with a visual analog scale. Thresholds for pain and sensory ratings at higher pressures of distention (36 and 48 mm Hg above baseline operating pressure) are most reproducible (Figure 12.20 and Table 12.5).

Reproducibility of Colonic Sensation Testing

Testing of compliance, tone and pain, and gas sensation in the left colon is associated with adequate performance to assess these functions in humans (Table 12.6). The coefficient of variation for sensation tests is lower

Figure 12.8 Discomfort Thresholds in Male and Female Patients With IBS Normalize Over Time While IBS Symptoms Persist

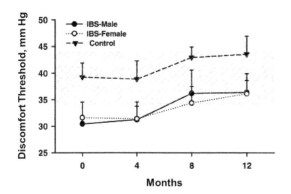

Longitudinal changes in discomfort thresholds for healthy controls, male patients with IBS, and female patients with IBS. Hatched area represents +95% CI of the initial discomfort threshold for the controls. Bars represent +1 SEM. IBS indicates irritable bowel syndrome.

(From Naliboff BD, Berman S, Suyenobu B, Labus JS, Chang L, Stains J, et al. Longitudinal change in perceptual and brain activation response to visceral stimuli in irritable bowel syndrome patients. Gastroenterology. 2006;131(2):352-65; used with permission.)

among women, a finding that is relevant to plan studies in functional GI disorders.

Measurements of Cerebral Blood Flow

Changes in cerebral blood flow during viscus stimulation require further study. Positron emission tomography and fMRI are the most widely used measurement techniques. After intravenous injection of a radioactive compound, positron emission tomography assesses blood flow or regional cerebral metabolism in brain areas. fMRI detects increases in oxygen concentration in areas of heightened neuronal activity without administration of radioactive compounds.

Brain regions have been shown to consistently exceed a false discovery rate threshold of $P<.05$ during supraliminal rectal balloon inflation in healthy controls and in patients with IBS (Table 12.7), and some brain areas have greater or lesser activations in patients with IBS than in healthy controls (Tillisch 2011; see suggested reading).

The precise relationship between general pain experience with gut distention or clinically recorded pain and imaging findings is not completely resolved, and in some instances there is little correlation between results, such as in response to placebo (Figure 12.21).

The functional connectivity between the various regions that seem to be activated in patients with IBS has been studied. Visceral sensitivity associated with hypervigilance and hyperalgesia in IBS seems related to changes in functional connectivity within networks associated with interoception, salience, and sensory processing (Figure 12.22).

Relationship of Altered Intestinal Permeability and Pain

The intestinal barrier has multiple components (see Figure 11.10). Alteration of mucosal permeability

Table 12.2 Prevalence of Hypersensitivity in IBS in Different Research Studies

Author, Year of Publication	Center	Threshold Definition	Increased Sensation (Including Viscerosomatic Referral), %
Mertz et al, 1990	UCLA, United States	Discomfort 3 on 5-point scale	95%
Bouin et al, 2002	Montreal, Canada	Pain 3 on 10-point scale	88% at 40 mm Hg
Posserud et al, 2007	Gothenburg, Sweden	Pain button	61% total, 39% by thresholds
Dorn et al, 2007	UNC, United States	Pain 3 on 5-point scale	About 50%, only thresholds
Van der Veek et al, 2008	Leiden, the Netherlands	Thresholds >10 mm on VAS	33%; thresholds and VAS ratings
Camilleri et al, 2008	Mayo Clinic, United States	First pain	21% hyper-, 16.5% hyposensitive by thresholds and VAS ratings

Abbreviations: IBS, irritable bowel syndrome; VAS, visual analog scale.

Figure 12.9   Rectal Sensory Thresholds

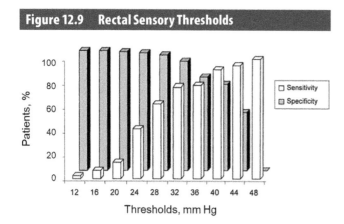

Sensitivity and specificity of barostat rectal distention to identify IBS (n=86 patients) and non-IBS (n=103 participants). Values are depicted at each distention level (pressure distention in mm Hg) tested. IBS indicates irritable bowel syndrome.

(From Bouin M, Plourde V, Boivin M, Riberdy M, Lupien F, Laganiere M, et al. Rectal distention testing in patients with irritable bowel syndrome: sensitivity, specificity, and predictive values of pain sensory thresholds. Gastroenterology. 2002 Jun;122(7):1771-7; used with permission.)

may lead to local inflammation and stimulation of pain pathways; immune activation results in increased mast cells in the gut mucosa in IBS. Higher levels of mediators from mast cells, such as histamine, tryptase, and trypsin, have been documented in colonic and jejunal biopsy supernatants of both patients with IBS-D and those with IBS-C. Similarly, substantially higher

total immunocytes and CD3+, CD4+, and CD8+ T cells were identified in biopsies from the same patients. Tryptase and proteases are associated with increased permeability; abnormal expression of tight junctions in the barrier is associated with the development of abdominal pain in IBS (Figures 12.23 through 12.28; see Figures 11.5 and 11.10).

Current Approaches to Management of Visceral Pain in Patients With IBS

Treatments for the relief of symptoms in IBS are summarized in Table 12.8.

Dietary Interventions

Food triggers vagally mediated reflexes that can stimulate painful contractions in the colon on the arrival of food in the upper gut or with inhibition of colonic water absorption and stimulation of colonic transit and high-amplitude propagated contractions by carbohydrates and their products that reach the colon. Deficiency of dietary fiber leads to constipation, which may cause pain.

Figure 12.10   Urge and Pain Perception in IBS

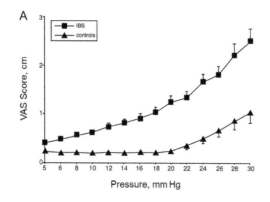
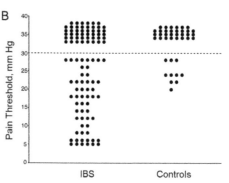

Hypersensitivity to balloon distention occurs in 33% of patients with IBS and is predicted by symptom severity but not by psychologic factors or demographics. A, Ratings: Intensity of urge perception in 101 patients with IBS and 40 controls. Urge did not differ between patients and controls. Data are expressed as mean ± SEM. B, Thresholds: Individual pain thresholds in patients with IBS and healthy controls. Substantially more patients (n=55, 54%) than controls (n=10, 25%) reached the pain threshold before the end of the ramp distention (dotted line, 30 mm Hg). IBS indicates irritable bowel syndrome; VAS, visual analog scale.

(From van der Veek PP, Van Rood YR, Masclee AA. Symptom severity but not psychopathology predicts visceral hypersensitivity in irritable bowel syndrome. Clin Gastroenterol Hepatol. 2008 Mar;6(3):321-8; used with permission.)

Table 12.3   Rectal Sensation Measurements of Patients With IBS Evaluated at Mayo Clinic

IBS Type	No. of Patients	Total, %	Hypersensitive, %	Hyperalgesia, %	Both Hypersensitive and Hyperalgesic, %	Hyposensitive, %
IBS-C	49	40	15	15	0	23
IBS-D	44	36	2.5	11.5	2.5	26
IBS-M	29	24	4	16	0	8
All IBS	122	100	7.6	13	2	17

Abbreviations: IBS, irritable bowel syndrome; IBS-C, constipation-predominant IBS; IBS-D, diarrhea-predominant IBS; IBS-M, mixed IBS.

Data from Camilleri M, McKinzie S, Busciglio I, Low PA, Sweetser S, Burton D, et al. Prospective study of motor, sensory, psychologic, and autonomic functions in patients with irritable bowel syndrome. Clin Gastroenterol Hepatol. 2008;6(7):772-81.

Fiber Supplementation

Different forms of fiber that are recommended for the treatment of constipation include psyllium, methylcellulose, calcium polycarbophil, and wheat dextrin. Bran, ispaghula, and unspecified fiber treatments are not more efficacious than control treatments for abdominal pain relief (relative risk, 0.87; 95% CI, 0.76-1.00).

Low-FODMAP Diet

Intake of FODMAPs (fermentable oligosaccharides, disaccharides, monosaccharides, and polyols) results in osmotic effects and production of gas and short-chain fatty acids with distention, pain, bloating, and stimulation of abnormal motility. The gas and short-chain fatty acid production results from rapid fermentation by intestinal bacteria.

Meta-analyses lend some support to the efficacy of a low-FODMAP diet for the treatment of abdominal pain and bloating because it reduces colonic fermentation or greater microbial diversity and reduces total bacterial abundance. These effects are associated with decreased markers of inflammation such as serum interleukin-6 and interleukin-8 and reduced fecal total short-chain fatty acids and n-butyric acid compared with baseline. Nevertheless, the use of a low-FODMAP diet remains controversial. Long term, a high level of restriction may result in nutritional deficiencies and, therefore, the need for oversight and monitoring by an expert dietitian. In addition to potential nutritional deficiencies,

there may be changes in gut microbiota with unclear consequences. Overall, there is still no clear method to predict positive response, and relative efficacy compared with other dietary, psychological, or pharmacologic interventions for IBS requires further study.

Probiotics

Bowel function and bloating are affected in IBS-D treated with individual probiotics such as *Bifidobacterium infantis* or combination probiotics. There is some benefit for global symptom or abdominal pain scores, although these effects seem to be strain-dependent and may be more significant in children. Further studies are required to address which bacterial strains and which patients are most likely to respond.

Classes of Available Pharmacologic Agents for Visceral Pain

Classes of pharmacologic agents for visceral pain are listed in Box 12.1 and detailed in Table 12.9.

Nonabsorbed Antibiotic: Rifaximin

Rifaximin, administered for 2 weeks, was efficacious for providing adequate relief of global IBS symptoms over

Figure 12.11   Increased Colonic Sensitivity in IBS Is Strongly Influenced by a Psychologic Tendency to Report Pain and Urge Rather Than Increased Neurosensory Sensitivity

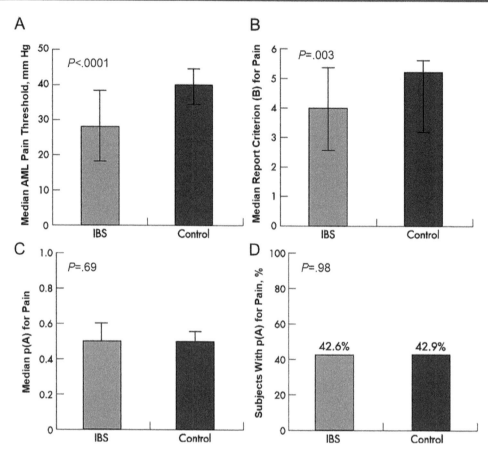

A, Median ascending method of limits (AML) pain thresholds: Thresholds were significantly higher in healthy controls than in patients with IBS. B, The pain report criterion (B) across both 30 mm Hg and 34 mm Hg stimuli: Patients with IBS had a lower criterion, which reflects their increased tendency to report pain irrespective of stimulus intensity. C, The median pain neurosensory sensitivity [p (A)]. There were no differences between the 2 groups. D, The percentage of patients whose ability to discriminate painful sensations between 30 mm Hg and 34 mm Hg stimuli was better than chance [p (A) >0.5]: There was no difference between the 2 groups. The bars on each graph represent the interquartile range. IBS indicates irritable bowel syndrome.

(From Dorn SD, Palsson OS, Thiwan SI, Kanazawa M, Clark WC, van Tilburg MA, et al. Increased colonic pain sensitivity in irritable bowel syndrome is the result of an increased tendency to report pain rather than increased neurosensory sensitivity. Gut. 2007 Sep;56(9):1202-9; used with permission.)

a subsequent 10 weeks in 2 studies. However, the durability of benefit in patients with IBS-D responding to 2 weeks of rifaximin treatment was 50% at 10 weeks and 10% at 20 weeks. The most significant benefit was for bloating, and the benefit was only borderline for abdominal pain (P=.055) and stool consistency (P=.08).

Antispasmodics

Antispasmodics reduce GI contractility. According to a Cochrane review (Quartero 2005; see suggested reading), some antispasmodics may be beneficial for

abdominal pain and global symptom relief. A meta-analysis (Ford 2008; see suggested reading) of 22 randomized, controlled trials of antispasmodics in IBS showed their superiority over placebo for relieving IBS symptoms (number needed to treat [NNT]=5), but there was noteworthy heterogeneity between studies. The strongest data were for otilonium bromide, which targets L- and T-type calcium channels and muscarinic type 2 and tachykinin neurokinin (NK)-2 receptors. Otilonium considerably improved the severity of abdominal pain and bloating, well-being, and global assessment compared with placebo, but there was no effect on bowel symptoms. Otilonium was associated

Figure 12.12   Psychosensory Modulation: Perception During Colonic Distentions: Effects of Unpleasant Stress and Relaxation

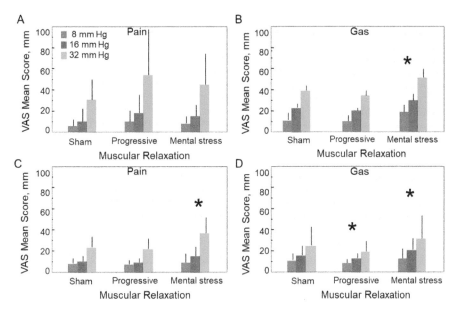

Effects of colonic distention on the sensation of pain and gas in the transverse (n=20) (A and B) and sigmoid (n=22) (C and D) colon in healthy volunteers. Stimulus intensity was related to symptom scores. Asterisks indicate increased sensations of pain in association with sigmoid distention and of gas in association with distention of both sigmoid and transverse colon during mental stress or decreased sensation of gas during distentions of sigmoid colon during progressive muscular relaxation.

(From Ford MJ, Camilleri M, Zinsmeister AR, Hanson RB. Psychosensory modulation of colonic sensation in the human transverse and sigmoid colon. Gastroenterology. 1995;109(6):1772-80; used with permission.)

Figure 12.13   Visceral Sensation in IBS: Hyperalgesia

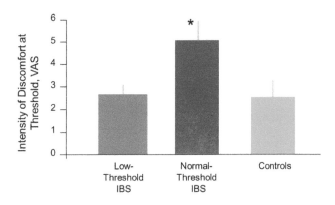

Figure shows intensity of discomfort sensation (based on a visual analog scale ranging from no sensation [0] to severe [9]). During phasic rectal distention, patients with IBS and normal thresholds perceived threshold stimuli more intensely than patients with IBS and low thresholds or controls. IBS indicates irritable bowel syndrome; VAS, visual analog scale. *$P<.01$.

(From Mertz H, Naliboff B, Munakata J, Niazi N, Mayer EA. Altered rectal perception is a biological marker of patients with irritable bowel syndrome. Gastroenterology. 1995;109(1):40-52; used with permission.)

Figure 12.14   Activation and Inactivation of Mechanotransducers in Series and in Parallel to Muscle Fibers in the Colon

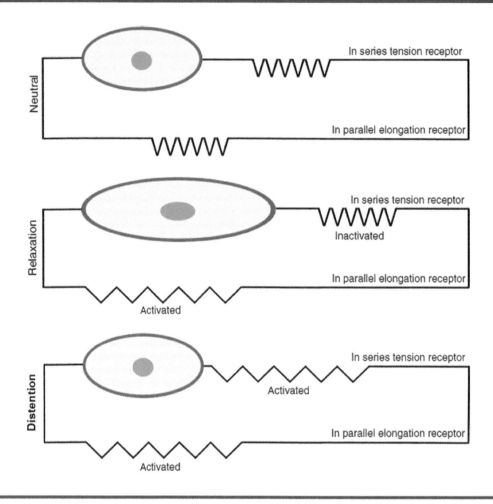

with a higher probability of remaining relapse-free during 10 weeks' follow-up. Antispasmodics are generally well tolerated, apart from the anticholinergic agents, which can cause atropine-like adverse effects, including constipation.

Peppermint Oil

Peppermint oil and its active ingredient, l-menthol, are calcium-channel antagonists (that may cause muscle relaxation), κ-opioid agonists (that alter gut sensitivity), serotonergic (serotonin type 3) antagonists, and activators transient receptor potential ion channel melastatin subtype 8, which has antinociceptive properties. Peppermint oil also has an anti-inflammatory effect.

A meta-analysis of 5 small trials (Khanna 2014; see suggested reading) showed peppermint oil resulted in global improvement of IBS symptoms and improvement in abdominal pain compared with placebo. Peppermint oil may cause adverse events such as heartburn, dry

Figure 12.15   Visceral Sensation: Methods for Measurement

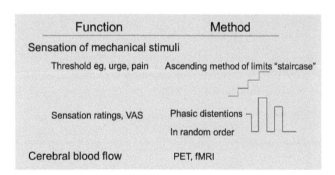

fMRI indicates functional magnetic resonance image; PET, positron emission tomogram; VAS, visual analog scale.

Figure 12.16   Brain Responses to Visceral Stimuli Reflect Visceral Sensitivity Thresholds in Patients With IBS

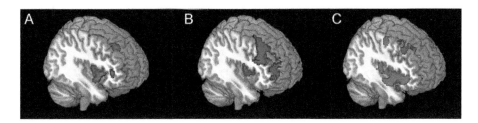

Hypersensitive patients with IBS had greater activation of insula and reduced deactivation in pregenual anterior cingulate cortex during noxious rectal distentions. Blood oxygen level–dependent (BOLD) responses (<0.01) within the regions of interest in A, healthy controls (n=18), B, normosensitive patients with IBS (n=18), and C, hypersensitive patients with IBS (n=15) during high rectal distention (45 mm Hg). Blue indicates decreased BOLD signal; IBS, irritable bowel syndrome; red, increased BOLD signal.

(From Larsson MB, Tillisch K, Craig AD, Engstrom M, Labus J, Naliboff B, et al. Brain responses to visceral stimuli reflect visceral sensitivity thresholds in patients with irritable bowel syndrome. Gastroenterology. 2012 Mar;142(3):463-72; used with permission.)

mouth, belching, peppermint taste and peppermint smell. A new small bowel-release formulation of peppermint oil showed no superiority over placebo.

Antidepressants

The NNT for antidepressant relief of pain in IBS is thought to be 4, but there are flaws or inconsistencies in the study design, analyses of efficacy, NNT, and safety for this class of pharmacologic agents. About one-third of patients taking antidepressants presented with adverse effects compared with 16.5%

of those given placebo, and the number needed to harm was 9.

Serotonin Type 3 Antagonists

Eight trials (Ford 2009; see suggested reading) that included 3,214 patients treated with alosetron and 1,773 with placebo documented relief of abdominal pain and discomfort, diarrhea, and urgency. The average number of participants for the alosetron trials was 10 times higher than that for the antidepressant trials. The overall pooled estimated RR for the relief of abdominal

Figure 12.17   Influence of Rectal Stimulus Intensity on Regional Cerebral Blood Flow in IBS, Not in Healthy Controls

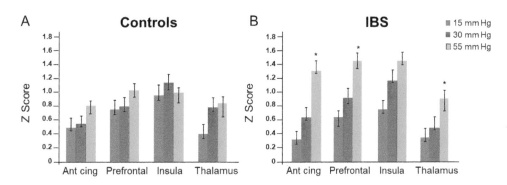

Central nervous system activation with rectal distention. Average activation of the anterior cingulate cortex (ant cing), insular cortex, prefrontal cortex, and thalamus in controls (A) and patients with IBS (B) in response to rectal distention at 15, 30, and 55 mm Hg. Activation of the anterior cingulate and thalamus is greater at 55 mm Hg than at 30 mm Hg for patients with IBS. * P<.05. IBS indicates irritable bowel syndrome.

(Modified from Mertz H, Morgan V, Tanner G, Pickens D, Price R, Shyr Y, et al. Regional cerebral activation in irritable bowel syndrome and control subjects with painful and nonpainful rectal distention. Gastroenterology. 2000 May;118(5):842-8; used with permission.)

Figure 12.18   Sex-Related Differences in Response to Gut-Directed Stimulus in Patients With Irritable Bowel Syndrome

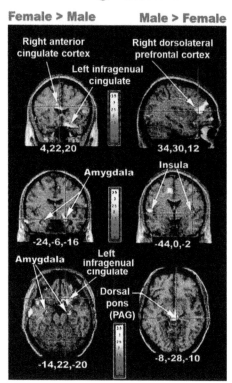

The responses are shown to the 45-mm Hg stimulus for male and female patients (compared with baseline). The left column shows voxels of significantly greater activation (*P*<.05) in female patients, and the right column shows voxels with appreciably greater activation in male patients (shown in radiologic orientation). PAG indicates periaqueductal gray.

(From Naliboff BD, Berman S, Chang L, Derbyshire SW, Suyenobu B, Vogt BA, et al. Sex-related differences in IBS patients: central processing of visceral stimuli. Gastroenterology. 2003 Jun;124(7):1738-47; used with permission.)

Figure 12.19   Activation of Brain Regions in Male and Female Patients in Response to Visceral (A) or Psychologic (B) Stressors

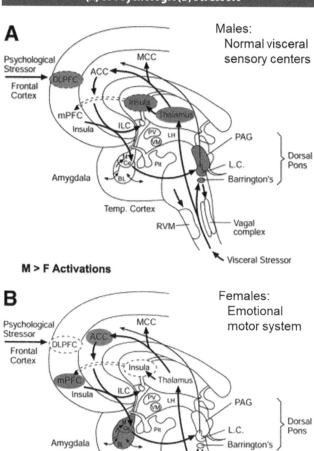

In general, men show activation of normal visceral sensory centers, whereas women show propensity to greater activation of emotional motor systems such as amygdala, insula, and anterior cingulate cortex. ACC indicates anterior cingulate cortex; DLPFC, dorsolateral prefrontal cortex; L.C., locus coeruleus; MCC, mid cingulate cortex; mPFC, medial prefrontal cortex; PAG, periaqueductal gray; RVM, rostral ventromedial medulla; Temp. cortex, temporal lobe cortex.

(From Naliboff BD, Berman S, Chang L, Derbyshire SW, Suyenobu B, Vogt BA, et al. Sex-related differences in IBS patients: central processing of visceral stimuli. Gastroenterology. 2003 Jun;124(7):1738-47; used with permission.)

pain and discomfort was 1.30 (95% CI, 1.22-1.39) in favor of serotonin type 3 antagonist treatment. The calculated NNT was 7.7. Results were consistent across studies.

These results for relief of abdominal pain and discomfort were confirmed in a separate meta-analysis of 10 trials (Andresen 2008; see suggested reading) of alosetron (6,232 patients): relative risk was 1.23 (95% CI, 1.15-1.32) for response and 1.55 (95% CI, 1.40-1.72) for global improvement for 4 trials (1,732 patients). Reports of ischemic colitis (about 1 in 800) and

complications from constipation led to restrictions in prescribing the drug. The precise effect of alosetron

Table 12.4   Comparison of Pressure Thresholds for Sensation in Health Across Published Studies Using Barostat-Delivered Ramp-like Distentions[a]

| Author | End Point | | | | | |
	First Sensation	Desire to Defecate/ Stool	Urge	Pain	Discomfort	Compliance, $Pr_{1/2}$
Bharucha et al (2004)	15 (2)	20 (2)	27 (2)	NR	NR	14 (1)
Bouin et al (2002)	NR	NR	NR	44 (5)	NR	NR
Hammer et al (1998)	6 (1)	14 (2)	21 (4)	NR	NR	NR
Lembo et al (1994)	NR	16 (1)	NR	NR	31 (3)	20
Mertz et al (1995)	NR	NR	NR	NR	30 (3)	NR
Naliboff et al (1997)	NR	34 (3)	37 (4)	39 (5)	38 (2)	NR
Cremonini et al (2005)	10 (1)	NR	20 (1)	37 (2)	25 (2)	12 (1)

Abbreviations: NR, not recorded; $Pr_{1/2}$, pressure at half maximum volume.

[a] Values are mean pressures, mm Hg (SEM).

From Cremonini F, Houghton LA, Camilleri M, Ferber I, Fell C, Cox V, et al. Barostat testing of rectal sensation and compliance in humans: comparison of results across two centres and overall reproducibility. Neurogastroenterol Motil. 2005;17(6):810-20; used with permission. Full reference citations for studies listed in this table can be found in the original source.

on ischemic colitis is unclear because there is an association between IBS and ischemic colitis independent of therapy. Ondansetron, which reduced symptom severity in IBS, was associated with higher adequate relief response than placebo. Ramosetron, which is efficacious in both male and female patients, has been approved and marketed in Japan.

Secretagogues

The chloride channel activator lubiprostone had efficacy for bowel function and reduced efficacy for relief of IBS pain and discomfort in a 3-month clinical trial in patients with IBS-C (Johanson 2008; see suggested reading). Linaclotide, a guanylate cyclase-C receptor agonist, relieves constipation, increases the proportion of adequate relief and global relief responders, and

reduces pain. Pain relief seems to result from inhibition of colonic nociceptors via extracellular cyclic guanosine 3′,5′-monophosphate, which reaches the visceral afferents in the lamina propria or submucosa from the colonocytes.

μ-Opioid Agonist

μ-Opioid agonists are used during acute exacerbations of abdominal pain, but they should not be used for the pain of IBS.

A Mixed Opioid Agent: Eluxadoline

Eluxadoline is a μ-opioid receptor and κ-opioid receptor agonist and a δ-opioid receptor antagonist with minimal oral

Figure 12.20   Mean Sensory Ratings (With 95% CI) for 2 Centers (M, Manchester, United Kingdom; R, Rochester, Minnesota) on Day 1 (A), Day 1 Post-4 h (B), and Day 15 (C)

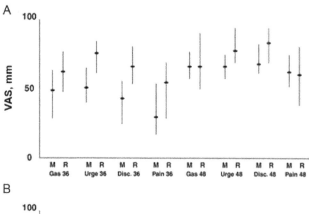

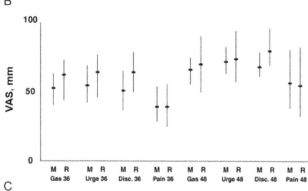

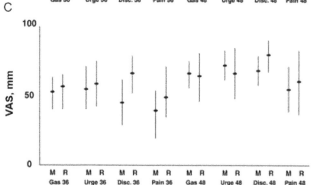

These observations show that rectal sensation tests can be replicated across centers with consensus equipment, methods, and parameters measured. Disc indicates discomfort; VAS, visual analog scale; 36 and 48, mm Hg of pressure applied during rectal distentions.

(From Cremonini F, Houghton LA, Camilleri M, Ferber I, Fell C, Cox V, et al. Barostat testing of rectal sensation and compliance in humans: comparison of results across two centres and overall reproducibility. Neurogastroenterol Motil. 2005 Dec;17(6):810-20; used with permission.)

bioavailability. Eluxadoline, at 100 and 200 mg, resulted in multiple improvements in global symptoms, IBS symptom severity score, IBS quality of life, adequate relief of IBS symptoms, and bowel dysfunction (Dove 2013; see suggested reading). Results for the primary efficacy end point (combined bowel function and pain) were associated with an NNT of approximately 8, although the abdominal pain scores were not substantial for either of 2 phase 3 randomized, placebo-controlled trials reported in a single article (Lembo 2016; see suggested reading) at 75-mg or 100-mg dosages. The adverse events of pancreatitis and sphincter of Oddi spasm each occurred in 0.3% of patients. The US Food and Drug Administration recommends exclusion of patients with a history of bile duct obstruction, pancreatitis, severe liver impairment, or severe constipation and of patients who drink more than 3 alcoholic beverages per day.

Histamine-1 Receptor Antagonist: Ebastine

Histamine sensitizes human submucosal neurons in rectal biopsies via activation of histamine-1 receptors. Ebastine, a non-sedating antagonist of histamine-1 receptors, reduces visceral hypersensitivity, overall IBS symptoms, and abdominal pain in patients with IBS.

NK2 Receptor Antagonist: Ibodutant

Neurokinins (eg, substance P) and NK2 receptors mediate long-lasting contractions of smooth muscle in the gut, stimulate sensory nerves, and activate visceral reflexes. Ibodutant, a highly selective NK2 antagonist with high oral bioavailability, resulted in improvement of abdominal pain, stool pattern, and overall symptoms in IBS-D in female patients, but not in male patients, with excellent tolerability.

γ-Aminobutyric Acid Agents

γ-Aminobutyric acid agents are α2δ ligands that reduce the release of several excitatory neurotransmitters from

Table 12.5   Intra- and Inter-Individual Coefficients of Variation of Pressure Thresholds for Sensation[a]

Sensation	Inter-Individual Day 1, %	Inter-Individual Day 1 + 4 hours, %	Inter-Individual Day 15, %	Intra-Individual Day 1 to Day 15, %
First sensation	56	77	64	43
Urgency	34	49	41	41
Discomfort	40	47	38	47
Pain	34	37	31	23

[a] Participants underwent sensation testing twice (4 hours apart) on Day 1 and repeated after 15 days.

From Cremonini F, Houghton LA, Camilleri M, Ferber I, Fell C, Cox V, Castillo EJ, et al. Barostat testing of rectal sensation and compliance in humans: comparison of results across two centres and overall reproducibility. Neurogastroenterol Motil. 2005;17(6):810-20; used with permission.

nerves. These transmitters include glutamate, noradrenaline, substance P, and calcitonin gene–related peptide, which are all involved in pain mechanisms. Two small studies suggested efficacy with gabapentin and pregabalin (Lee 2005, Houghton 2007; see suggested reading).

Future Visceral and Somatic Analgesics

Recent developments provide a new approach to address abdominal pain with peripheral visceral

Table 12.6   Intra- and Inter-Individual Coefficients of Variation in Colonic Motor and Sensory Testing

Function	All Participants (n=72), %		Men (n=38), %		Women (n=34), %	
	Mean (SD)	Inter/Intra	Mean (SD)	Inter/Intra	Mean (SD)	Inter/Intra
Compliance Pr$_{1/2}$, mm Hg	19.7 (4.5)	22.8/17.5	20.6 (4.9)	23.7/17.0	18.8 (3.9)	20.8/18.2
Pressure thresholds, mm Hg						
First	15.6 (14.4)	91.9/90.2	17.1 (15.6)	91.4/84.9	14.0 (12.9)	92.0/98.1
Gas	24.0 (17.5)	72.8/75.9	24.9 (18.5)	74.1/72.7	22.9 (16.5)	71.7/71.9
Pain	42.4 (13.2)	31.0/30.6	43.6 (14.4)	33.1/35.4	41.2 (11.7)	28.4/27.2
Sensation ratings at 36 mm Hg distention, VAS mm (scale 0-100)[a]						
Gas	53.3 (22.3)	41.9/36.6	53.8 (18.5)	34.5/43.1	52.8 (25.9)	49.1/29.1
Pain	48.6 (27.3)	56.3/33.0	49.4 (27.2)	55.1/38.3	47.9 (28.1)	58.6/27.1

Abbreviations: Pr$_{1/2}$, pressure at half maximum volume; VAS, visual analog scale.

[a] Sensation ratings were based on 100-mm VAS.

Modified from Odunsi ST, Camilleri M, Bharucha AE, Papathanasopoulos A, Busciglio I, Burton D, et al. Reproducibility and performance characteristics of colonic compliance, tone, and sensory tests in healthy humans. Dig Dis Sci. 2010;55(3):709-15; used with permission.

Table 12.7   Activation of Brain Regions During Supraliminal Rectal Balloon Inflation

Brain Region, by Study Group	Cluster No.	Volume, mm³	ALE Value	Hemisphere
Healthy controls				
Anterior insula	1	5,752	0.0025	Right
Anterior insula			0.0024	
Postcentral gyrus (BA 43)			0.0013	
Anterior insula	2	2,968	0.0029	Left
Thalamus	3	2,256	0.0027	Right
Inferior parietal lobule (BA 40)	4	1,744	0.0023	Left
Putamen	5	1,680	0.0025	Left
Anterior midcingulate cortex (BA 24)	6	1,320	0.0018/ 0.0017	Right/Left
Lateral prefrontal cortex (BA 9/46)	7	1,088	0.0019	Left
Inferior parietal lobule (BA 40)	8	408	0.0018	Right
Posterior anterior cingulate cortex (BA 32)	9	296	0.0013	Right
Anterior midcingulate cortex/ pACC (BA 32)	10	272	0.0013	Left
Medial prefrontal cortex (BA 9/32)	11	168	0.0013	Right
Patients with IBS				
Anterior midcingulate cortex	1	4,304	0.0034	Right
Superior temporal gyrus (BA 22)	2	1,960	0.0020	Left
Anterior midcingulate cortex (BA 32/24)	3	1,288	0.0021/ 0.0021	Left/Right
Midbrain	4	1,072	0.0025	Left
Cerebellum			0.0020	Right
Thalamus	5	960	0.0025	Right
Superior frontal gyrus (BA 6)	6	704	0.0019	Right
Thalamus	7	496	0.0021	Left
a/pMCC (BA 24)	8	312	0.0014	Left
Amygdala	9	264	0.0018	Left
pACC (BA 24)	10	192	0.0014	Right
Putamen	11	112	0.0015	Right

Abbreviations: ALE, activation likelihood estimate; aMCC, anterior midcingulate cortex; BA, Brodmann area; IBS, irritable bowel syndrome; pACC, perigenual anterior cingulate gyrus.

From Tillisch K, Mayer EA, Labus JS. Quantitative meta-analysis identifies brain regions activated during rectal distension in irritable bowel syndrome. Gastroenterology. 2011 Jan;140(1):91-100; used with permission.

Figure 12.21   Reduction of expected pain (A) and perceived pain intensity (B) on visual analog scale (VAS, 0-100 mm)

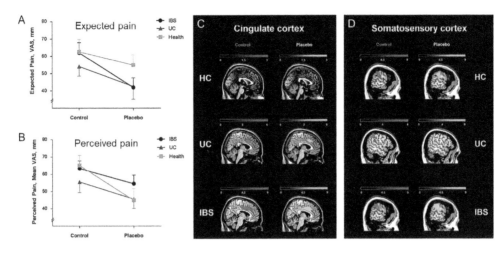

Placebo compared with control conditions in patients with irritable bowel syndrome (IBS), ulcerative colitis (UC) in remission, and in healthy controls (HC) matched to the IBS group. All *P*<.001 (analysis of variance), except for the UC vs HC analysis on expected pain (*P*>.05). No statistically significant differences between group means. C and D, Rectal distention-induced neural activation in the cingulate cortex (C) and the somatosensory cortex (S1/S2) (D) in the control (activation shown in red) and placebo (activation shown in green) conditions, respectively: HC (upper row), UC in remission (middle row), and IBS (lowest row). Results of within-group analyses on the contrast (placebo > control) using 1-sample *t* tests showed significant reductions in rectal pain–induced neural activation in HC (*P*<.05) and in patients with UC (*P*<.001, uncorrected). In contrast, patients with IBS actually had enhanced (rather than reduced) activation of the somatosensory cortex in the placebo condition (*P*<.001, uncorrected). Images overlaid on a structural T1-weighted magnetic resonance image used for spatial normalization.

(From Schmid J, Langhorst J, Gaß F, Theysohn N, Benson S, Engler H, et al. Placebo analgesia in patients with functional and organic abdominal pain: a fMRI study in IBS, UC and healthy volunteers. Gut. 2015 Mar;64(3):418-27; used with permission.)

Figure 12.22   Group Differences in Default Mode Network (DMN) Connectivity

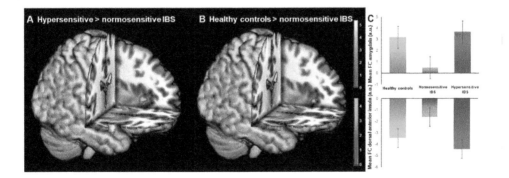

Results from region of interest analyses comparing functional connectivity within the DMN in (A) hypersensitive compared with normosensitive patients and (B) healthy controls relative to normosensitive IBS. C, Mean functional connectivity (FC) values in arbitrary units (a.u.) for each participant, extracted from 1-sample *t* test of DMN FC for amygdala (top) and dorsal anterior insula (bottom). Images were superimposed on a structural T1-weighted magnetic resonance image used for spatial normalization and thresholded at *P*<.001 uncorrected for visualization purposes. Positive correlations are shown in red-yellow, and negative correlations are depicted in blue-green. IBS indicates irritable bowel syndrome.

(From Icenhour A, Witt ST, Elsenbruch S, Lowen M, Engstrom M, Tillisch K, et al. Brain functional connectivity is associated with visceral sensitivity in women with Irritable Bowel Syndrome. Neuroimage Clin. 2017 Jun 2;15:449-457; Open access article licensed under Creative Commons Attribution CC-BY-NC-ND 4.0 [https://creativecommons.org/licenses/by-nc-nd/4.0/].)

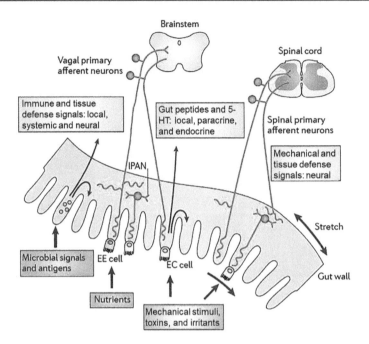

Information about luminal factors and conditions of the gut is signaled through extrinsic vagal and spinal afferents to the brainstem and spinal cord, respectively. Mechanical stimuli (stretch, pressure, distortion, and shearing forces) can activate spinal, vagal, and intrinsic primary afferents (IPANs) directly, without intermediary cells such as the enteroendocrine (EE) cells. Although no synaptic connections have been found between IPANs and extrinsic afferents, the latter form networks around myenteric ganglia (intraganglionic laminar endings), many of which receive synaptic input from IPANs. Signaling molecules (including proteases, histamine, serotonin [5-HT], and cytokines) that are produced by immune cells in Peyer patches and within the gut epithelium can activate their respective receptors on vagal and spinal afferents. Similarly, neuropeptides and hormones (gut peptides) that are released from EE cells in response to other luminal factors, such as nutrients, toxins, or antigens, can act both in an endocrine fashion, reaching targets in the brain (area postrema, dorsal vagal complex, and hypothalamus), and through receptor activation on spinal and vagal afferents, in a paracrine fashion. Enterochromaffin (EC) cells signal to both IPANs and vagal afferents.

(From Mayer EA. Gut feelings: the emerging biology of gut-brain communication. Nat Rev Neurosci. 2011;12(8):453-66; used with permission.)

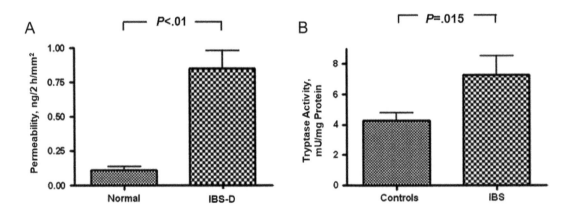

A, Permeability was significantly increased in patients with IBS-D compared with controls (0.109+0.091 vs 0.848+0.600 ng/2 h per mm² (n=14 and 21, respectively; P<.01). B, Tryptase activity of biopsy tissues from patients with IBS was significantly increased compared with that in normal controls (4.27±2.12 mU/mg protein and 7.24±4.07 mU/mg protein; n=18 and 10, respectively; P=.015). IBS-D indicates diarrhea-predominant irritable bowel syndrome.

(From Lee JW, Park JH, Park DI, Park JH, Kim HJ, Cho YK, et al. Subjects with diarrhea-predominant IBS have increased rectal permeability responsive to tryptase. Dig Dis Sci. 2010 Oct;55(10):2922-8; used with permission.)

Figure 12.25   Proteolytic activity in human colonic biopsies and present in colonic washes (A-C)

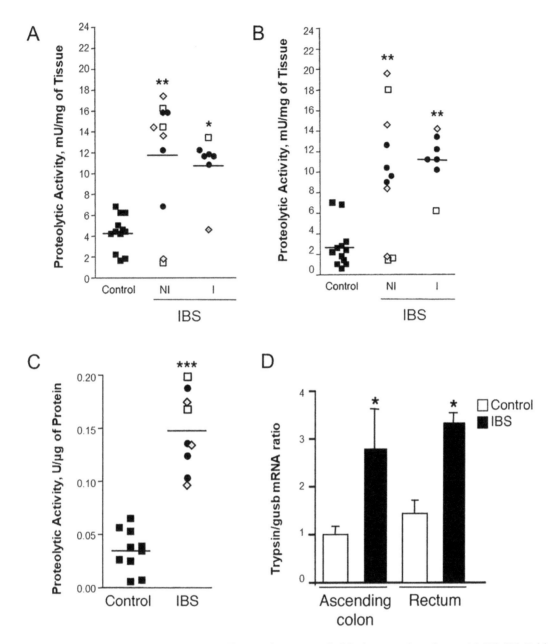

Arginine-directed protease activity in supernatants of biopsy from controls (black squares), patients with IBS (IBS-D, black circles; IBS-C, white squares; or IBS-D/C, diamonds). IBS biopsy supernatants were separated according to the presence of inflammatory (I) or non-inflammatory (NI) signs, and biopsies were harvested at the level of the ascending colon (A) or the rectum (B). C, Protease activity in colonic washes from control (black squares) and patients with IBS. Data are mean (SEM). *P<.05, **P<.01, ***P<.005 compared with control group. IBS indicates irritable bowel syndrome; IBS-C, constipation-predominant IBS; IBS-D, diarrhea-predominant IBS; IBS-D/C, diarrhea-constipation alternating IBS. D, Trypsin expression in human colonic biopsies and culture supernatants. Dual reverse transcription polymerase chain reaction of trypsin and β-glucuronidase (gusb) of biopsies from patients with irritable bowel syndrome and controls quantified by densitometry analysis of the gels. Data are mean (SEM); n=12. *P<.05 compared with control group.

(Modified from Cenac N, Andrews CN, Holzhausen M, Chapman K, Cottrell G, Andrade-Gordon P, et al. Role for protease activity in visceral pain in irritable bowel syndrome. J Clin Invest. 2007 Mar;117(3):636-47; used with permission.)

Figure 12.26   Relationship of Tight Junction Proteins and IBS: BMI, Abdominal Pain, and Duration

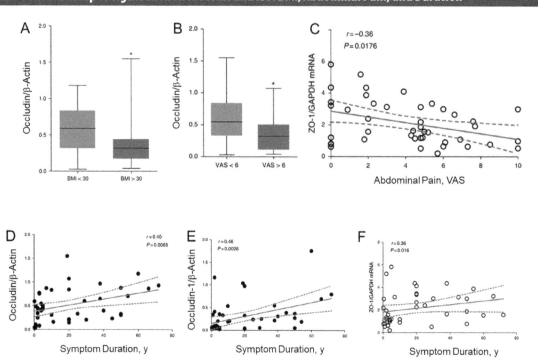

A, Expression of occludin in colonic mucosa according to BMI in patients with IBS (n=45) by BMI <30 kg/m² (n=29) or BMI >30 kg/m² (n=16). *P<.05 with Mann-Whitney test. B and C, Occludin expression and ZO-1 mRNA level in the colonic mucosa according to abdominal pain. Expression of occludin in colonic mucosa (B) (n=45) and mRNA level for ZO-1 (C) (n=43) according to abdominal pain in patients with IBS. B, Values are medians and interquartile ranges by VAS <6 (n=32) or VAS >6 (n=13). *P<.05 with Mann-Whitney test. C, Data were correlated with nonparametric Spearman test. D-F, Correlation between tight junction proteins and duration of symptoms. Correlation between the expression of occludin (D) or claudin-1 (E) in colonic mucosa and duration of symptoms in patients with IBS (n=45). Correlation between the mRNA level for ZO-1 in colonic mucosa and the duration of symptoms (F) in patients with IBS (n=43). Data were correlated with nonparametric Spearman test. BMI indicates body mass index; GADPH, glyceraldehyde 3-phosphate dehydrogenase; IBS, irritable bowel syndrome; VAS, visual analog scale; ZO-1, zonula occludens-1.

(From Bertiaux-Vandaele N, Youmba SB, Belmonte L, Lecleire S, Antonietti M, Gourcerol G, et al. The expression and the cellular distribution of the tight junction proteins are altered in irritable bowel syndrome patients with differences according to the disease subtype. Am J Gastroenterol. 2011 Dec;106(12):2165-73; used with permission.)

analgesics (Table 12.9) through modulation of opioid receptors, for example, through biased ligands that activate the G-protein pathway without activating β-arrestin, which is responsible for the adverse GI and respiratory effects of opioids. Other compounds target nonopioid mechanisms, including cannabinoid, N-methyl-D-aspartate, calcitonin gene–related peptide, estrogen, and adenosine A2B receptors and transient receptor potential channels (TRPV1, TRPV4, and TRPM8). Although current evidence is based predominantly on animal models of visceral pain, early human studies also support the evidence from the basic and animal research. This augurs well for the development of non-addictive, visceral analgesics for treatment of chronic abdominal pain, an unmet clinical need (Camilleri 2018, see suggested reading).

Figure 12.27   Fecal Serine Proteases, Increased Permeability, and Pain in IBS

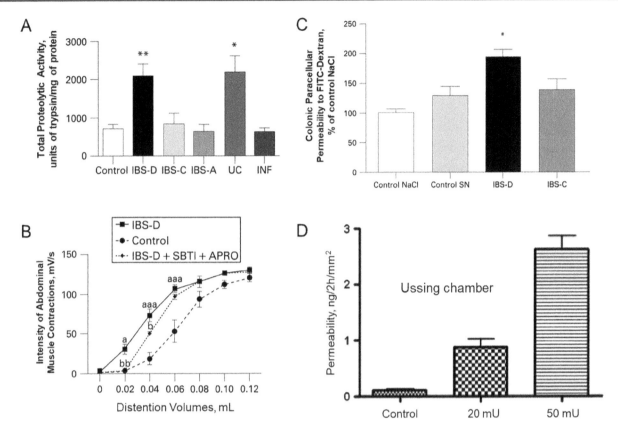

A, Fecal total protease activity in healthy controls; patients with IBS-D, IBS-C, and IBS-A; patients with active UC; and patients with acute infectious diarrhea. *P<.05 and **P<.01 compared with healthy controls. Error bars represent SEM. B, Supernatants of patients with IBS-D–induced allodynia and visceral hypersensitivity in wild-type mice at low distention volumes compared with supernatants of controls (0.02, 0.04, 0.06 mL; [a], P<.05, [aaa] P<.001, respectively), an effect that was partially prevented by the administration of serine protease inhibitors (at 0.02 and 0.04 mL distention volumes; [bb] P<.01 and [b] P<.05, respectively). C, Colonic paracellular permeability to FITC–dextran in Ussing chambers 60 minutes after administration of fecal supernatants (SN) of patients with IBS-D and IBS-C and healthy controls on colonic mucosal strips of wild-type mice (*P<.05 compared with control SN). D, Tryptase (dose in mU on x axis) increases basolateral permeability of normal rectal mucosa. APRO indicates aprotinin; FITC, fluorescein isothyocyanate; IBS, irritable bowel syndrome; IBS-A, alternating IBS; IBS-C, constipation-predominant IBS; IBS-D, diarrhea-predominant IBS; INF, infectious; SBTI, soybean trypsin inhibitor; UC, ulcerative colitis.

(A-C, Modified from Gecse K, Roka R, Ferrier L, Leveque M, Eutamene H, Cartier C, et al. Increased faecal serine protease activity in diarrhoeic IBS patients: a colonic lumenal factor impairing colonic permeability and sensitivity. Gut. 2008 May;57(5):591-9; used with permission. D, from Lee JW, Park JH, Park DI, Park JH, Kim HJ, Cho YK, et al. Subjects with diarrhea-predominant IBS have increased rectal permeability responsive to tryptase. Dig Dis Sci. 2010 Oct;55(10):2922-8; used with permission.)

Figure 12.28   Severity of Abdominal Pain in Patients With IBS

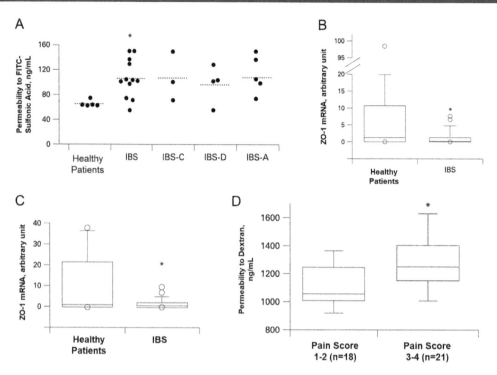

Patients show positive correlation with the degree to which their colonic supernatants induce paracellular permeability and downregulate ZO-1 mRNA expression in mucosal biopsies as well as Caco-2 monolayers in response to exposure to biopsy supernatants. A, Paracellular permeability to FITC-sulfonic acid in colonic biopsies. B, Reduced tight junction proteins (ZO-1, *not* occludin) mRNA expression in mucosal biopsies. C, Reduced (ZO-1, *not* occludin) mRNA expression in Caco-2 + supernatant. D, Paracellular permeability of Caco-2 cells as a function of severity of abdominal pain in 39 patients with IBS (* *P*=.006). Caco-2 indicates a cell line that spontaneously differentiates to express morphologic and functional characteristics of mature small intestinal columnar epithelial cells (enterocytes); FITC, fluorescein isothiocyanate; IBS, irritable bowel syndrome; IBS-A, alternating IBS; IBS-C, constipation-predominant IBS; IBS-D, diarrhea-predominant IBS; ZO-1, zonula occludens-1.

(From Piche T, Barbara G, Aubert P, Bruley des Varannes S, Dainese R, Nano JL, et al. Impaired intestinal barrier integrity in the colon of patients with irritable bowel syndrome: involvement of soluble mediators. Gut. 2009 Feb;58(2):196-201; used with permission.)

Table 12.8   Efficacy of Interventions for Relief of Symptoms in IBS Based on Systematic Reviews and Meta-analyses

Intervention	Parameter	RR or OR (95% CI)
Dietary or probiotics or antibiotics		
Bran, ispaghula, and unspecified fiber	Abdominal pain	RR, 0.87 (0.76-1.00)
Low FODMAP diet	Abdominal pain	OR, 1.81 (1.13-2.88)
Probiotics	Global improvement	−0.25 (−0.36 to −0.14)
Probiotics: combination of *Escherichia coli* and *Enterococcus faecalis* or *E coli* alone	Abdominal pain	RR, 1.96 (1.14-3.36)
Rifaximin	Global improvement	OR, 1.57 (1.22-2.01)
Rifaximin	Bloating	OR, 1.55 (1.23-1.96)
Antispasmodics		
Peppermint oil	Global improvement	RR, 2.23 (1.78-2.81)
Antidepressant therapy	Global improvement	RR, 0.66 (0.57-0.78)
	Abdominal pain	RR, 0.62 (0.43-0.88)
Antidepressant therapy	Global improvement	RR, 0.67 (0.58-0.77)
Antidepressant therapy	Abdominal pain	RR, 0.62 (0.43-0.88)
Drugs targeting specific gastrointestinal receptors		
Alosetron	Abdominal pain and discomfort	RR, 1.30 (1.22-1.39)
	Overall risk difference	RR, 0.13 (0.1-0.16)
Alosetron	Abdominal pain and discomfort	RR, 1.23 (1.15-1.32)
	Global improvement	RR, 1.5 (1.40-1.72)
Ondansetron	Adequate relief response	RR, 4.7 (2.6-8.5)
Linaclotide	Adequate relief response	RR, 1.95 (1.3-2.9)
	Abdominal pain	RR, 1.58 (1.02-2.46)

Abbreviations: FODMAP, fermentable oligosaccharides, disaccharides, monosaccharides, and polyols; OR, odds ratio of achieving significant relief; RR, relative risk of not achieving relief.

Modified from Camilleri M, Boeckxstaens G. Dietary and pharmacological treatment of abdominal pain in IBS. Gut. 2017;66(5):966-74; used with permission. Full references for the reviews and meta-analyses can be found in the original source.

Box 12.1

Classes of Pharmacologic Agents for Visceral Pain

Antidepressants (tricyclic agents, selective serotonin reuptake inhibitors)

Peppermint oil

5-HT_3 receptor antagonists (alosetron, ondansetron, ramosetron)

Nonabsorbed antibiotic (rifaximin)

Secretagogues (lubiprostone, linaclotide)

μ-Opioid receptor (OR) and κ-OR agonist and δ-OR antagonist (eluxadoline)

$Histamine_1$ receptor antagonist (ebastine)

Neurokinin-2 receptor antagonist (ibodutant)

GABAergic agents (gabapentin and pregabalin)

Abbreviations: GABA, γ-aminobutyric acid; 5-HT, 5-hydroxytryptamine (serotonin).

From Camilleri M, Boeckxstaens G. Dietary and pharmacological treatment of abdominal pain in IBS. Gut. 2017;66(5):966-74; used with permission.

Table 12.9   Classes of Novel Peripheral Visceral Analgesics

Class of Peripheral Visceral Analgesic	Examples	Summary of Mechanism of Action
Novel μ-Opioid Agents		
Novel biased ligand of the μ-opioid receptor	TRV130 PZM21	Activates G-protein without β-arrestin pathway
Targeting μ-opioid receptor under acidic conditions	NFEPP	A fluorinated derivative of fentanyl exclusively activated at acidic sites, eg, inflammation
NOP receptor modulation	SCH 221510	NOP ligand may reverse a possible deficiency of endogenous nociceptin in IBS
Dual action on NOP and μ-opioid receptor	Cebranopadol, BU08070	Peripherally active mixed μ-opioid peptide/NOP receptor agonist
Buprenorphine analogs	ORP-101	Combines analgesia from μ-opioid receptor agonism and the anti-addictive effects of a κ-opioid receptors antagonist
Morphiceptin analog	P-317	Cyclic pentapeptide derivative of morphiceptin with indirect evidence of peripheral action
Novel CB_2R receptor agonists	LY3038404; PF-03550096; APD371 (olorinab)	Selective CB_2 agonists; may have superior analgesic effects devoid of the centrally mediated CB_1 effects
N-methyl-D-aspartate receptor antagonists	Ketamine	Prevent central sensitization to opioid analgesics, improving effectiveness of opioids
Calcitonin gene–related peptide receptor antagonists	$CGRP_{8-37}$	Blocks endosomal signaling of the calcitonin receptor–like receptor to pain transmission
Drugs targeting TRP channels		
TRPV1	JYL1421	TRPV1 receptor antagonist reduces mechanical but not chemical hyperalgesia
TRPV4	RN1734	Selective TRPV4 antagonist reduced chemical-induced hyperalgesia
TRPM8	Peppermint and caraway oil	Agonists that reduce colonic hypersensitivity to mechanical stimuli
GPER and ER ligands	G-1, estradiol	Nonselective GPER agonist or ER ligand inhibit muscle contractility and chemical-induced colonic hyperalgesia
Adenosine A2B receptor antagonist	Aminophylline	Antagonizes A2B receptors that are involved in the control of intestinal secretion, motility, and sensation

Abbreviations: CB_2R, cannabinoid receptor 2; ER, estrogen receptor; GPER, G-protein–coupled estrogen receptor; IBS, irritable bowel syndrome; NOP, nociceptin/orphanin FQ opioid peptide; TRP, transient receptor potential.

From Camilleri M. Toward an effective peripheral visceral analgesic: responding to the national opioid crisis. Am J Physiol Gastrointest Liver Physiol. 2018 Jun 1;314(6):G637-46; used with permission.

Suggested Reading

Andresen V, Montori VM, Keller J, West CP, Layer P, Camilleri M. Effects of 5-hydroxytryptamine (serotonin) type 3 antagonists on symptom relief and constipation in nonconstipated irritable bowel syndrome: a systematic review and meta-analysis of randomized controlled trials. Clin Gastroenterol Hepatol. 2008 May;6(5):545–55. Epub 2008 Jan 31.

Blackshaw LA, Brookes SJ, Grundy D, Schemann M. Sensory transmission in the gastrointestinal tract. Neurogastroenterol Motil. 2007 Jan;19(1 Suppl):1–19. Epub 2007 Feb 7.

Camilleri M. Toward an effective peripheral visceral analgesic: responding to the national opioid crisis. Am J Physiol Gastrointest Liver Physiol. 2018 Jun 1;314(6):G637–46. Epub 2018 Feb 22.

Camilleri M, Boeckxstaens G. Dietary and pharmacological treatment of abdominal pain in IBS. Gut. 2017 May;66(5):966–74. Epub 2017 Feb 25.

Camilleri M, McKinzie S, Busciglio I, Low PA, Sweetser S, Burton D, et al. Prospective study of motor, sensory, psychologic, and autonomic functions in patients with irritable bowel syndrome. Clin Gastroenterol Hepatol. 2008 Jul;6(7):772–81. Epub 2008 May 5.

Delgado-Aros S, Camilleri M. Visceral hypersensitivity. J Clin Gastroenterol. 2005 May-Jun;39(5 Suppl 3):S194–203. Epub 2005 Mar 31.

Dove LS, Lembo A, Randall CW, Fogel R, Andrae D, Davenport JM, et al. Eluxadoline benefits patients with irritable bowel syndrome with diarrhea in a phase 2 study. Gastroenterology. 2013 Aug;145(2):329–38. Epub 2013 Apr 9.

Ford AC, Brandt LJ, Young C, Chey WD, Foxx-Orenstein AE, Moayyedi P. Efficacy of 5-HT3 antagonists and 5-HT4 agonists in irritable bowel syndrome: systematic review and meta-analysis. Am J Gastroenterol. 2009 Jul;104(7):1831–43. Epub 2009 May 26.

Ford AC, Talley NJ, Spiegel BM, Foxx-Orenstein AE, Schiller L, Quigley EM, et al. Effect of fibre, antispasmodics, and peppermint oil in the treatment of irritable bowel syndrome: systematic review and meta-analysis. BMJ. 2008 Nov 13;337:a2313.

Houghton LA, Fell C, Whorwell PJ, Jones I, Sudworth DP, Gale JD. Effect of a second-generation alpha2delta ligand (pregabalin) on visceral sensation in hypersensitive patients with irritable bowel syndrome. Gut. 2007 Sep;56(9):1218–25. Epub 2007 Apr 19.

Johanson JF, Drossman DA, Panas R, Wahle A, Ueno R. Clinical trial: phase 2 study of lubiprostone for irritable bowel syndrome with constipation. Aliment Pharmacol Ther. 2008 Apr;27(8):685–96. Epub 2008 Jan 28.

Khanna R, MacDonald JK, Levesque BG. Peppermint oil for the treatment of irritable bowel syndrome: a systematic review and meta-analysis. J Clin Gastroenterol. 2014 Jul;48(6):505–12.

Lee KJ, Kim JH, Cho SW. Gabapentin reduces rectal mechanosensitivity and increases rectal compliance in patients with diarrhoea-predominant irritable bowel syndrome. Aliment Pharmacol Ther. 2005 Nov 15;22(10):981–8.

Lembo AJ, Lacy BE, Zuckerman MJ, Schey R, Dove LS, Andrae DA, et al. Eluxadoline for Irritable Bowel Syndrome with Diarrhea. N Engl J Med. 2016 Jan 21;374(3):242–53.

Quartero AO, Meineche-Schmidt V, Muris J, Rubin G, de Wit N. Bulking agents, antispasmodic and antidepressant medication for the treatment of irritable bowel syndrome. Cochrane Database Syst Rev. 2005 Apr 18;(2):CD003460.

Tillisch K, Mayer EA, Labus JS. Quantitative meta-analysis identifies brain regions activated during rectal distension in irritable bowel syndrome. Gastroenterology. 2011 Jan;140(1):91–100. Epub 2010 Aug 11.

References Listed in Table 12.2

Bouin M, Plourde V, Boivin M, Riberdy M, Lupien F, Laganiere M, et al. Rectal distention testing in patients with irritable bowel syndrome: sensitivity, specificity, and predictive values of pain sensory thresholds. Gastroenterology. 2002 Jun;122(7):1771–7.

Camilleri M, McKinzie S, Busciglio I, Low PA, Sweetser S, Burton D, et al. Prospective study of motor, sensory, psychologic, and autonomic functions in patients with irritable bowel syndrome. Clin Gastroenterol Hepatol. 2008 Jul;6(7):772–81. Epub 2008 May 5.

Dorn SD, Palsson OS, Thiwan SI, Kanazawa M, Clark WC, van Tilburg MA, et al. Increased colonic pain sensitivity in irritable bowel syndrome is the result of an increased tendency to report pain rather than increased neurosensory sensitivity. Gut. 2007 Sep;56(9):1202–9. Epub 2007 May 4.

Mertz H, Naliboff B, Munakata J, Niazi N, Mayer EA. Altered rectal perception is a biological marker of patients with irritable bowel syndrome. Gastroenterology. 1995 Jul;109(1):40–52.

Posserud I, Syrous A, Lindstrom L, Tack J, Abrahamsson H, Simren M. Altered rectal perception in irritable bowel syndrome is associated with symptom severity. Gastroenterology. 2007 Oct;133(4):1113–23. Epub 2007 Jul 25.

van der Veek PP, Van Rood YR, Masclee AA. Symptom severity but not psychopathology predicts visceral hypersensitivity in irritable bowel syndrome. Clin Gastroenterol Hepatol. 2008 Mar;6(3):321–8. Epub 2008 Feb 7.

Implications of Pharmacogenomics for Irritable Bowel Syndrome

Introduction

The pharmacogenomics effect on the metabolism of medications typically used in irritable bowel syndrome (IBS) is predominantly through cytochrome P450 (CYP) metabolism. Genetic variations of receptors or pathways involved in IBS-related mechanisms affect responses to treatments, as best found with serotonergic agents. Thus, pharmacogenomics factors affect both pharmacokinetics and pharmacodynamics. Unfortunately, to date, large clinical trials have not incorporated testing for genetic variations that could affect the efficacy of medications in IBS. Pharmacogenomics testing for patients with IBS seems to be particularly relevant for treatments with central neuromodulators, in psychiatry practice, aided by commercially available tests focused on drug metabolism. Specific mechanisms or pathways in IBS are still poorly characterized compared with those in cancer and inflammatory bowel disease. However, pharmacogenomics tests related to metabolism of medications are available.

Definition

Pharmacogenomics is the study of genetic variation and effects of pharmacologic agents, typically through alterations in pharmacokinetics (absorption, distribution, metabolism, and elimination) or pharmacodynamics (effectiveness or adverse effects).

A glossary of terms relevant to pharmacogenomics is included in Box 13.1, and characterization of DNA sequence variants is included in Box 13.2.

Genetic Variation in Drug-Metabolizing Enzymes

There are 2 common pathways whereby DNA variants alter drug metabolism. First, pathways occur when there is a narrow margin between doses that determine efficacy compared with doses that cause adverse effects or toxicity. The second pathway may result from gene variants affecting the single predominant pathway for elimination of a drug (eg, CYP2D6, CYP3A4) or when the gene variation affects drug transport molecules or the transcriptional regulation of proteins such as enzymes or transporters involved in determining the biologic effects (efficacy or toxicity) of a drug. In patients with IBS, variants in germline variants, rather than somatic genomic variants, are usually the cause of DNA-related health issues.

Drug-metabolizing enzymes modify functional groups of a drug, and gene variants may alter an enzyme's ability to modify the function of a drug. The CYP450 enzymes (which are controlled by a family of 58 human *CYP* genes) are responsible for 5% or more of the phase 1 drug-metabolizing reactions. For example, hydroxylation in phase 1 reactions makes lipophilic molecules more water soluble. Phase 2 enzyme reactions involve conjugation with endogenous substituents and complete the process to form nontoxic substances that can be excreted in bile or urine (Figure 13.1). Typical examples of phase 2 drug-metabolizing enzymes are transferases, such as glucuronosyltransferases, and catechol *O*-methyl transferases.

Drug metabolism by CYP enzymes is the most common alteration of phase 1 drug metabolism in patients with IBS, particularly CYP2D6 and CYP2C19. Examples of drugs commonly used in IBS

Box 13.1

Glossary of Terms Relevant to Pharmacogenomics

Genome is the entire set of genetic instructions found in a cell. In humans, the genome consists of 23 pairs of chromosomes, found in the nucleus, and a small chromosome found in each cell's mitochondria. Each set of 23 chromosomes contains approximately 3.1 billion bases of DNA sequence

Somatic DNA: A somatic cell refers to any cell in the body except sperm and egg cells. Somatic cells are diploid, having 2 sets of chromosomes, 1 inherited from each parent. The DNA in those chromosomes is called somatic DNA. Mutations in the somatic DNA may result in disease, typically in cancers. However, such somatic mutations are not passed on to the offspring

Germline DNA is the DNA in germline cells (egg and sperm cells) used by sexually reproducing organisms to pass on genes from generation to generation

DNA variation is a general term to indicate diversity of genomes in a species

DNA variants: There are 2 main types of DNA variants: polymorphisms and histone variants

Polymorphism involves 1 of 2 or more variants of a particular DNA sequence. The most common type of polymorphism involves variation at a single base pair, such as a change from threonine (T) to cytosine (C). Such a variation is called a single nucleotide polymorphism, which occurs in at least 1% of the population and may correlate with disease, drug response, and other phenotypes. Polymorphisms can also be much larger in size and involve long stretches of DNA, which may be present (inserted) or absent (deleted). Deletions and insertions tend to be especially harmful when the number of missing or extra base pairs is not a multiple of 3

Histone is a protein that provides structural support to a chromosome. Given the length of DNA molecules, they are able to wrap around complexes of histone proteins, giving the chromosome a more compact shape that can fit in the cell nucleus. Some variants of histones are associated with the regulation of gene expression

DNA sequencing identifies an individual's variants by comparing the DNA sequence of an individual with the DNA sequence of a reference genome maintained by the Genome Reference Consortium. In addition to single nucleotide polymorphisms, and insertions and deletions (mentioned above), there may be substitutions when multiple nucleotides are altered from the reference sequence or structural variants in which large sections of a chromosome or even whole chromosomes are duplicated, deleted, or rearranged in some manner

From Camilleri M. Implications of pharmacogenomics to the management of IBS. Clin Gastroenterol Hepatol. 2019 Mar;17(4):584-94; used with permission.

and consequences of genetic variation are listed in Table 13.1.

The geographic and racial distributions of variants that alter CYP2 activity are illustrated in Figure 13.2. The highest prevalence of poor drug metabolism, affecting about 33% of a cohort in a hospital in New York (Finklestein 2016; see suggested reading), is in the CYP3A4/5 grouping. However, variants in the CYP3 genes are less relevant in IBS because the main substrates of CYP3A4 are immunosuppressive, chemotherapeutic, and antimicrobial (including antifungal) agents.

Nevertheless, CYP3A4 is relevant to treatment with prokinetics, such as cisapride (serotonin-receptor agonist) and erythromycin, which may result in cardiac arrhythmias, if the metabolizing CYP3A4 enzymes are inhibited by concomitantly administered drugs.

The newer, more specific serotonin-receptor agonist prucalopride is not metabolized by CYP3A4.

The nomenclature of CYP enzyme genes, including family, subfamily, isoenzyme, and allele, is shown in Figure 13.3.

The outcomes of drug metabolism vary significantly between poor metabolizers and ultrametabolizers (Table 13.2). In the United States, there are 20 to 30 million poor metabolizers and 15 to 20 million ultrametabolizers for CYP2D6 (Table 13.3) or, in summary, 8% each. The effect on active drug or prodrugs according to ultrarapid, extensive, intermediate, and poor metabolizer status is given in Table 13.2.

Codeine has 200-fold weaker affinity for the μ-opioid receptor than morphine. Therefore, codeine is a prodrug, and it cannot exert its clinical effects unless it is metabolized by CYP2D6 to morphine. CYP2D6

Box 13.2

Characterization of DNA Sequence Variants (Guideline From American College of Medical Genetics and Genomics)

Pathogenic

> A sequence variant that is previously reported and is a recognized cause of a disorder

Likely pathogenic

> A sequence variant that is previously unreported and is of the type which is expected to cause a disorder

Variant of unknown significance

> A sequence variant that is previously unreported and is of the type which may or may not be causative of a disorder

Likely benign

> A sequence variant that is previously unreported and is probably not causative of disease

Benign

> A sequence variant that is previously reported and is a recognized neutral variant

Sequence Variant

> A sequence variant that is previously not known or expected to be causative of disease but is found to exist in people with a particular disease or disorder. As a result of mutations, a gene can differ among individuals in terms of its DNA sequence. The differing sequences are referred to as alleles. A gene's location on a chromosome is termed a *locus* (from the Latin word for *place*). If a person has the same allele on both members of a chromosome pair, that person is a homozygote. If the alleles differ in DNA sequence, that person is a heterozygote. The combination of alleles that is present at a given locus is termed the *genotype*

> All genetic variation originates from the process known as mutation, which is defined as a change in DNA sequence. Mutations can affect either germline cells or somatic cells

> One type of single-gene mutation is the base-pair substitution, in which 1 base pair is replaced by another. This mutation can result in a change in the amino acid sequence. However, because of the redundancy of the genetic code, many of these mutations do not change the amino acid sequence (silent substitutions) and, therefore, they usually have no effect

> Base-pair substitutions that alter amino acids may be 1 of 2 basic types: missense mutations, which produce a change in a single amino acid, and nonsense mutations, which produce 1 of the 3 stop codons (UAA, UAG, or UGA) in the mRNA, thereby terminating translation of the mRNA (shorter polypeptide chain). Conversely, if a stop codon is altered so that it encodes an amino acid, an abnormally elongated polypeptide can be produced. These alterations of amino acid sequences can have profound consequences

> Because codons consist of groups of 3 base pairs, insertions or deletions can alter the downstream codons, resulting in a frameshift mutation

> Other types of mutation can alter the regulation of transcription or translation. A promoter mutation can decrease the affinity of RNA polymerase for a promoter site, often resulting in reduced production of mRNA and, thus, decreased production of a protein

> Mutations can also interfere with the splicing of introns, as mature mRNA is formed from the primary mRNA transcript. Splice-site mutations, those that occur at intron–exon boundaries, alter the splicing signal that is necessary for proper excision of an intron

From Camilleri M. Implications of pharmacogenomics to the management of IBS. Clin Gastroenterol Hepatol. 2019 Mar;17(4):584-94; used with permission.

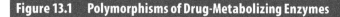

Figure 13.1   Polymorphisms of Drug-Metabolizing Enzymes

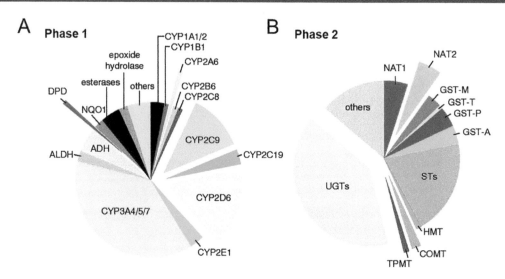

Polymorphisms modify functional groups (A) (phase 1 reactions, eg, hydroxylation) or conjugate with endogenous substituents (B) (phase 2 reactions). ADH indicates alcohol dehydrogenase; ALDH, aldehyde dehydrogenase; COMT, catechol O-methyl transferase; CYP, cytochrome P450; DPD, dihydropyrimidine dehydrogenase; GST, glutathione S-transferase; HMT, histamine methyltransferase; NAT, N-acetyltransferase; NQO1, NADPH:quinone oxidoreductase or DT diaphorase; STs, sulfotransferases; TPMT, thiopurine methyltransferase; UGTs, uridine 5′-triphosphate glucuronosyltransferases.

(From Evans WE, Relling MV. Pharmacogenomics: translating functional genomics into rational therapeutics. Science. 1999 Oct 15;286(5439):487-91; used with permission.)

ultrarapid metabolizers have more than 2 functional copies of the *CYP2D6* gene. They result in the generation of excess morphine with a risk for toxicity, including respiratory depression and death.

Examples of specific alterations in drug pharmacokinetics and efficacy of treatment that are relevant in functional gastrointestinal and motility disorders (specifically with tricyclic antidepressants, proton pump inhibitors, and histamine$_2$ blockers) are provided in Table 13.1, and they involve particularly CYP2D6 and CYP2C19.

Specific alleles in the *CYP2D6* and *CYP2C19* genes determine the enzymatic activity and, therefore, the metabolizer phenotypes of the carrier: ultrarapid, extensive, intermediate, or poor metabolizer. For example, *CYP2C19* *2 and *11 are null alleles associated with no enzyme activity, whereas *9, *1, and *17 are associated with decreased, normal, or increased enzyme activity, respectively (Table 13.4). It follows that the presence of 2 *17 alleles results in ultrametabolizer, 2 *1 alleles with extensive metabolizer, the combination *1 and *2 or 2 *9 alleles with intermediate metabolizer status, and 2 null alleles (*2 or *11) with poor metabolizer status.

If the drug requires bioconversion by an enzyme for efficacy, the activation of such a prodrug is reduced in slow metabolizers. Conversely, the effects of the enzyme may result in the inactivation of directly acting drugs in ultrarapid metabolizers. Similarly, the risk of adverse effects is affected by the metabolizer status or the coadministration of a drug that activates or inactivates the enzyme. Thus, a slow metabolizer of a directly acting drug or the coadministration of a drug that inhibits enzyme activity may result in high tissue levels and adverse effects.

Relevant drug interactions resulting from changes in drug metabolism are listed in Table 13.5. Given that the genes for drug metabolism do not change, genetic testing can be performed once and information included in a patient's medical record to document the relevant drug metabolic pathways.

Pharmacogenetic alert algorithms (Figure 13.4) within electronic health records can now inform providers regarding metabolizer status in reference to a specific prescription and can inform the prescriber in time to facilitate selecting an alternative medication.

Medications used in the treatment of IBS may also compete for the same CYP enzymes that

Table 13.1   Drugs Used in Treatment of IBS and Common Genetic Variations in Drug Metabolism

CYP	Prevalence of Poor-Metabolizing Phenotype	Examples of Drugs Commonly Used in IBS	Example of Drug Metabolized	Effect of Poor Metabolizer Polymorphism on Drug's Efficacy
2D6	6.8% in Sweden; 1% in China	Central neuromodulators: TCA: *amitriptyline, nortriptyline, desipramine*; Tetracyclic: *mianserin*; SSRI: *citalopram, fluoxetine, paroxetine*; SNRI: *venlafaxine*; Mixed: *mirtazapine* Analgesics: opioids (*codeine, oxycodone*) Antinausea: *dolasetron, ondansetron, fluphenazine, promethazine, tropisetron* Antispasmodics (Ca^{2+} blockers): *diltiazem, nicardipine, nifedipine*	Nortriptyline Codeine	Enhanced Decreased (codeine is a prodrug that is converted to morphine to be effective)
2C19	~3% in white United States and Sweden; ~16% in China, Japan	PPIs (except rabeprazole [CYP3A4]) Histamine$_2$ blockers Central neuromodulators: *clomipramine, imipramine* Anxiolytics: *diazepam*	Omeprazole Ranitidine	Enhanced Enhanced

Abbreviations: CYP, cytochrome P450; IBS, irritable bowel syndrome; PPI, proton pump inhibitor; SNRI, serotonin-norepinephrine reuptake inhibitor; SSRI, selective serotonin reuptake inhibitor; TCA, tricyclic antidepressant.

From Camilleri M. Implications of pharmacogenomics to the management of IBS. Clin Gastroenterol Hepatol. 2019 Mar;17(4):584-94; used with permission.

impact the pharmacokinetics of concomitantly administered drugs.

To facilitate interpretation, color coding is used in the alerts, such as that provided in GeneSight psychotropic reports: green (use as directed), yellow (use with caution), and red (use with increased caution and frequent monitoring) (Figure 13.5).

Commercially available gene assays for *TPMT; CYPs 2D6, 2C9, 2C19* and *3A5; VKORC1; CFTR; HLA-B; G6PD; UGT1A1; DPYD; SLCO1B1;* and *IL28B* identify actionable genetic variations that can inform important therapeutic decisions. A study of prescribed medications conducted at 5 US medical centers (Rautio 2008; see suggested reading) estimated that 7% of the 1,200 US Food and Drug Administration–approved medications and 18% of prescriptions written in the United States could be affected by these actionable pharmacogenes (Figure 13.6).

CYP Enzyme Inhibitors and Inducers

Many commonly used medications potently inhibit or induce CYP enzymes (Table 13.5) and affect their efficacy or adverse effects. However, the current literature does not identify reports of drug trials documenting the association of alteration of CYP enzymes with altered efficacy or toxicity in IBS.

Evidence of Clinical Effect of Pharmacogenomics Testing of Drug Metabolism

Pharmacogenomic testing has been reported to have clinical value when applied in patients prescribed antidepressants or central neuromodulators. In fact, patients given antidepressants on the basis of pharmacogenomics testing compared with treatment-as-usual approach have considerably higher odds (odds ratio, 2.26) for achieving clinical response and greater relative benefits (1.71-fold).

The current guidance is that pharmacogenomics testing may be of value for selecting an optimal neuromodulator in functional gastrointestinal disorders and for avoidance of potentially deleterious drug interactions.

Figure 13.2   Distribution Maps of *CYP2* Altered Activity Variants

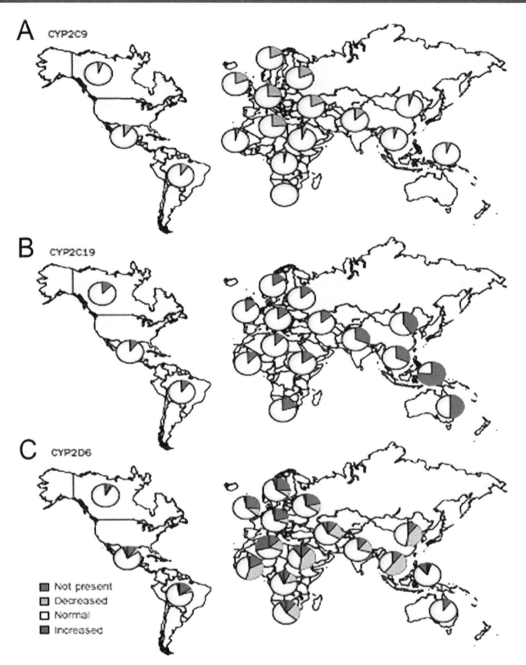

A, CYP2C9. B, CYP2C19. C, CYP2D6. The darker region in each pie chart shows the proportion of people residing in that region with documented genetic variants. CYP indicates cytochrome P450.

(Modified from Sistonen J, Fuselli S, Palo JU, Chauhan N, Padh H, Sajantila A. Pharmacogenetic variation at *CYP2C9*, *CYP2C19*, and *CYP2D6* at global and microgeographic scales. Pharmacogenet Genomics. 2009 Feb;19(2):170-9; used with permission.)

Figure 13.3   Nomenclature of Cytochrome P450 Enzyme Genes, Including Family, Subfamily, Isoenzyme, and Allele

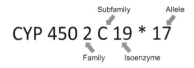

(From Camilleri M. Implications of pharmacogenomics to the management of IBS. Clin Gastroenterol Hepatol. 2019 Mar;17(4):584-94; used with permission.)

Pharmacogenomics Related to Drug Targets or Pathways, not Drug Metabolism, in IBS

The literature on genetic variation in receptor or transporters in IBS is summarized in Table 13.6.

One of the best examples of the effect of genetic variation of targets or pathways on the effects of medications in the treatment of IBS with diarrhea and IBS with constipation is provided by alosetron, a serotonin type 3 antagonist, and tegaserod, a serotonin

Table 13.2   The Effect of Polymorphisms on Drug Metabolism

Metabolizer Status	Active Drugs	Prodrugs: Opposite Effect to That of Active Drug
Ultrarapid	No drug response at ordinary dosage (nonresponders)	May have adverse events
Extensive[a]	Expected response to standard dose	
Intermediate	+/− Lesser consequences than poor metabolizers	
Poor	Too slow or no drug metabolism: • Too high drug levels at usual doses • High risk for adverse drug reactions (toxicity)	May not respond

[a] Note that "extensive" reflects the "normal" or expected response and does not imply excessive or ultrarapid metabolism.

From Camilleri M. Implications of pharmacogenomics to the management of IBS. Clin Gastroenterol Hepatol. 2019 Mar;17(4):584-94; used with permission.

Table 13.3   *CYP2D6* Phenotypes for 1,013 RIGHT Protocol Participants

CYP2D6 Metabolizer Phenotype	No. of Patients (%)
Ultrarapid	83 (8)
Extensive to ultrarapid	162 (16)
Extensive	203 (20)
Intermediate to ultrarapid	1 (<1)
Intermediate to extensive	199 (20)
Intermediate	217 (21)
Poor to intermediate	71 (7)
Poor	77 (8)

Abbreviation: RIGHT, Right Drug, Right Dose, Right Time—Using Genomic Data to Individualize Treatment protocol.

From Bielinski SJ, Olson JE, Pathak J, Weinshilboum RM, Wang L, Lyke KJ, et al. Preemptive genotyping for personalized medicine: design of the right drug, right dose, right time-using genomic data to individualize treatment protocol. Mayo Clin Proc. 2014 Jan;89(1):25-33; used with permission.

type 4 agonist. Variations in the genetic control of the serotonin-transporter protein (SERT), which affect serotonin neurotransmission, influence the response to alosetron and tegaserod. Variants in serotonin

Table 13.4   Predicted Enzyme Activity for *CYP2D6* and *CYP2C19*[a]

Predicted Enzyme Activity	*CYP2D6*	*CYP2C19*
Increased activity	*2A[b]	*17
Normal activity	*1, *35	*1
Decreased activity	*2,[b] *9, *10, *14B, *17, *29, *41	*9
No activity or null alleles	*3, *4, *5, *6, *7, *8, *11, *12, *13, *14A, *15, *36, *68	*2, *3, *4, *5, *6, *7, *8, *10, *11[c]

[a] Phenotyping was derived from the Human Cytochrome P450 (CYP) Allele Nomenclature Committee website (Sim 2010) and the PharmGKB website for the related Clinical Pharmacogenetics Implementation Consortium guidelines (Whirl-Carrillo 2012).[d]

[b] *CYP2D6*2A* and *CYP2D6*2* as described in Black et al (2012).[d]

[c] *CYP2C19*11* is found in cis with the *2 variants; therefore, it is classified as a no activity or null allele (Skierka 2014).[d]

[d] Full reference citation for studies listed in this table can be found in the original source.

From Nassan M, Nicholson WT, Elliott MA, Rohrer Vitek CR, Black JL, Frye MA. Pharmacokinetic pharmacogenetic prescribing guidelines for antidepressants: a template for psychiatric precision medicine. Mayo Clin Proc. 2016 Jul;91(7):897-907; used with permission.

Table 13.5　Medications That Potently Inhibit or Induce Cytochrome P450 Enzymes

CYP	Potent Inhibitors: Slow Down Substrate Drug Metabolism and Increase Drug Effect	Potent Inducers: Speed Up Substrate Drug Metabolism and Decrease Drug Effect
2C9	Amiodarone Fluconazole Fluoxetine Metronidazole Ritonavir Trimethoprim/sulfamethoxazole	Carbamazepine Phenobarbital Phenytoin Rifampin
2C19	Fluvoxamine Isoniazid Ritonavir	Carbamazepine Phenytoin Rifampin
2D6	Amiodarone Cimetidine Diphenhydramine Fluoxetine Paroxetine Quinidine Ritonavir Terbinafine	No significant inducers
3A4/5	Clarithromycin Diltiazem Erythromycin Grapefruit juice Itraconazole Ketoconazole Nefazodone Ritonavir Telithromycin Verapamil	Carbamazepine *Hypericum perforatum* (St. John's wort) Phenobarbital Phenytoin Rifampin

Modified from Lynch T, Price A. The effect of cytochrome P450 metabolism on drug response, interactions, and adverse effects. Am Fam Physician. 2007 Aug 1;76(3):391-6; used with permission.

Figure 13.4　Pharmacogenetic Alert Algorithm

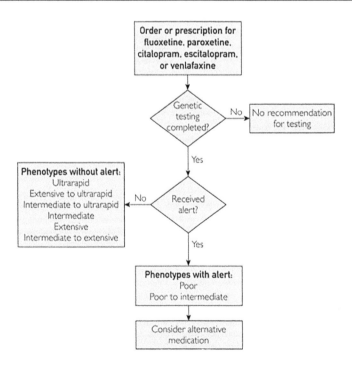

(From Nassan M, Nicholson WT, Elliott MA, Rohrer Vitek CR, Black JL, Frye MA. Pharmacokinetic pharmacogenetic prescribing guidelines for antidepressants: a template for psychiatric precision medicine. Mayo Clin Proc. 2016 Jul;91(7):897-907; used with permission.)

Figure 13.5   Sample of the GeneSight Psychotropic Report

ANTIDEPRESSANTS

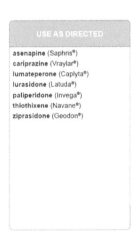

USE AS DIRECTED	MODERATE GENE-DRUG INTERACTION		SIGNIFICANT GENE-DRUG INTERACTION	
desvenlafaxine (Pristiq®)	trazodone (Desyrel®)	1	selegiline (Emsam®)	2
levomilnacipran (Fetzima®)	venlafaxine (Effexor®)	1	mirtazapine (Remeron®)	1,6
vilazodone (Viibryd®)	fluoxetine (Prozac®)	1,4	sertraline (Zoloft®)	2,4
	bupropion (Wellbutrin®)	1,6	amitriptyline (Elavil®)	3,8
	citalopram (Celexa®)	3,4	clomipramine (Anafranil®)	1,6,8
	escitalopram (Lexapro®)	3,4	desipramine (Norpramin®)	1,6,8
			doxepin (Sinequan®)	1,6,8
			duloxetine (Cymbalta®)	1,6,8
			imipramine (Tofranil®)	1,6,8
			nortriptyline (Pamelor®)	1,6,8
			vortioxetine (Trintellix®)	1,6,8
			fluvoxamine (Luvox®)	1,4,6,8
			paroxetine (Paxil®)	1,4,6,8

CLINICAL CONSIDERATIONS

1: Serum level may be too high, lower doses may be required.
2: Serum level may be too low, higher doses may be required.
3: Difficult to predict dose adjustments due to conflicting variations in metabolism.
4: Genotype may impact drug mechanism of action and result in reduced efficacy.
6: Use of this drug may increase risk of side effects.
8: FDA label identifies a potential gene-drug interaction for this medication.

ANTIPSYCHOTICS

USE AS DIRECTED	MODERATE GENE-DRUG INTERACTION		SIGNIFICANT GENE-DRUG INTERACTION	
asenapine (Saphris®)	fluphenazine (Prolixin®)	1	chlorpromazine (Thorazine®)	1,6
cariprazine (Vraylar®)	olanzapine (Zyprexa®)	1	aripiprazole (Abilify®)	1,6,8
lumateperone (Caplyta®)	quetiapine (Seroquel®)	1	brexpiprazole (Rexulti®)	1,6,8
lurasidone (Latuda®)	clozapine (Clozaril®)	1,8	iloperidone (Fanapt®)	1,6,8
paliperidone (Invega®)	haloperidol (Haldol®)	1,8	perphenazine (Trilafon®)	1,6,8
thiothixene (Navane®)			risperidone (Risperdal®)	1,6,8
ziprasidone (Geodon®)			thioridazine (Mellaril®)	1,6,9

CLINICAL CONSIDERATIONS

1: Serum level may be too high, lower doses may be required.
6: Use of this drug may increase risk of side effects.
8: FDA label identifies a potential gene-drug interaction for this medication.
9: Per FDA label, this medication is contraindicated for this genotype.

All psychotropic medications require clinical monitoring.
This report is not intended to imply that the drugs listed are approved for the same indications or that they are comparable in safety or efficacy. The brand name is shown for illustrative purposes only; other brand names may be available. The prescribing physician should review the prescribing information for the drug(s) being considered and make treatment decisions based on the patient's individual needs and the characteristics of the drug prescribed. Propranolol and oxcarbazepine might be considered off-label when being used for neuropsychiatric disorders. Please consult their respective FDA drug labels for specific guidelines regarding their use.

Assurex

Medications categorized into the green section do not have any identified gene–drug interactions; yellow and red sections include footnotes that indicate the clinical consideration as to what gene–drug interactions are affecting each specific medication.

(From GeneSight [Internet]. 2019 [cited 2020 Jan 27]. Available from: https://genesight.com/wp-content/uploads/2017/05/GeneSight.Psychotropic.Report.pdf; used with permission.)

Figure 13.6 Actionable Germline Genetic Variation and Associated Treatment

A

Genetic Variation	Medications
TPMT	Mercaptopurine, thioguanine, azathioprine
CYP2D6	Codeine, tramadol, tricyclic antidepressants
CYP2C19	Tricyclic antidepressants, clopidogrel, voriconazole
VKORC1	Warfarin
CYP2C9	Warfarin, phenytoin
HLA-B	Allopurinol, carbamazepine, abacavir, phenytoin
CFTR	Ivacaftor
DPYD	Fluorouracil, capecitabine, tegafur
G6PD	Rasburicase
UGT1A1	Irinotecan, atazanavir
SLCO1B1	Simvastatin
IFNL3 (IL28B)	Interferon
CYP3A5	Tacrolimus

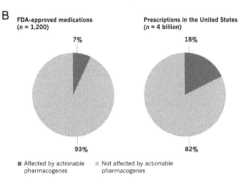

B

A, Medications affected by actionable pharmacogenes: several pharmacogenetically high-risk drugs are commonly prescribed in clinical practice. B, In the United States, 7% of approved medications and 18% of all prescriptions are affected by actionable pharmacogenes. FDA indicates US Food and Drug Administration.

(Data from CPIC. 2019 [cited 2020 Jan 27]. Available from: https://cpicpgx.org/genes-drugs/. B, From Relling MV, Evans WE. Pharmacogenomics in the clinic. Nature. 2015 Oct 15;526(7573):343-50; used with permission.)

Table 13.6 Summary of the Literature on Genetic Variation in Receptor or Transporters That Have Been Investigated in Treatment Trials Specifically Conducted in Patients With IBS

Pathway	Gene	Mechanism	Drug and Receptor Target	Clinical Applicability	Study (year)[a]
Serotonergic pathway	5-HTTLPR	Short (S) variant of 5-HTTLPR associated with reduced SERT function, reduced 5-HT reuptake, and increased synaptic 5-HT, compared with long (L) variant	Tegaserod (5-HT$_4$ receptor agonist)	S/S and L/S genotypes may predict better response to tegaserod in IBS-constipation	Li et al (2007)
			Alosetron (5-HT$_3$ receptor antagonist)	L/L genotype may predict better response to alosetron in IBS with diarrhea	Camilleri et al (2002)
	TPH1	Polymorphism predicts response to 5-HT$_{3R}$ antagonists	Ramosetron (5-HT$_3$ antagonist)	Genotypes rs4537731 T/T, rs7130929 C/C, and rs211105 T/T may predict higher response to ramosetron in IBS with diarrhea	Shiotani et al (2015)
Cannabinoid pathway	CNR1	CNR1 rs806378 genotype associated with colonic transit in IBS with diarrhea with symptom rating of gas	Dronabinol (nonselective cannabinoid agonist)	Genotype rs806378 CT/TT may predict more delay in colonic transit in response to dronabinol in IBS with diarrhea	Wong et al (2012)
Bile acid pathway	KLB and FGFR4	Variants in KLB and FGFR4 modulate negative feedback on hepatocyte bile acid synthesis	Chenodeoxy-cholic acid	Genetic variations in KLB and FGFR4 may predict response to chenodeoxycholic acid in IBS-constipation	Rao et al (2010)
			Colesevelam (bile acid sequestrant)	Genetic variations in KLB and FGFR4 may predict response to colesevelam in IBS with diarrhea	Wong et al (2012)

Abbreviations: 5-HT, 5-hydroxytryptamine (serotonin); IBS, irritable bowel syndrome; SERT, serotonin-transporter protein.

[a] Full reference citations for studies listed in this table can be found in the original source.

Modified from Halawi H, Camilleri M. Pharmacogenetics and the treatment of functional gastrointestinal disorders. Pharmacogenomics. 2017 Jul;18(11):1085-94; used with permission.

Figure 13.7   Ligand-Receptor Interaction at Synapse (eg, Serotonin)

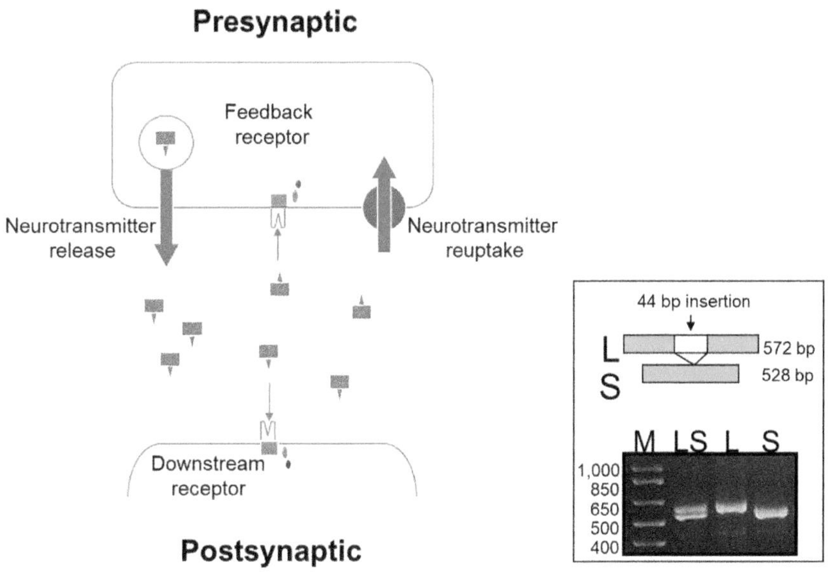

Serotonin transporter (SERT) is central to fine-tuning brain serotonin neurotransmission, is abundant in cortical and limbic areas, and affects emotional aspects of behavior. There is a polymorphism in the promoter region upstream of serotonin coding sequence (SERT-P): long and short variants of polymorphic region. bp indicates base pairs; L, homozygous long allele; LS, heterozygous long-short allele; M, molecular weight marker; S, homozygous short allele.

(From Camilleri M, Atanasova E, Carlson PJ, Ahmad U, Kim HJ, Viramontes BE, et al. Serotonin-transporter polymorphism pharmacogenetics in diarrhea-predominant irritable bowel syndrome. Gastroenterology. 2002 Aug;123(2):425-32; used with permission.)

transporter (*5-HTTR*) influence synthesis of SERT-P and control effects of serotonin and serotonergic agents in the colon. The promoter region (SERT-P) upstream of the serotonin coding sequence for SERT is affected by long and short variants (44 base pairs long), constituting a polymorphic region in the gene (*5-HTTLPR*) for SERT. The long variant, *5-HTTLPR* or serotonin transporter long polymorphic repeat, is associated with normal promoter-mediated transcription and synthesis of SERT, which result in reuptake of serotonin from synaptic cleft. With less serotonin in the synapse, there is reduced risk of overstimulation of postsynaptic serotonergic receptors. Conversely, a single short allele in *5-HTTLPR* is sufficient to reduce SERT synthesis, resulting in more 5-HT in the synaptic cleft (Figure 13.7). Thus, clinical research studies showed *5-HTTLPR* was associated with enhanced colonic transit response to alosetron

in IBS with diarrhea and reduced global response to tegaserod based on a patient-reported outcome (Figures 13.8 and 13.9).

Pharmacogenomics in IBS and Precision Medicine

Currently, the greatest pharmacogenomics application in IBS is in the use of neuromodulators, including analgesics and antidepressants, for the visceral hypersensitivity component of IBS.

As specific pathophysiologic mechanisms of IBS are better characterized, the effect of pharmacogenomics on precision medicine may be enhanced by application of drugs to specific transporters and receptors.

Figure 13.8   Reduced 5-HT at Synapse Associated With Effective 5-HT Reuptake Enhances Response to the 5-HT₃ Antagonist Alosetron

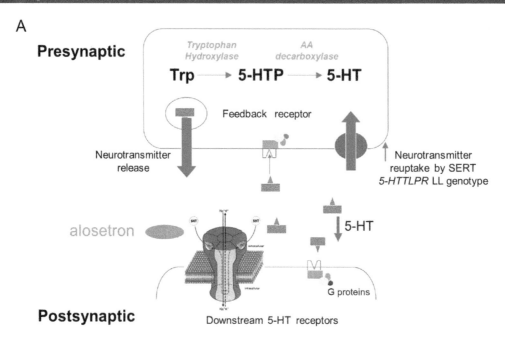

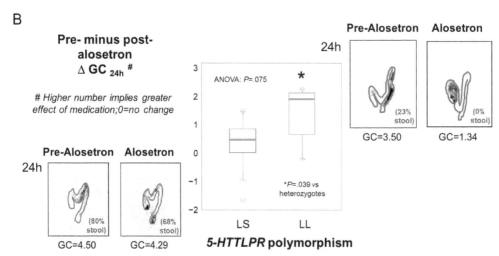

A, Theoretical basis for increased reuptake of 5-HT at synapse to be associated with enhanced response to 5-HT₃ antagonist. 5-HT indicates 5-hydroxytryptamine (serotonin); 5-HTP, hydroxytryptophan; SERT, serotonin transporter. B, Observations in pharmacogenetic trial using colonic transit as phenotype of interest. The *5-HTTLPR* polymorphism is associated with colonic transit response to alosetron in irritable bowel syndrome with diarrhea. ANOVA indicates analysis of variance; GC, geometric center; LL, homozygous long allele; LS, heterozygous long-short allele.

(From Camilleri M, Atanasova E, Carlson PJ, Ahmad U, Kim HJ, Viramontes BE, et al. Serotonin-transporter polymorphism pharmacogenetics in diarrhea-predominant irritable bowel syndrome. Gastroenterology. 2002 Aug;123(2):425-32; used with permission.)

Figure 13.9   Reduced 5-HT at Synapse Associated With Effective 5-HT Reuptake Reduces Response to the 5-HT₄ Agonist Tegaserod

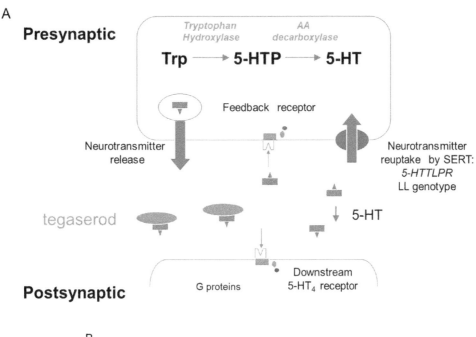

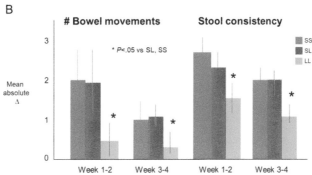

A, Theoretical basis for increased reuptake of 5-HT at synapse to be associated with reduced response to 5-HT₄ agonist. 5-HT indicates 5-hydroxytryptamine (serotonin); 5-HTP, 5-hydroxytryptophan; LL, homozygous long allele; SERT, serotonin transporter; Trp, tryptophan. B, Effect of *5-HTTLPR* genotype on clinical efficacy of tegaserod, a 5-HT₄ agonist, in irritable bowel syndrome with constipation. LL indicates homozygous long allele; SL, heterozygous short-long allele; SS, homozygous short allele.

(From Li Y, Nie Y, Xie J, Tang W, Liang P, Sha W, et al. The association of serotonin transporter genetic polymorphisms and irritable bowel syndrome and its influence on tegaserod treatment in Chinese patients. Dig Dis Sci. 2007 Nov;52(11):2942-9; used with permission.)

Suggested Reading

Black JL 3rd, Walker DL, O'Kane DJ, Harmandayan M. Frequency of undetected CYP2D6 hybrid genes in clinical samples: impact on phenotype prediction. Drug Metab Dispos. 2012 Jan;40(1):111–9. Epub 2011 Oct 17.

Camilleri M. Implications of pharmacogenomics to the management of IBS. Clin Gastroenterol Hepatol. 2019 Mar;17(4):584–94. Epub 2018 May 2.

Camilleri M, Atanasova E, Carlson PJ, Ahmad U, Kim HJ, Viramontes BE, et al. Serotonin-transporter polymorphism pharmacogenetics in diarrhea-predominant irritable bowel

syndrome. Gastroenterology. 2002 Aug;123(2):425–32. Epub 2002 Jul 30.

Finkelstein J, Friedman C, Hripcsak G, Cabrera M. Pharmacogenetic polymorphism as an independent risk factor for frequent hospitalizations in older adults with polypharmacy: a pilot study. Pharmgenomics Pers Med. 2016 Oct 14;9:107–16.

Li Y, Nie Y, Xie J, Tang W, Liang P, Sha W, et al. The association of serotonin transporter genetic polymorphisms and irritable bowel syndrome and its influence on tegaserod treatment in Chinese patients. Dig Dis Sci. 2007 Nov;52(11):2942–9. Epub 2007 Mar 31.

Nassan M, Nicholson WT, Elliott MA, Rohrer Vitek CR, Black

JL, Frye MA. Pharmacokinetic pharmacogenetic prescribing guidelines for antidepressants: a template for psychiatric precision medicine. Mayo Clin Proc. 2016 Jul;91(7):897–907. Epub 2016 Jun 13.

National Human Genome Research Institute [Internet]. [cited 2019 Apr 1]; Available from: https://www.genome.gov.

Rautio J, Kumpulainen H, Heimbach T, Oliyai R, Oh D, Jarvinen T, et al. Prodrugs: design and clinical applications. Nat Rev Drug Discov. 2008 Mar;7(3):255–70. Erratum in: Nat Rev Drug Discov. 2008 Mar;7(3):272.

Relling MV, Evans WE. Pharmacogenomics in the clinic. Nature. 2015 Oct 15;526(7573):343–50. Epub 2015 Oct 16.

Sim SC, Ingelman-Sundberg M. The human cytochrome P450 (CYP) allele nomenclature website: a peer-reviewed database of CYP variants and their associated effects. Hum Genomics. 2010 Apr;4(4):278–81.

Whirl-Carrillo M, McDonagh EM, Hebert JM, Gong L, Sangkuhl K, Thorn CF, et al. Pharmacogenomics knowledge for personalized medicine. Clin Pharmacol Ther. 2012 Oct;92(4):414–7.

Gastrointestinal Physiologic and Motility Problems in Older Persons: Constipation, Irritable Bowel Syndrome, and Diverticulosis

Esophagus

Aging affects motor and sensory functions throughout the gut. In the pharynx and esophagus, the changes can result in dysphagia and aspiration. As people age, swallow is slower as a result of abnormalities in the oral phase of swallowing, reduced lingual propulsive force, dry mouth with diminished pharyngeal lubrication, and delayed upper esophageal sphincter opening. The term *presbyesophagus* describes disorganized and inefficient peristalsis, typically in nonagenarians. It is characterized by non-propagated contractions occurring as frequently as well-propagated, normal-amplitude contractions (Figure 14.1).

Stomach and Small Bowel

Gastric emptying of solids in older persons is normal, but liquid emptying may be delayed or accelerated. Even healthy older people have decreased perception of gastric distention without any change in fasting gastric compliance. They also have reduced gastric tone late in the postprandial period, and this may contribute to discomfort or satiety and to the anorexia that frequently occurs in older persons.

There are minor changes of unclear clinical significance in small bowel motility in the seventh and eighth decades. Propagation velocity of interdigestive migrating motor complexes is slower, and contraction frequency after feeding is modestly reduced.

Colonic and Rectoanal Motor Functions

The effects of aging on colonic transit and biomechanical properties of the colon in asymptomatic older persons are incompletely documented. Most reports document normal overall colonic transit but delayed rectosigmoid transit, which may result from abnormal motility in specific regions or from the frequently found dysfunction of the defecatory mechanisms. Thus, older patients experience incomplete evacuation or longer time to expel content from the rectum. A form of rectal evacuation disorder that is more prevalent in older persons and especially in multiparous women results from descending perineum syndrome.

Aging is associated with a decline in skeletal muscle mass and strength and increased fatigability. Thus, anal sphincter pressures during voluntary squeeze decline with aging even in the absence of rectoanal symptoms. In addition, in asymptomatic women, aging has been reported to be associated with reduced anal resting and squeeze pressures, reduced rectal compliance, reduced rectal sensation, and perineal laxity. All of these factors may predispose to fecal incontinence in older women.

The effects of sex, parity, and obstetric trauma on rectoanal function are compounded by the

Figure 14.1   Presbyesophagus

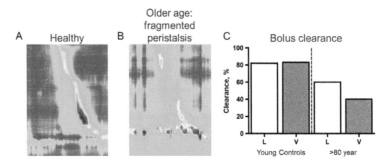

Comparison of peristalsis in a healthy patient (A) and fragmented peristalsis in older patient (B) without clearance of the bolus (C). L indicates liquid; V, viscous.

(From Cock C, Besanko L, Kritas S, Burgstad CM, Thompson A, Heddle R, et al. Impaired bolus clearance in asymptomatic older adults during high-resolution impedance manometry. Neurogastroenterol Motil. 2016 Dec;28(12):1890-1901; used with permission.)

presence of other risk factors, including hormonal changes associated with menopause, concomitant diseases or medications, and long-standing constipation with excessive straining that may lead to stretch injury of the pudendal nerves, denervation of the external anal sphincter, and reduced rectal sensation leading to incontinence of stool (and sometimes of urine due to denervation of the urethral sphincter).

Aging has been associated with changes in smooth muscle function and loss of excitatory (cholinergic) neurons, effects leading to constipation and possibly loss of inhibitory neurons, which cause uncoordinated contractions and discomfort.

Pelvic floor and anal sphincter dysfunction are reviewed in greater detail below.

Small Bowel Absorptive Functions

Aging does not alter small bowel anatomy, enterocyte height, intraepithelial lymphocyte counts, or permeability of lactose and mannitol. Changes in the absorptive function for carbohydrates, fats, and vitamin B_{12} result from disease rather than age-related processes. Declining calcium absorption after 60 years of age is associated with decreased intestinal responsiveness to vitamin D, and this change contributes to increased bone loss with aging. Multiple small, probably clinically insignificant, changes in nutrient absorption have been described, as summarized in Box 14.1.

Epidemiologic Studies of Gastrointestinal Symptoms

Functional Gastrointestinal Disorders

There is a high prevalence of symptoms consistent with functional gastrointestinal (GI) disorders in older persons. The age- and sex-adjusted prevalences (95% CI) of these symptoms per 100 persons were as follows: frequent abdominal pain, 24.3 (95% CI, 19.3-29.2); irritable bowel syndrome (IBS), 10.9 (95% CI, 7.2-14.6); chronic constipation, 24.1 (95% CI, 19.1-29.0); chronic diarrhea, 14.2 (95% CI, 10.1-18.2); and fecal incontinence more than 1 time per week, 3.7 (95% CI, 1.6-5.9). When compared with Olmsted County, Minnesota, adults aged 30 to 64 years, 65- to 93-year-old residents had a higher prevalence of constipation and, to a lesser extent, fecal incontinence and no difference in the prevalence of frequent abdominal pain, IBS, and chronic diarrhea (Figure 14.2). In 704 Olmsted County, Minnesota, residents older than 65 years, functional bowel disorders interfered with daily living and quality of life.

In a Danish cohort, prevalence data for diarrhea and constipation were only slightly higher in older than in younger adults, but functional dyspepsia and IBS reduced functional ability at baseline and 5 years later (Kay 1993; see suggested reading).

Box 14.1

Changes in Absorptive Functions of Carbohydrates, Fats, and Vitamin B$_{12}$

Reduced Absorption

 Carbohydrate

 Protein

 Triglycerides

 Folate, vitamin B$_{12}$

 Vitamin D, calcium

No Change

 Thiamine

 Riboflavin

 Niacin

 Vitamin K

 Zinc, magnesium, iron

Increased Absorption

 Cholesterol

 Vitamin A

 Vitamin C

From Morley JE. The aging gut: physiology. Clin Geriatr Med. 2007 Nov;23(4):757-67; used with permission.

Several factors predispose to constipation in the older persons, including inactivity, inappropriate diet, depression, medications, neuromuscular disorders, and poor rectal sensation and evacuation dynamics.

Diverticulosis

Diverticulosis is more prevalent with increasing age. About 56% of people older than 70 years have diverticulosis on postmortem examination and a greater density of diverticula on colonoscopic examination. The increase in diverticula with older age suggests that the disease is progressive, although the mechanisms are unclear. Predominant locations of diverticula differ by country: diverticula are predominantly in the sigmoid and left colon in Western countries, whereas 70% to 80% of people in Japan with diverticulosis have predominance of right-sided diverticula. A study of US black persons showed a greater percentage of the diverticula in the proximal colon and fewer in the distal colon than in white persons.

Foregut Diseases of Motility

Gastroesophageal Reflux Disease

Gastroesophageal reflux disease (GERD) is highly prevalent (daily symptoms in 8% of men and 15% of women) and poses special diagnostic and therapeutic challenges in older persons. GERD symptoms at least once a month are reported by 54% of men and 66% of women. Increasing age and coexisting upper abdominal symptoms influence consultation behavior in patients with GERD. Patients may not report classic symptoms such as dysphagia, chest pain, and heartburn and may, therefore, present with a severe disease and complications (ie, esophageal ulceration and bleeding).

GERD symptoms in older persons are more commonly regurgitation, dysphagia, dyspepsia, vomiting, or noncardiac chest pain rather than heartburn. There may often be associated atypical symptoms, such

Figure 14.2   Epidemiology of Gastrointestinal Symptoms

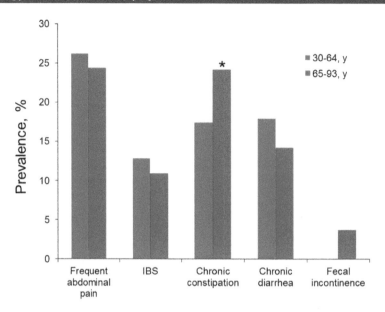

Prevalence of common gastrointestinal symptoms in residents of Olmsted County, Minnesota, by age: frequent abdominal pain 6 or more times in prior year; irritable bowel syndrome (IBS), frequent abdominal pain, and 3 or more Manning criteria; chronic constipation, straining at stool, and hard stools often or less than 3 stools per day; chronic diarrhea, loose, watery stools often or more than 3 stools per day; and clinically significant fecal incontinence once a week or more or the need to wear a pad for protection. Among these symptoms, chronic constipation is the only one more prevalent in the elderly residents (*).

(Data from Talley NJ, Zinsmeister AR, Van Dyke C, Melton LJ 3rd. Epidemiology of colonic symptoms and the irritable bowel syndrome. Gastroenterology. 1991 Oct;101(4):927-34 and Talley NJ, O'Keefe EA, Zinsmeister AR, Melton LJ 3rd. Prevalence of gastrointestinal symptoms in the elderly: a population-based study. Gastroenterology. 1992 Mar;102(3):895-901.)

as abdominal symptoms, chest pain, or respiratory symptoms (eg, hoarseness, chronic cough, wheezing). When older patients have sufficiently severe heartburn to require upper GI endoscopy, they tend to have more significant esophageal mucosal disease (eg, erosive esophagitis, Barrett esophagus) than patients younger than 60 years.

Pill Esophagitis

Pill-induced erosive esophagitis in older persons has been associated with ingestion of more than 70 drug types, including antibacterials (eg, doxycycline, tetracycline, and clindamycin, which together account for >50% of cases of pill esophagitis), aspirin, potassium chloride, ferrous sulfate, bisphosphonates, quinidine, alprenolol, corticosteroids, and nonsteroidal anti-inflammatory drugs. The passage of capsules or tablets through the esophagus is often slower in older persons, and may cause damage from the caustic contents of the drug in contact with the esophagus for a sufficient

time. Additional common risk factors for pill esophagitis are ingestion of medications at bedtime or without fluids. Given the high prevalence of pill esophagitis, drug-related damage should be suspected in all older patients presenting with esophagitis, chest pain, and dysphagia.

Midgut and Hindgut Diseases

Weight Loss, Protein-Energy Malnutrition, and Anorexia

Weight loss in older persons is associated with functional decline, sarcopenia, and mortality, especially when there is a 10% loss in body weight over 10 years. For patients with 4% or more body weight loss over 1 year, underlying causes should be sought, including depression, benign GI conditions, medication toxicity, or cancer.

Protein-energy malnutrition is relatively common in older persons and, yet, even grossly undernourished patients may have normal results of hematologic and biochemical indices of nutritional status (eg, serum transferrin, transthyretin [pre-albumin], and retinol-binding protein).

There is a decline in food intake, or physiologic anorexia, with aging, and this may be multifactorial: alterations in the GI satiating system, increased levels of leptin (especially in men) or cytokines (causing protein wasting), changes in central nervous system neurotransmitters, loss of adipose tissue, sarcopenia, depression, and dieting leading to loss of skeletal tissue and fat mass. Even in healthy older people, the perception of gastric distention can be decreased without a change in fasting gastric compliance. Gastric tone is reduced late in the postprandial period, and this effect may contribute to discomfort or satiety and to the anorexia that is frequent in older persons (Figure 14.3).

The cause for early satiation in older persons is unclear. The effects of aging on gastric accommodation after ingestion of food and satiation (postprandial fullness and appetite) have not been adequately studied. There is evidence of decreased gastric perception and greater gastric accommodation, which may either reduce the pleasurable sensation associated with eating or, paradoxically, allow for greater intake of food due to increased gastric accommodation and reduced perception of gastric distention.

Malabsorption

The most common causes of malabsorption in older persons are celiac disease, chronic pancreatic exocrine insufficiency, and small intestinal bacterial overgrowth (SIBO), even in the absence of an anatomical defect of the small bowel such as dilatation or diverticulosis. The result of the lactulose-hydrogen breath test is often positive in people 65 years or older, particularly in women. One study of 791 patients reported that 54% had a positive result on the lactulose-hydrogen breath test, although it is not clear whether this represented true SIBO or accelerated delivery of the substrate to the colon (Newberry 2016; see suggested reading). Patients with a methane-positive lactulose breath test have slower small bowel and colonic transit (Figure 14.4), a finding suggesting that there is a subset of patients with SIBO who do have an underlying motility disorder.

Tests of absorptive capacity may have normal results, but empiric antibiotic treatment may positively affect nutritional state.

Constipation, IBS, and Diverticulosis

Constipation, IBS, and diverticulosis are all manifestations of colonic dysmotility, and all 3 conditions are regarded as complications of low fiber in the diet. Extracolonic pelvic floor muscles also contribute to the development of these syndromes.

Mechanisms

The mechanisms leading to colonic dysmotility, IBS, and diverticulosis are not definitely proved in the elderly. Possibly, uncoordinated colonic activity and colonic segmentation result from disorders of inhibitory control of neuromuscular function. The total number of neurons in the myenteric plexus is decreased, and collagen deposited in the distal colon is increased with aging in humans. However, one study reported preserved nitrergic but not cholinergic neuromuscular transmission (Wade 2004; see suggested reading). In vitro studies conducted with sigmoid colon muscle strips showed an altered motor pattern with reduced spontaneous motility and enhanced neutrally mediated colonic responses involving both excitatory and inhibitory motor pathways. Conversely, smooth muscle (circular and longitudinal layers), interstitial cells of Cajal, glial cells, and myenteric neuron densities remained unaltered in one study (Bernard 2009; see suggested reading).

The mechanisms involved in constipation and IBS are detailed in Chapters 10 and 11 ("Chronic Constipation" and "Irritable Bowel Syndrome: Peripheral Mechanisms, Biomarkers, and Management"). Factors contributing to constipation in older persons include inactivity, inappropriate diet, depression, medications, neuromuscular disorders, poor rectal sensation, and evacuation dynamics that may lead to fecal impaction.

Diverticulosis

The effects of diverticulosis (Figures 14.5 and 14.6) on colonic motility and transit in the absence of a stricture are unclear. Morphologically, interstitial cells of Cajal and glial cells are decreased in colonic diverticular disease, whereas enteric neurons seem to be normally represented (Figures 14.7 through 14.9).

Figure 14.3   Physiologic Anorexia of Aging

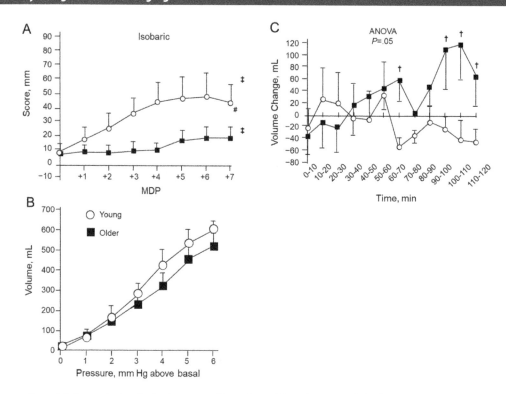

Decreased perception of fullness during isobaric gastric distention with an intragastric balloon (A). This altered perception occurs without a change in fasting gastric compliance, shown by the similarity of the pressure-volume curves (B). The decreased perception of balloon distention is associated with greater gastric accommodation late in the postprandial period, and the reduced perception cannot be explained by reduced gastric tone, which is reflected in the greater gastric accommodation (C). ANOVA indicates analysis of variance; MDP, minimal distention pressure to obtain apposition of the balloon to the gastric wall; †, $P<.05$ young vs older; ‡, $P<.05$ change from baseline; #, $P<.01$.

(From Rayner CK, MacIntosh CG, Chapman IM, Morley JE, Horowitz M. Effects of age on proximal gastric motor and sensory function. Scand J Gastroenterol. 2000 Oct;35(10):1041-7; used with permission.)

Diverticula are thought to develop as a result of isometric contraction of individual haustrations causing high intraluminal pressure and segmentation, with pulsion diverticula developing at points of weakness in the colonic wall at the sites of perforating arteries. Because compliance of the colon is lowest in the sigmoid region, it is conceivable that the sigmoid region is the zone with the highest intraluminal pressure and, therefore, the area of predilection for the development of diverticulosis. The high intraluminal pressures lead to hypertrophy of the circular muscle layers and greater collagen and elastin deposition, further luminal narrowing, stiffening or further reduction of colonic compliance (See Figure 12.6), and increased likelihood of pulsion diverticulum formation (Figure 14.10). Intraluminal pressure patterns are normal under resting conditions, but they are augmented in response to a meal or neostigmine in patients with diverticulosis (Figure 14.11).

Pelvic Floor and Sphincter Dysfunctions: Effects on Colonic Symptoms

The resting pressure (the internal anal sphincter tone) and the voluntary contractile anal pressure (the external anal sphincter pressure) decrease insignificantly with age and are lower in women than in men. Anorectal function in older persons compared with that in younger persons includes decreased anal pressures, lower rectal volume required to cause

Figure 14.4 Alteration of Small Bowel and Colon Transit on Basis of Presence and Type of SIBO

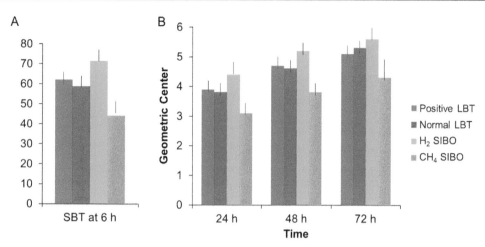

CH_4 SIBO indicates methane-type small intestinal bacterial overgrowth; H_2 SIBO, hydrogen-type SIBO; LBT, lactulose breath test; SBT, small bowel transit.

(Data from Suri J, Kataria R, Malik Z, Parkman HP, Schey R. Elevated methane levels in small intestinal bacterial overgrowth suggests delayed small bowel and colonic transit. Medicine (Baltimore). 2018 May;97(21):e10554.)

desire to defecate, inability to expel a solid 18-mm sphere or 50-mL balloon (Figure 14.12), and lower maximum tolerated volume. Anal resting and, to a lesser extent, squeeze pressures both decline with age in asymptomatic women. Rectal compliance is also lower with aging and may predispose to urge incontinence (Figures 14.13 and 14.14).

The degree of perineal descent is also greater in older women (Figure 14.15) and predisposes to descending perineum syndrome. The anorectal and evacuation characteristics of a series of patients with descending perineum syndrome evaluated at Mayo Clinic are summarized in Table 14.1. In this relatively young cohort of patients, the predominant clinical presentation

Figure 14.5 Dense Sigmoid Diverticulosis

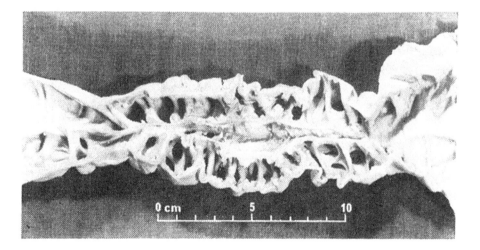

Thickened circular muscle bands are branching.

(From Hughes LE. Postmortem survey of diverticular disease of the colon: II: the muscular abnormality of the sigmoid colon. Gut. 1969 May;10(5):344-51; used with permission.)

Figure 14.6   Diverticulosis in Sigmoid Colon

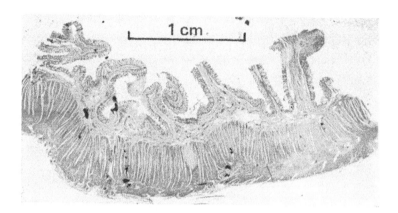

Circular muscle has uniform thickening.

(From Hughes LE. Postmortem survey of diverticular disease of the colon: II: the muscular abnormality of the sigmoid colon. Gut. 1969 May;10(5):344-51; used with permission.)

Figure 14.7   Neural Elements in Control and Diverticular Disease

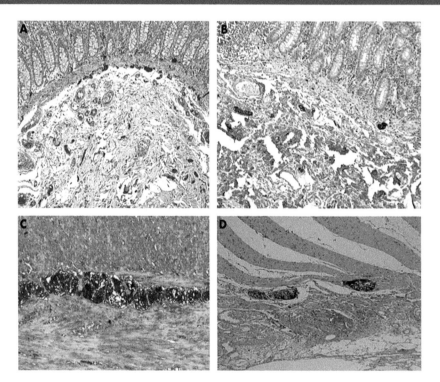

Photomicrographs of submucosal and myenteric plexus of controls (A and C) and patients with diverticular disease (B and D). PGP 9.5; original magnification, ×20 (A, B) and ×40 (C, D).

(From Bassotti G, Battaglia E, Bellone G, Dughera L, Fisogni S, Zambelli C, et al. Interstitial cells of Cajal, enteric nerves, and glial cells in colonic diverticular disease. J Clin Pathol. 2005 Sep;58(9):973-7; used with permission.)

Figure 14.8   Submucosal and Myenteric Plexus of Glia in Control (A) and Diverticular Disease (B)

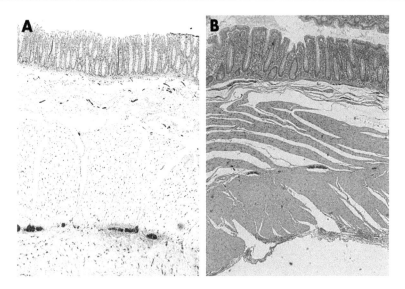

(S-100; original magnification, ×20.)

(From Bassotti G, Battaglia E, Bellone G, Dughera L, Fisogni S, Zambelli C, et al. Interstitial cells of Cajal, enteric nerves, and glial cells in colonic diverticular disease. J Clin Pathol. 2005 Sep;58(9):973-7; used with permission.)

Figure 14.9   Interstitial Cells of Cajal in Control (A and C) and Diverticular Disease (B and D)

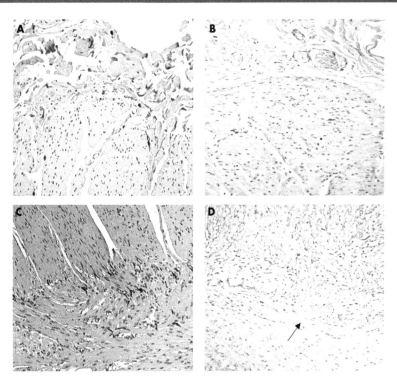

Expression of Kit in the submucosal and myenteric plexus of controls (A and C) and patients with diverticular disease (B and D). Original magnification, ×10. Reduced function of interstitial cells of Cajal might be responsible for significant decrease in rhythmic contractile patterns in colon of patients with diverticulosis (arrow indicates paucity of Kit-positive cells in myenteric plexus).

(From Bassotti G, Battaglia E, Bellone G, Dughera L, Fisogni S, Zambelli C, et al. Interstitial cells of Cajal, enteric nerves, and glial cells in colonic diverticular disease. J Clin Pathol. 2005 Sep;58(9):973-7; used with permission.)

Figure 14.10   Segmentation Produces Pulsion Force That Distends Colonic Diverticula and Probably Causes Initial Mucosal Herniation

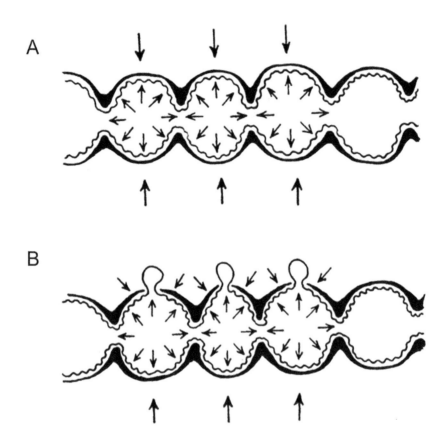

A, Segmentation of colon. B, Intraluminal pressure increase from segmentation results in pulsion diverticula at weakened sites of entry of perforating arteries in colon.

(From Painter NS, Truelove SC, Ardran GM, Tuckey M. Segmentation and the localization of intraluminal pressures in the human colon, with special reference to the pathogenesis of colonic diverticula. Gastroenterology. 1965 Aug;49:169-77; used with permission.)

was defecatory disorder, with relatively maintained sphincter pressures despite the excessive perineal descent. The Mayo cohort consisted of 39 patients (38 women, 1 man), mean age (SD) 53 (14) years, who presented with constipation (38, 97%), incomplete rectal evacuation (36, 92%), excessive straining (38, 97%), digital rectal evacuation (15, 38%), and fecal incontinence (6, 15%).

Other cohorts with higher mean age tend to have greater disorders of continence, presumed to result from excessive straining over the years that produces stretch neuropathy of the pudendal nerves and external sphincter denervation. Thus, among a cohort of 53 patients from Sheffield, United Kingdom (Bartolo 1983; see suggested reading), 32 patients (31 women

and 1 man; mean age, 66 years, range, 38-93 years) had incontinence to rectally infused saline, low resting and squeeze sphincter pressures, and neurophysiologic evidence of sphincter denervation, and 21 patients (16 women and 5 men; mean age, 58 years, range, 39-79 years) presented with obstructed defecation but no incontinence. There were no differences in obstetric history or the presence of anterior mucosal prolapse between the continent and incontinent groups. Consistent with the Mayo Clinic cohort, there was greater opening of the rectoanal angle with straining in the continent group with excessive perineal descent.

In summary, excessive perineal descent is associated with laxity of the perineum and typically occurs in multiparous women. Evacuatory functions should be tested

Figure 14.11   Effect of Neostigmine, 1 mg, in Male With Diverticulosis

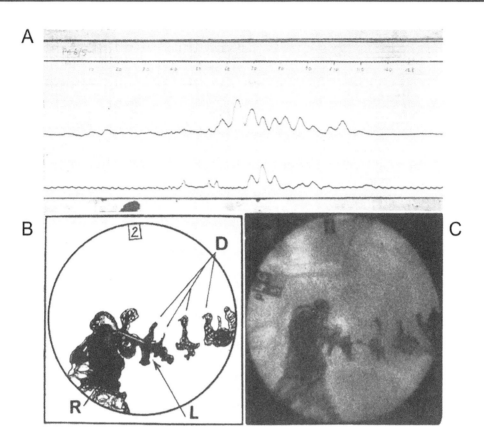

Sigmoid segmentation occurs with high intraluminal pressure. A, Pressure tracing from the colon of a man with diverticulosis who had been given 1 mg of neostigmine half an hour before. B, Anatomical drawing showing marked segmentation. D indicates diverticula; L, site of recording tip; R, rectum. C, Marked segmentation of sigmoid colon on barium enema.

(From Painter NS, Truelove SC, Ardran GM, Tuckey M. Segmentation and the localization of intraluminal pressures in the human colon, with special reference to the pathogenesis of colonic diverticula. Gastroenterology. 1965 Aug;49:169-77; used with permission.)

Figure 14.12   Effect of Age on Ability to Pass an Object Out of the Anorectum

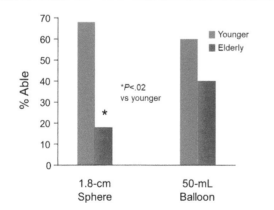

(From Bannister JJ, Abouzekry L, Read NW. Effect of aging on anorectal function. Gut. 1987 Mar;28(3):353-7; used with permission.)

rather than assuming constipation is a consequence of aging because retraining of the pelvic floor muscles with biofeedback may be safe and effective, although not as effective as in younger patients with spastic (dyssynergic) rectal evacuation disorders.

Fecal Incontinence

Subtypes of fecal incontinence are summarized in Table 14.2. Examples of sphincter weakness are shown in Figures 14.16 and 14.17. High-resolution manometry alone and together with measurement of anorectal descent during evacuation may identify rectal prolapse (Figure 14.18) and large rectoceles, which sometimes

Figure 14.13   Lesser Effect of Age on Anal Squeeze Pressure Than Resting Pressure

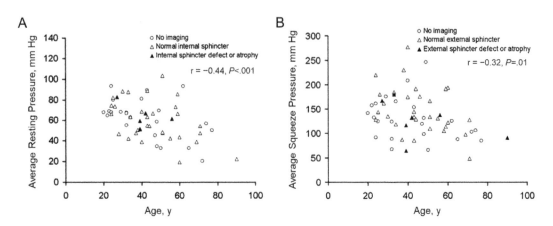

A, Anal resting pressures. B, Anal squeeze pressures.

(From Fox JC, Fletcher JG, Zinsmeister AR, Seide B, Riederer SJ, Bharucha AE. Effect of aging on anorectal and pelvic floor functions in females. Dis Colon Rectum. 2006 Nov;49(11):1726-35; used with permission.)

occur in patients with fecal incontinence, especially in older persons and multiparous women. Combined anatomical imaging (magnetic resonance imaging or endoanal ultrasonography) is critical for identifying surgically remediable problems such as rectal mucosal prolapse or intussusception and anal sphincter defects (Figure 14.19).

Conclusion

Aging affects the functional reserve of the proximal esophagus, anus, and pelvic floor and leads to motility disturbances in older persons, manifesting mainly as high dysphagia, constipation, and fecal incontinence, especially in the presence of prior obstetric damage.

Figure 14.14   Stiffening of Rectum in Older Women

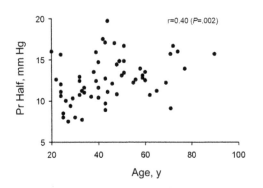

Pr half is reciprocal of compliance. The graph shows the effect of age on rectal compliance. The higher Pr half (ie, pressure corresponding to half-maximum volume) suggests that the rectum is stiffer in older women (the only sex included in the study).

(From Fox JC, Fletcher JG, Zinsmeister AR, Seide B, Riederer SJ, Bharucha AE. Effect of aging on anorectal and pelvic floor functions in females. Dis Colon Rectum. 2006 Nov;49(11):1726-35; used with permission.)

Figure 14.15   Effects of Age and Sex on Pelvic Floor Function: Rectoanal Angle to Pubococcygeal Line (cm)

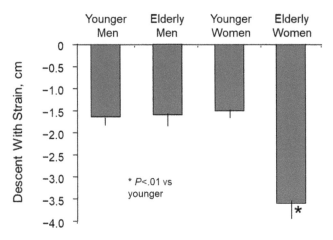

Degree of perineal descent is greater in elderly women than in younger women.

(Data from Bannister JJ, Abouzekry L, Read NW. Effect of aging on anorectal function. Gut. 1987 Mar;28(3):353-7.)

Table 14.1 Characteristics of Anorectal and Evacuation Functions in Descending Perineum Syndrome

Anorectal and Evacuation Tests	Mean (SD)
Mean anal sphincter pressure, mm Hg	
At rest	54 (26)
During squeeze	96 (35)
Added weight required to empty balloon from rectum, g[a]	492 (132) (normal, <200)
Rectal evacuation of radiolabeled Veegum[b]/30 s, %	61 (24) (normal, >54)
Increase in rectoanal angle from rest to straining during defecation, degrees	14.0 (11) (normal, >14)
Perineal descent, cm	4.4 (1) (normal, <4)

[a] Applies only to patients unable to expel balloon from rectum.

[b] Magnesium aluminum silicate.

Data from Harewood GC, Coulie B, Camilleri M, Rath-Harvey D, Pemberton JH. Descending perineum syndrome: audit of clinical and laboratory features and outcome of pelvic floor retraining. Am J Gastroenterol. 1999 Jan;94(1):126-30.

Table 14.2 Subtypes of Fecal Incontinence

Type	Clinical Description	Potential Mechanism(s)
Passive incontinence	The involuntary discharge of stool or gas without awareness	Weak IAS and EAS
		Neuropathy
		Rectal hyposensitivity
Urge incontinence	The discharge of fecal matter despite active attempts to retain bowel contents	Weak IAS and EAS
		Rectal hypersensitivity
		Impaired rectal compliance
Fecal seepage	The leakage of stool following otherwise normal evacuation	Dyssynergia
		Rectal hyposensitivity
		Neuropathy

Abbreviations: EAS, external anal sphincter; IAS, internal anal sphincter.

Data from Rao SS; American College of Gastroenterology Practice Parameters Committee. Diagnosis and management of fecal incontinence. Am J Gastroenterol. 2004 Aug;99(8):1585-604.

Figure 14.16   Examples of Anal Sphincter Weakness on High-Resolution Manometry

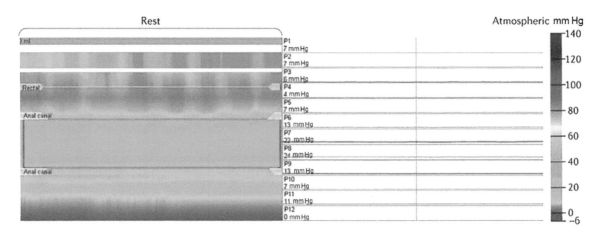

Sphincter hypotonia in a patient with fecal incontinence, visualized in the color contour plot as a band of pale green (20-25 mm Hg) set between normal blue (about 5 mm Hg) rectal (superiorly) and atmospheric (inferiorly) pressures.

(From Carrington EV, Scott SM, Bharucha A, Mion F, Remes-Troche JM, Malcolm A, et al; International Anorectal Physiology Working Group and the International Working Group for Disorders of Gastrointestinal Motility and Function. Expert consensus document: advances in the evaluation of anorectal function. Nat Rev Gastroenterol Hepatol. 2018 May;15(5):309-323; open access article distributed under the Creative Commons Attribution License [https://creativecommons.org/licenses/by-nc/4.0/legalcode].)

Figure 14.17   Standard and High-Definition Anorectal Manometry and Pressure Topography During Rest and Voluntary Squeeze

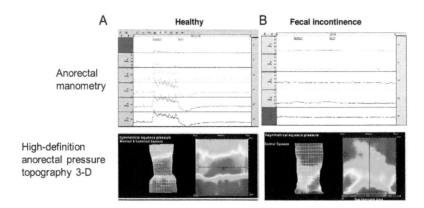

In the healthy patient (A), sphincter pressure is normal, and the increase observed during squeeze is normal. In the incontinent patient (B), the sphincter is weak during squeeze. Color reflects the strength of the pressure: green is weaker than red.

(From Rao SS. Advances in diagnostic assessment of fecal incontinence and dyssynergic defecation. Clin Gastroenterol Hepatol. 2010 Nov;8(11):910-9; used with permission.)

Figure 14.18 High-Resolution Manometry (HRM) and Magnetic Resonance Imaging (MRI) Findings in Rectal Prolapse

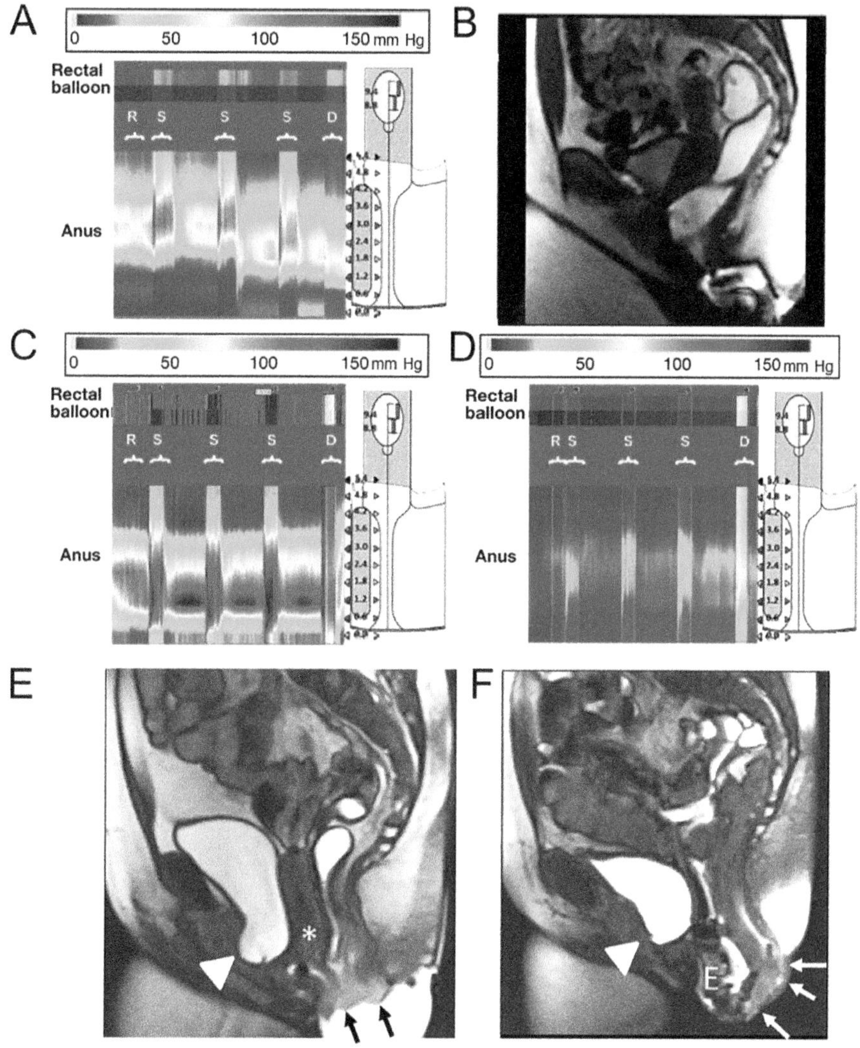

(A) HRM and (B) MRI results for patient with low risk of prolapse because the anal pressures were normal at rest (R) and during squeeze (S), and defecation (D) was associated with increased rectal pressure, anal relaxation, and rectal evacuation. C through F, HRM and MRI features of 2 rectal prolapse phenotypes. In contrast to results in A, pressures are increased during defecation (D) throughout rectum and anus in C and D, and the corresponding MRI images in E and F show small (E) and large (F) rectal prolapse (arrows), a cystocele (arrowhead), enterocele (E), and uterine prolapse (asterisk).

(From Prichard DO, Lee T, Parthasarathy G, Fletcher JG, Zinsmeister AR, Bharucha AE. High-resolution Anorectal Manometry for Identifying Defecatory Disorders and Rectal Structural Abnormalities in Women. Clin Gastroenterol Hepatol. 2017 Mar;15(3):412-420; used with permission.)

Figure 14.19   Endoanal Ultrasound Images for Patients With Fecal Incontinence

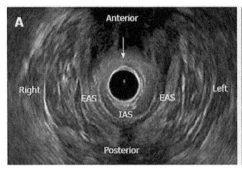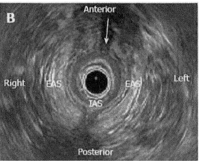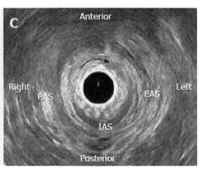

A, A combined defect (arrow) of the external anal sphincter (EAS) from 10- to 2-o'clock and of the internal anal sphincter (IAS) from 9- to 3-o'clock positions in a woman with an obstetric anal sphincter injury. B, An anterior EAS defect (arrow) in a woman with an obstetric anal sphincter injury. C, An IAS defect in a man who had complication after previous anorectal surgery for fistula. The IAS defect is indicated by the lack of continuity of the IAS, which extends from 8- to 4-o'clock position (indicated in part by the curved black arrow from 11- to 1-o'clock).

(From Albuquerque A. Endoanal ultrasonography in fecal incontinence: Current and future perspectives. World J Gastrointest Endosc. 2015 Jun 10;7(6):575-81; open access article distributed under the Creative Commons Attribution License [https://creativecommons.org/licenses/by-nc/4.0/legalcode].)

Older patients may have reversible, nonmalignant disease and can be restored to health through proper management.

Suggested Reading

Bartolo DC, Read NW, Jarratt JA, Read MG, Donnelly TC, Johnson AG. Differences in anal sphincter function and clinical presentation in patients with pelvic floor descent. Gastroenterology. 1983 Jul;85(1):68–75. Epub 1983 Jul 1.

Bernard CE, Gibbons SJ, Gomez-Pinilla PJ, Lurken MS, Schmalz PF, Roeder JL, et al. Effect of age on the enteric nervous system of the human colon. Neurogastroenterol Motil. 2009 Jul;21(7):746–e46. Epub 2009 Feb 8.

Fox JC, Fletcher JG, Zinsmeister AR, Seide B, Riederer SJ, Bharucha AE. Effect of aging on anorectal and pelvic floor functions in females. Dis Colon Rectum. 2006 Nov;49(11):1726–35. Epub 2006 Oct 17.

Harewood GC, Coulie B, Camilleri M, Rath-Harvey D, Pemberton JH. Descending perineum syndrome: audit of clinical and laboratory features and outcome of pelvic floor retraining. Am J Gastroenterol. 1999 Jan;94(1):126–30. Epub 1999 Feb 6.

Kay L, Jorgensen T, Schultz-Larsen K. Colon related symptoms in a 70-year-old Danish population. J Clin Epidemiol. 1993 Dec;46(12):1445–9.

Newberry C, Tierney A, Pickett-Blakely O. Lactulose hydrogen breath test result is associated with age and gender. Biomed Res Int. 2016;2016:1064029. Epub 2016 Mar 17.

Peery AF, Keku TO, Martin CF, Eluri S, Runge T, Galanko JA, et al. Distribution and characteristics of colonic diverticula in a United States screening population. Clin Gastroenterol Hepatol. 2016 Jul;14(7):980–5. Epub 2016 Feb 14.

Prichard DO, Lee T, Parthasarathy G, Fletcher JG, Zinsmeister AR, Bharucha AE. High-resolution anorectal manometry for identifying defecatory disorders and rectal structural abnormalities in women. Clin Gastroenterol Hepatol. 2017 Mar;15(3):412–20. Epub 2016 Oct 11.

Talley NJ, O'Keefe EA, Zinsmeister AR, Melton LJ 3rd. Prevalence of gastrointestinal symptoms in the elderly: a population-based study. Gastroenterology. 1992 Mar;102(3):895–901.

Wade PR, Cowen T. Neurodegeneration: a key factor in the ageing gut. Neurogastroenterol Motil. 2004 Apr;16 Suppl 1:19–23.

Index

Tables, figures, and boxes are indicated by *t*, *f*, and *b* following the page number